A

L

E

A

P

I

N

T

H

E

D

A

R

K

——

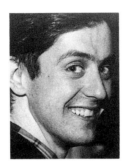

In Memoriam
François Laliberté

A LEAP IN THE DARK

AIDS, ART AND CONTEMPORARY CULTURES

edited by
Allan Klusaček and Ken Morrison

Véhicule Press

an artextes edition

1992

AN ARTEXTES EDITION

Published with the assistance of The Canada Council.

Cover photo: U.S. Presidential Commission members Theresa Crenshaw and Admiral James Watkins gown up for a tour of the HIV lab at Mt. Sinai Medical Center in Miami, 1987. Photo by Jane Rosett.

Cover and book design by Rodolfo Borello and Don Anderson, Associés Libres.
Imaging by ECW Type & Art.
Printed by Les Editions Marquis Ltée.

CANADIAN CATALOGUING IN PUBLICATION DATA

Main entry under title:

A Leap in the dark : AIDS, art and contemporary cultures

Included bibliographical references.
ISBN 1-55065-020-3

1. AIDS (Disease) — Social aspects. 2. AIDS (Disease)
3. AIDS (Disease) in art. I. Klusacek, Allan
II. Morrison, Ken

ISBN 1-55065-020-3 Véhicule
ISBN 2-9800632-7-4 Artexte

RA644.A25L43 1992   362.1'969792   C91-090599-1

Véhicule Press, P.O.B. 125, Place du Parc Station, Montreal, Quebec H2W 2M9.
Artexte Information Centre, 3575 St-Laurent Blvd., Suite 303, Montreal, Quebec H2X 2T7.
Distributed in Canada by Artexte and University of Toronto Press; and in the U.S. by University of Toronto Press (Buffalo, NY), Inland Book Company (New Haven, CT), and Bookslinger Inc. (St. Paul, MN).

Printed in Canada on acid-free paper.

CONTENTS

S IDART, out of which this book grew, was conceived as a specific event, for a specific audience: the Fifth International Conference on AIDS which took place in Montréal, June 1989.

SIDART was a series of cultural events and exhibitions from around the world that dealt with AIDS-related themes. It included eight exhibitions: several of which were international (photography, children's drawings from an International Red Cross competition, contemporary AIDS posters, World Health Organization Global Programme on AIDS logo competition, Names project quilts), some of which were local (Montréal artists' posters and paintings) and one historical (posters from previous epidemics). The five days of activities included a week of film and video presentations, eight plays by theatre companies from four continents, musicians and dancers, several exhibits on communications technology and AIDS, and information kiosks for the general public.

SIDART was an attempt to bring the world of the conference and community together — to bring a closed scientific exchange into the community in which it took place so that the citizens might participate. SIDART also attempted, through cultural practices, to set the abstractions of scientific exchange in the context of the world around us — the world of the young and old, black and white, 'developed' and 'developing,' and gay and straight.

We wish to thank the following individuals for their efforts and contributions for SIDART: Elyse Boivin, Claude Paul Boivin, Lyse Lavictoire, Ivan L. Head, David Nostbakken, Paulin, Michel René Labelle, Denis Poitras, Alexandre Marsolais, Karine Chassagne, Richard A. Morisset, Tom Netter, Jonathan M. Mann, Katheline Kay, Richard Preston, Kevin Orr, Ken Mews, Barbara Wallace, Marlon Montenegro Montelban, Ormond McKague, René Lavoie, Francis Bates, Catherine Hankins, Michel R. Morissette, Margaret A. Somerville, Pierre Dionne, Richard Burzynski, Donald De Gagné, Anne Usher, Pierre Viens, Andy Fabo, John Greyson, Bernard Dagenais, Tom Elmslie, Colette Lachance, Anne Kern, James Miller, Carole Peacock, Georges Tarjan, Jean Robert, Tom Waugh, Serge Turgeon, Christa Brunswicher, Lyne Champoux, Jan Zita Grover, Nora Ritchie, Len Hilgermann, Maurice Arguin, Manfred Sahlsberg, Carmen Chevalier, Wieland Speck, Jacques Vandembourghe, Sophie Lussier, Simon Watney, Jon Baggaley, Lucy Felicissimo, and Guy Lonergan.

We gratefully acknowledge the editorial assistance of Lesley Johnstone, Kathleen Fleming, Simon Dardick, ARTEXTE, and the design contributions of Daniel Anderson and Rodolfo Borello of Associés Libres. We wish also to thank our co-workers and friends for their patience and understanding while we worked on this project. Salut to Diffusions gaies et lesbiennes du Québec, René Lavoie, Jacques Perron, Groupe Intervention Vidéo, Tony Bergeron, le Centre communautaire des gais et lesbiennes de Montréal, Michael Bailey, Canadian AIDS Society, C-SAM, and Tom.

ACKNOWLEDGEMENTS

A *Leap in the Dark* grew out of a personal as well as a social reality. Both of the editors have lived close to AIDS since the beginning of the 1980s. Although we had already met on several occasions, we really got to know each other at the funeral of a close friend and former lover. From this point on, AIDS was no longer an abstract threat but a very personal and physical one. Since then many friends we have in common have succumbed to AIDS; several who were integral to this anthology.

Caught between an indifferent, if not openly hostile society, and our own social community — the Montréal gay community, (whose response to this epidemic is still largely characterized by apathy and denial) — we were compelled to do something about our frustration, sadness and anger. As a result we have worked in community action projects and became involved in international conferences, research projects, local speaking engagements and prevention programs in the gay community. This anthology developed out of our ongoing examination of alternative approaches to AIDS prevention, sensitization, and activism.

AIDS 101

AIDS is a focal point for many of the social ills that plague modern society, as well as being what many countries have declared their major public health problem. It challenges and defies our institutions, our communities and for many of us, our lives and bodies. AIDS is a health condition without a cure. Little exists in terms of medical treatment. As has been pointed out time and time again, prevention is all we have.

AIDS is a condition not, as such, a disease. It has, medical science presumes, a primary cause, HIV, which is a retrovirus; a virus that undergoes continual transformations. The virus, a parasite, has a host, a specific kind of cell that is central to the functioning of the immune system. This particular virus spreads slowly in the body, eventually rendering the immune system totally dysfunctional and no longer able to fight off infections. When a person who has been infected with HIV develops one or more opportunistic infections the medical establishl-ment calls this condition AIDS, Acquired Immune Deficiency Syndrome.

HIV must get into the blood stream of a person in order to be a problem. In and of itself this should be a difficult thing to do. The virus, however, is carried by blood, vaginal fluids, and sperm. Other bodily fluids such as saliva and tears do not have sufficient quantities of HIV to make them a problem. Other than an infected mother transmitting the virus to her unborn or newborn baby, the major routes of transmission between adults in order of efficacy are: sharing intravenous needles, unprotected anal intercourse, and unprotected vaginal intercourse.

This Book

A Leap in the Dark includes a diverse selection of ways this basic AIDS information and AIDS related issues have been communicated. In different contexts and in many countries this simple information is politically suppressed.

We make no apologies about the sense of specificity inherent to this collection. We do not claim in any way to speak for Others. We are presenting efforts that contain their own power and legitimacy largely within the context in which they were produced and for whom they were intended. We are responding to Larry Kramer's declaration concerning the Fifth International Conference on AIDS, "We came to teach not to learn." As participants and editors we believe the opposite. We need to learn in order to teach.

This book is not organized according to any hierarchy of aesthetic expression (a debate that surprisingly in the late twentieth century still inspires controversy) nor in order to give particular legitimacy to any one culture, form of expression, or author.

The first section sets AIDS in a historical context. It illustrates that many of the social responses to AIDS, including stigmatization and discrimination, are not new but merely contemporary manifestations of earlier reactions to other epidemics. The response to AIDS, like them, reflects the general fear of the unknown, in this case fear of sex and death. This section also chronicles the changing role of community medicine and epidemiology in modern society. Finally, it illustrates how the gay community, in particular, has been affected by this epidemic and how it has affected change.

The second section provides different examples of how the visual arts have been used as a strategy in reacting to AIDS. Drawn specifically from the North American visual arts community response to AIDS, these articles examine and depict how Western theories of representation employ image re-making to challenge existing concepts of power, science, life and death. They all offer us ways and means to see how in different contexts images convey different meanings.

Expanding the discussion to mass media, the next section places AIDS within the context of Western television, video, and print. Many people see these media as "entertainment" and consequently as a preferred means of communication. The media are therefore subject to enormous social and political pressures revolving around issues of morality, prejudice, panic, and censorship.

The next theme revolves around the issue of behaviour change within a specific frame of reference: gay culture and it's porn representation in North America and Western Europe. Gay porn, by definition, is doubly marginalized and has consistently taken into consideration issues of control around both it's production and distribution because of censorship. These articles suggest ways in which to use this tradition to promote safer sex while at the same time preserving pleasure and lives.

The process of naming is a first step towards self-affirmation, particularly within a context of death and denial. Literature has traditionally performed this role. The works included in the fifth section are about the diversity and range of coming to terms with AIDS.

The final section of the book reflects on theatre as a means of expressing cultural specificity and interactive education. Theatre has a long tradition of transmitting history and ideas throughout many cultures. Realized in the frame of ceremony, theatre is a means of socializing as well as a means of educating.

We wish to express our appreciation for the generosity and commitment of the many contributors to this collection. Their patience and talent shines through a world of hate, indifference, and confusion.

Allan Klusaček and Ken Morrison
rue St-Urbain, Montréal, July 1991.

Un virus n'est pas un signe*

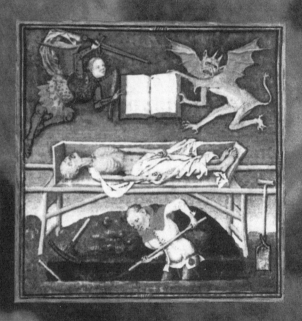

*NI UNE BÊTE ENRAGÉE
NI UNE ÉPÉE CELLULAIRE
NI UN PUITS EMPOISSONÉ
NI UNE TROMPETTE MILLÉNAIRE

HISTORY TEACHES:
WHAT HAVE
WE LEARNED?

Fear of the Other, Condemned and Damned: AIDS, Epidemics and Exclusions

Mikhaël Elbaz & Ruth Murbach

This essay grew out of the shared reflections of an anthropologist working on exclusion models, and a lawyer who studies how new ethical, scientific and socio-legal rules have emerged since the advent of AIDS. The object of our study is the field of representations that mark the outcast in various legal and cultural orders. The salient point is that AIDS has brought back panic, fear and terror of the Other, condemned and damned, at a time when our Western societies, armed with the miracle of antibiotics, sanitary hygiene, self-surveillance and the presence of the providential state, seemed to have repressed the fear of death.

AIDS, however, gives no credence to such tenets. It expresses the contingency of men who, like Job, ignore the reasons for the unleashing of Gods' furies and revert to a cultural repertoire which has delimited possible reactions to "diabolical" diseases since the beginning of time: denial, escape, fear, aggression, projection, guilt designation, conspiracy theories, exclusion and stigmatization and appeals for salvation to moralism and mysticism.

Faced with an enemy whose law is unknown but which no one can ignore, and which furthermore unites eros and thanatos in a society obsessed with pleasure, people remain divided on whether to change deeply rooted behaviours, blame "deviant" minorities — homosexuals and IV drug users — or appeal to the providential state and medical authority.

AIDS appeared among a constellation of disorders such as menacing nuclear war, environmental pollution, a stock market crash, long term threats which did not interfere with the individual's dream of a continued existence. At the same time, AIDS has catalyzed our memory of all past epidemics by condensing both the representations of evil and its inscription in the body, and the social reactions to them (see table). History, admittedly, does not repeat itself and fear finds its expression according to the collective imagination and the *Zeitgeist* of each society. Besides, AIDS assembles elements which, symbolically, men have always invested with particular powers: blood, sex and sperm.[1]

We believe that a reexamination of the past might lead to a reorientation of present debates and caution against any vilification of people with AIDS, and against any retreat from human rights. AIDS represents a frightful disaster for societies which have gradually adapted to ideologies of hygiene and individual security, inherited from the past and from the supreme power of the medical profession. The anxiety aroused by AIDS evokes the fear and terror of bygone days, but in a more specific sense. It is the loss of all immune system defenses that is at stake in cultures that have constructed their social and legal rules on risk control and a fascination with technology. Will the fragile balance between individual and collective rights be sustained, or will we be confronted with a new kind of "panoptism" from which procedures designed to maintain the social bond will emerge? To find answers to these questions, we will evoke forms of exclusion and stigmatization, first within theocracy, then in states governed by the rule of law.

Although the facts may vary in each era, portrayals of epidemic diseases have changed little over time. Public reaction has never been either calm or rational. Attitudes tended rather to express powerlessness when faced with the unknown and the uncontrollable. Societies have always tried to unburden their disasters on the strange and the stranger,[2] oscillating between blaming divine wrath, rumour, and conspiracy. Knowledge concerning the modes of transmission and the spread of contagion becomes entangled with beliefs; appeals are directed towards theological, scientific or governmental references, eventually hiding other interests. In the Middle Ages, the inability to domesticate disease led to the creation of scapegoats: lepers, plague victims, Jews, and witches. The exclusions and stigmatizations of these groups drew from cultural patterns which can be invoked alone or in various combinations:

1. **The body as the signature of evil**: this condemns lepers, witches and prostitutes as living incarnations of sin. Expurgating the evil means separating designated groups from society: ritually, for the sick, and violently for witches, in the inquisitorial scene created by priests;

2. **Religion and identity**: this stigmatizes heretics, Jews and, occasionally, strangers;

3. **Socio-economic status**: particularly concerning trade and craft associated with blood, money and filth; but this also widens the gap between the rich and the poor.

During what Braudel termed "this long sixteenth century" — from the fourteenth through the sixteenth centuries — Western Europe fell prey to political and social upheavals, to famine and all the other "disasters of the times."[3] However, the main cause for the drastic decrease of its population was the plague, considered the greatest recurring catastrophe of the past. It created a real "culture of death" that found its expression in theatrical dramatizations of existence, a celebration of excess and a frenzy of living for the moment. There was also a macabre exhibitionism depicted on objects decorated with grinning skeletons and iconography dominated by the *danse macabre*. Appropriated by the Church, these themes served an orthodox theology of death and salvation.

Leprosy was also judged to be the result of a breakdown of moral values and was seized upon as divine punishment for sexual transgression. Until the fourteenth century, leprosy resisted alchemy, incantation for miraculous healings as well as penitence. A slow developing disease marked by disfiguration, it was "controlled" by the theocracy by excluding lepers through rituals that symbolized their passage from this world to the anticipated next. At the same time, extermination programs were implemented, notably in England under Henry II, and in France, under Phillip V, where lepers were segregated in thousands of leprosaria.

At that time, the body and its treatment mirrored a society that prescribed the exclusion or ritual marking of the Other. The body also expressed codes of purity and impurity, of what was permitted and what was forbidden. What is revealing in this context is the concentration of the anti-Judaic movement during the epidemics between the twelfth and fourteenth centuries (even though it was not the consequence of them), as historians Poliakov and Delumeau have shown.[4] This involved a diabolic causality and an actively created demonology within the fictitious war taking place in the Western world between Gentiles and Jews.

Jews were required to wear the yellow star and to live segregated in ghettos. They became the scapegoat archetype during the Black Plague in France, with the Toulon pogrom of 1348, and with the Bubonic Plague in Rome where 20 percent of the 4000 Jews confined in the ghetto perished.[5] Expelled from most Western European countries between the twelfth and the fourteenth centuries, these nomads came to symbolize, contrary to evidence, the very idea of contamination in a world where exchanges and encounters with the Other were limited.

The Cagots are also important in a discussion of the theological state's inability to protect those whose body is signed and written by collective imagination. Until the seventeenth century, this mysterious medieval peasant population of southwestern France was considered to be descendant of lepers, Cathar heretics, Jews or Arabs. Without being lepers, but treated as such, they were marked with a distinctive sign: a piece of red cloth sewn on the chest in the form of a goose's leg. They were barred from contaminating agricultural land. They were forbidden to possess arms, own land, marry outside of their group or be buried close to the majority population.[6]

These cases demonstrate how rumour and suspicion are capable, in situations of fear and terror, of designating a population to disgrace. Since the appearance of AIDS, it is well known how receptive the general population is to rumours and conspiracy theories, in spite of constant access to information. One need only recall the first name for the disease: GRID (Gay-Related Immunodeficiency), as well as recurrent proposals in different regions of the world to tattoo carriers of the virus or mark their identity papers.

This rapid overview indicates the conjunction, during this era, of physical exclusions (leprosaria, lazaretto, ghetto, sealed urban areas such as the Trastevere in Rome in 1656), with symbolic exclusions, manifested through distinctive marks (the leper's clothing, the red goose leg on the Cagot's chest, the yellow Star of David worn by the Jews), and increasingly, expulsion, inquisition and extermination of the sick.

In opposition, the formation of the Modern States introduced a separation of the state from religion, being replaced by legal process and the declaration of equal rights for all citizens. The priests cede their healer's role to physicians, while the bureaucrats and the police try to delimit disorder in times of epidemics.[7]

The history of the terror wrought by syphilis, which lasted five centuries until the end of World War II, is comparable to the present AIDS pandemic on many levels. The first medical reports in the West appear at the time of Charles VIII's withdrawal from Italy in 1495 and describe the revolting nature of this slow and extremely contagious sexually-transmitted disease. Known as the Neapolitan disease to the French, the French disease to the Italians, the Christian disease to the Persians, the German disease to the Polish, the Polish disease to the Russians, the Chinese disease to the Japanese, and the New World disease to everyone after Christopher Columbus's return — all these designations express the meaning of *epidêmos*: the arrival, the appearance of the foreigner within a people. The name and the clinical description of the disease were not specified until much later.

From the very first wave of syphilis, an accusatory discourse appeared, while exclusionary measures were meant to redress both the therapeutic and preventive impasses. It was during the nineteenth century that the medical world developed its normative discourse the furthest, despite evidence that syphilis had a lower mortality rate than other contemporary epidemics like cholera and tuberculosis, and represented less of a financial burden to the State. Anti-syphilis hygiene came to mean moral hygiene, producing a wave of regulations to eradicate, or at least limit prostitution.[8] Half a century later, World War I offered the occasion to decree emergency measures confining prostitutes to camps. However, as proof that syphilis was equally distributed in all social classes contemporary literature presented another argument and fashioned the compensatory myth of creative evil. This myth, as well as the fear and the moralizing discourse, did not come to an end until after World War II when antibiotics were discovered, even though the number of new reported cases has continued to increase since the 1960s.

In the case of tuberculosis, the romantic image of consumption created in literature has overshadowed the reality of what is still a social disease in developing countries, with eight million new cases and three million deaths reported each year. Tuberculosis has become the disease of others, and fear and memory have been overcome since the victorious discovery of a cure. Indeed, its depiction as a sublimation of soul and spirit from a decaying body involves forgetting a social reality which has been considered the curse of modernity, industrialization and massive urbanization. Tuberculosis, however, also represents a century of discord between theoretical and therapeutic knowledge and the cleavage between "guilty" victims — workers with ill-adapted customs, or alcoholics — and those who are "innocent," having inherited the disease or been contaminated by the former. Furthermore, these categories of blame or compassion have determined the extent of, and access to, treatment. As was the case with other epidemics, the debates revolving around the origin and transmission of the disease were embedded in the fight for medical power. This is demonstrated by the institution of various sanitary measures towards the end of the nineteenth century and the beginning of the twentieth century, culminating in a triumphant hygienism over individual rights.

In the nineteenth century, which saw the outbreak of so many contagious diseases, it was cholera that provoked the most spectacular public reaction. This was due to the very public spectacle it offered: almost immediate death by physical decomposition, dehumanization/disfiguration, and the inability of both the medical establishment and governmental authorities to contain the disaster, because they remained divided on what the germ's modes of transmission were.[9] Abundant iconographic materials and pamphlet tracts testify to the conflicts which shook the industrial world and the colonial empire, the local and national political scenes at the time.[10] A comparable staging and portrayal of decimated populations, not hidden from public view, is absent from the present pandemic.[11] Mass communication has allowed us to follow the evolution of scientific discoveries in the fight against AIDS, but has also, on occasion, helped propagate rumour and the virus of fear by transmitting the message of certain moral entrepreneurs.

Richard Evans' monumental sociological work[12] illustrates another unique feature of the cholera epidemic, particularly in the last European wave, which struck only Hamburg, among all European cities, in 1892: popular blame for the massive casualties was then directed toward the State, expected to be henceforth a Welfare State.

The AIDS phenomenon has erupted in a world where risk management is conceived of differently, according to nations, state structures, the relation to the body, disease and the sacred. Although much is known about the virus, it still incites suspicion of generalized or selective contamination, thus reanimating the secular concern about the circulation of human beings. Carriers of the virus conjure up the spectre of eventual pollution through sperm and blood, which themselves have been transformed into commodities subjected to new controls in postmodern societies. "Cursed" minorities, primarily homosexuals and IV drug users, but increasingly the North American urban poor — Blacks and Hispanics in particular — are blamed, and bear the stigmatization and the symbolic confusion between identity and behaviour, which alone explains the transmission.[13]

Located between damnation and salvation, science and the medical world, by accepting to be the repository of collective anxieties, have become the ultimate reference. Although cautious, due to the lack of effective therapies, scientists collaborate nonetheless in a competitive context characterized by a tangled web of national glory, corporate interests and researchers' personal prestige. Indeed, the history of epidemics shows that medical science is woven into a social and political fabric and that its power is not unlimited. Each epidemic is produced by and reveals society, and challenges its social cohesion. The Black Plague decimated 40 percent of Europe's population and accelerated political and social transformation. This was not as evident in the case of cholera. The extent of the AIDS disaster remains uncertain, but it could, if the most dismal prognosis becomes a reality, lead to inquisitorial or totalitarian excesses which governments, adhering to the rule of law have thus far spared us. Nevertheless, there have been outbreaks of panic and people with AIDS have been, and continue to be, subjected to humiliation and rejection, notably in the areas of work, housing, insurance, and schools.

History has also taught us that blaming the victims of an epidemic disease is much easier when they can be conceived of as "different." The distance established between the self and the Other, condemned and damned, allows rumour to persist long after factual information is provided. This distance does not disappear, generally, until the discovery of a cure. Note however that, beyond compassion for the sick, their state of latent death that calls into question the lives of the healthy, as well as the medical and sanitary ideologies we inherited from the nineteenth century. AIDS has sent a tremor through references and social defences; it is the unexpected event in a civilization where speed and contagion go together in so many areas of social life.

People with AIDS (after a period of accepting designation, stigmatization and marginalization) have been pushed to organize and defend life, however fragile. Beyond norms, out-laws, subject to medical experimentation, they have banded together to break the silence, define different medical and legal rules, and introduce into their struggle for life new reflections on our relation to the body, to health, to sexuality and to self-care. New social and behavioral norms are emerging right in front of us, even if we ignore, as yet, how the epidemic will be subdued. By speaking out, they remind us that scientific and social models and standards are neither neutral nor immutable. Furthermore, the AIDS epidemic takes post-industrial societies back to fatalities they believed were past, or at least limited to societies in the Third World. The internalization of this contagious and absolute evil demonstrates the uncertainty of humanity, and indicates, more than ever before in history, the need for concerted measures and medical ethics that are not confined to indifference toward the developing world, but are, rather, concerned with prevention and treatment for the majority.

It is impossible to conclude. After a decade of AIDS we have still not developed beyond our limited cultural repertory in responding to the disorder that arises from the threat of transmittable death. Between yesterday's order of God and today's order of Science, we tinker with temporary responses — waiting for time to deliver us from evil and uncertainty.

Table: *Comparison of the major epidemics in the Western World*

	SOCIAL REPRESENTATIONS:		SOCIAL RESPONSES
	THE EVIL	THE SIGNED BODY	
LEPROSY 14th century	sin; wrath of God;	disfiguration; slow death;	rejection; stigmatization; ritual exclusion; extermination; role of the Church; rumour and conspiracy theories; quackery;
PLAGUE 14th-18th century (recurrent)	wrath of God; catastrophe; from abroad;	fast death;	escape; quarantine; closing of borders; scapegoats: persecution of Jews, lepers, witches; extermination; role of the Church; sanitary police; culture of death; rumour and conspiracy theories; quackery;

7

SYPHILIS 16th-20th century	sin; wrath of God; vice; shame; "guilty" and "innocent" victims; hereditary evil; army (ambulant city); from abroad;	disfiguration; slow death;	confinement in camps; compensatory myth of "creative evil" in arts and literature; role of the medical power; moralizing discourse; quackery;
CHOLERA 19th century (recurrent)	poverty; filth; alcohol; urban environment	decomposition of the body; fast death;	escape; closing of borders; sanitary measures; role of local (city) authorities; role of the medical power; moralizing discourse; iconography;
TUBERCULOSIS 19th-20th century	shame; alcohol; urban environment; hereditary evil; industrialization;	consumption; slow death;	confinement; compensatory myth of "creative evil" in literature; role of the medical power; moralizing discourse; quackery;
AIDS 20th-? century	"perverted" sex; drugs; shame; wrath of God; "guilty" and "innocent" victims urban environment; from abroad; hereditary evil.	disfiguration; decomposition; consumption; fast or slow death.	silence; stigmatization; compulsory or voluntary sanitary measures; closing of some borders; confinement in Cuba; role of the medical, scientific and governmental powers; role of community organizations; role of people with AIDS; role of the media; international cooperation/competition; rumour and conspiracy theories; moralizing discourse; quackery.

NOTES

1. Jean-Pierre Bardet, et al., eds., *Peurs et terreurs face à la contagion: Choléra, tuberculose, syphilis, XIXe-XXe siècles* (Paris: Fayard, 1988); Elizabeth Fee, and Daniel M. Fox, eds., *AIDS: The Burdens of History* (Berkeley: University of California Press, 1988). See especially Guenter B. Risse, "Epidemics and History: Ecological Perspectives and Social Responses," in this anthology, 33-66; Goudsblom, J., "Public Health and the Civilizing Process," *The Milbank Quarterly* 64:2, 161-88, and "Les grandes épidémies et la civilisation des moeurs," *Actes de la recherche en sciences sociales* 68, 3-14.

2. Jean Delumeau, *Le péché et la peur: La culpabilisation en occident* (Paris: Fayard, 1983); Jean Delumeau and Yves Lequin, *Les malheurs des temps: Histoire des fleaux et des calamités en France* (Paris: Librairie Larousse, 1987).

3. Delumeau and Lequin, ibid.

4. Leon Poliakov, *Histoire de l'antisémitisme*, 1 (Paris: Calmann-Lévy, 1981); Delumeau, *Le péché*, op. cit.

5. Risse, op. cit.

6. C. Delacampagne, *L'invention du racisme* (Paris: Fayard, 1981).

7. Jacques Attali, *L'ordre cannibale: Vide et mort de la medecine* (Paris: Grasset, 1979).

8. Bardet, op. cit.

9. Bardet, ibid.; Patrice Bourdelais, and Jean-Yves Raulot, *Une peur bleue: Histoire du choléra en France* (Paris: Payot, 1987); Richard J. Evans, *Death in Hamburg: Society and Politics in the Cholera Years, 1830-1910* (Oxford: Oxford University Press, 1987); Fee and Fox, eds., op. cit.; Charles E. Rosenberg, *The Cholera Years: The United States in 1832, 1849 and 1866* (Chicago: University of Chicago Press, 1962).

10. Patrice Bourdelais and André Dodin, *Visages du choléra* (Paris: Éditions Bélin, 1987).

11. Susan Sontag, *AIDS and its Metaphors* (New York: Farrar, Strauss and Giroux, 1988).

12. Evans, op. cit.

13. Mary Catherine Bateson and Richard Goldsby, *Thinking AIDS: The Social Response to the Biological Threat* (Reading, Mass.: Addison-Wesley, 1988); Ronald Bayer, *Private Acts, Social Consequences: AIDS and the Politics of Public Health* (New York: The Free Press, 1989); Douglas Feldman and Thomas Johnson, eds., *The Social Dimensions of AIDS: Methods and Theory* (New York: Praeger, 1986); Ruth Murbach, "Le grand désordre: Le sida et les normes," *Anthropologie et Sociétés*, 13:1, 77-102.

Translated from the French by Michael Bailey.

New Diseases

Alfred W. Crosby

N ew diseases appear when microorganisms mutate and acquire pathological qualities, and when either pathogens migrate and find human populations not previously exposed to said organisms, or when humans move into areas with pathogens to which they have not previously been exposed. All of these happened soon after Christopher Columbus crossed the Atlantic in 1492. The bulk of the evidence that exists on the history of venereal syphilis suggests that it was an American Indian disease before 1492 and crossed the Atlantic to Europe the next year, or shortly after, or that the germs of an American Indian syphilis crossed the Atlantic and "hybridized" with similar but not identical Old World germs, producing a "new" infection. Either way, an unprecedented dangerous venereal infection appeared in Europe in the 1490s and spread throughout the Eastern Hemisphere in the sixteenth century.

Syphilis, in its earliest manifestation was a particularly hideous infection:

> "There were byles, sharpe, and standing out, havying the similitude and quantite of acornes, from which came so foule humours, and so great stench, that who so ever smelled it, thought hym selfe to be enfect" — and it killed in a matter of weeks or months. Fortunately, within a few decades it evolved into the syphilis we know today, a relatively mild infection that usually takes years to wreak its damage.[1]

The impact of venereal syphilis among the populations of the Old World after 1492 was considerable, but minor when compared to what Old World diseases accomplished in the Americas (and afterward in Australia, South Africa, New Zealand, the islands of the Pacific, and similarly isolated spots). The micro-organisms that infect human beings had rarely, if ever, crossed the Atlantic and Pacific oceans before Columbus because their hosts — humans and certain other organisms — had rarely done so. Therefore, circa 1492, the disease environments of the Old and New Worlds were quite different. The Americas, where humans were comparatively recent arrivals, and where dense populations were a comparatively recent development, had few infectious diseases. There were pinta,

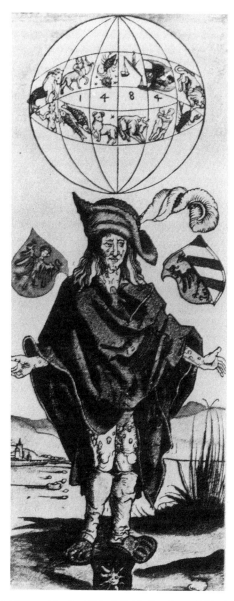

Albrecht Dürer, *The Syphilitic*. 1496 is the date of this depiction of a man afflicted with what was a new disease in Europe at the time. The '1484' on the globe over the zodiac refers to the year of an astrological conjunction blamed for being the cause of this new disease.

yaws, syphilis, hepatitis, encephalitis, polio, some varieties of tuberculosis, Oroya fever, and perhaps not many more. The distinctly American ones, like Oroya fever, were, for one reason or another, usually inexportable.[2]

In the Old World, dense sedentary populations of humans, their direct ancestors and similar species, had lived in close association with domesticated animals for millennia, creating a very large pool of humans and animals for the generation of infections. The Old World had a long menu of devastating infections to offer the New World, including smallpox, measles, diphtheria, trachoma, whooping cough, chicken pox, bubonic plague, malaria, typhoid fever, cholera, yellow fever, amoebic dysentery, influenza, and others.[3]

The most spectacularly devastating among them was smallpox, which apparently underwent a radical change in the sixteenth century. It was an old disease in Europe and not particularly lethal, as you might expect of an old disease. Smallpox is mentioned many times in the records of medieval and Renaissance Europe, but almost always as what we would call a "childhood disease," as an inevitable infection for the young, but not one that commonly ended in death. Some time in the sixteenth century, not long after the beginning of the history of European imperialism, smallpox became quite deadly. It remained so right through what we in America often call "colonial history" and until the spread of vaccination and the appearance of variola minor (a mild form of smallpox) in the nineteenth century.

Smallpox is of special interest to historians of the Americas because it was the most important single ally of the European imperialists. In the myths of the Kiowa of the plains of North America, this disease is personified, significantly, as wearing the black suit and tall hat of missionaries:

I come from far away, across the Eastern Ocean. I am one with the white men — they are my people. Sometimes I travel ahead of them, and sometimes I lurk behind. But I am always their companion and you will find me in their camps and in their houses.[4]

Smallpox first arrived in the New World on board one or more European ships in the waters off Santo Domingo at the end of 1518 or the beginning of 1519. It quickly decimated the Taino Indians of the Greater Antilles, possibly dealing them the *coup de grâce* — they slipped over the brink of extinction shortly thereafter. The disease soon crossed the Gulf of Mexico to the mainland of Central America and Mexico. It arrived there some months after the Hernando Cortés expedition, immediately after the Aztecs had driven him and his men out of Tenochtitlan (Mexico City). Some years later Francisco de Aguilar, one of Cortés' followers, described this event: "When the Christians were exhausted from war, God saw fit to send the Indians smallpox, and there was a great pestilence in the city."

The degree of mortality will never be known. In modern times strains of smallpox have often killed 20 and 30 percent of populations at risk, and we must consider that the Aztecs had no conception of quarantine nor of how to provide supportive therapy. They were in the midst of a battle for their very existence. A mortality rate of half of the citizens of Tenochtitlan is not impossible.

We do have testimony from Indian eye witnesses from which we can derive some idea of the psychological impact of the epidemic:

> It was (the month of) Tepeihuit when it began, and it spread over the people as great destruction. Some of it covered (with pustules) on all parts — their faces, their heads, their breasts, etc. There was great havoc. Very many died of it. They could not walk; they only lay in their resting places and beds. They could not move; they could not stir; they could not change position, nor lie on one side; not face down, nor on their backs. And if they stirred, much did they cry outs. Great was its destruction. Covered, mantled with pustules, very many people died of them.[5]

Without smallpox, the Spaniards, enormously inferior to the Aztecs in the size of their force, would never have attracted and been able to control Indian allies in the numbers they did, nor would they have been able to capture Tenochtitlan that year or for years to come.

When the Spanish conquistadors were conquering the Aztec empire, word of their existence may not have even arrived in the realms of the Inca, far to the south in present-day Ecuador, Peru, Bolivia and northern Chile. But not long after, an epidemic of an unknown, lethal disease characterized by pustules, almost certainly smallpox, spread through the Inca Empire, killing many, including the Inca (Emperor) and his chosen successor. Civil war between claimants to the crown followed, killing more. When Francisco Pizarro and his conquistadors arrived in 1532, Atalhualpa had just won the civil war, but the Incan Empire had not yet recovered. Pedro Pizarro, brother of Francisco, wrote that had the old Inca, Huayna Capac "been alive when we Spaniards entered this land, it would have been impossible for us to win it."[6]

Such stories can be told of epidemics that cleared the way for the English in Virginia and Massachusetts, the *coureurs de bois* of Canada, the Charleston traders, the slave raiders moving from Sao Paulo, the Russians seeking furs in North America, and of the permanent settlers that followed all of them. The colonists of Roanke Island, off the coast of North Carolina, recorded that in the 1580s an infection spread among the Indians which "was so strange that they neither knew what it was, nor how to cure it; the like by report of the oldest men in the country never happened before, time out of mind." Another disease spread through the peoples of coastal New England, starting in 1616; around Boston Bay the bones of the dead were so plentiful that one European, travelling there a few years later, described the land as "a new found Golgotha."[7]

Old World diseases continue to eliminate Native Americans in our time. In 1952 measles infected ninety percent of the Indians and Eskimos of Ungava Bay, Québec, killing 7 percent in this one epidemic. Two years later the same disease swept Xingu National Park in Brazil, killing over a quarter of those Indians who had the benefit of only traditional therapies.[8] The Yanomamas of Brazil have decreased by 10 percent in the past few years, most of the loss due to disease. The Yanomama assessment of the cause is neither correct nor completely wrong: "White man causes illness; if the whites had never existed, disease would never have existed either."[9]

Colonists from the Old World, without the infections they brought with them, would never have conquered the Americas as rapidly or completely as they did. It is likely that the Euro-Americans of Canada and the United States, for instance, would have won their wars with the Indians through technological superiority, but they would never have accomplished a *demographic*, as well as a military, takeover without their arsenal of pathogens. In all likelihood, the Euro-Americans would currently be in the same situation as the whites in the Union of South Africa; that is to say, a numerically inferior elite precariously perched on top of a vast majority of angry indigenes.

A statement made long ago by a Maya of Yucatàn, similar to that of the Yanomama's above, describes what conditions were like among the Maya before the white invasion. It can be interpreted as wishful dreaming or a clinically accurate recollection:

> There was then no sickness; they had no aching bones; they had then no high fever; they had then no smallpox; they had then no burning chest; they had then no abdominal pain; they had then no consumption; they had then no headache. At that time the course of humanity was orderly. The foreigners made it otherwise when they arrived here.[10]

Does any of this have significance for us wrestling with the current AIDS crisis? Indeed, yes. A lesson can be drawn from the history of syphilis in the sixteenth century: pathogens are not necessarily stable and often change to the advantage of humanity, given time. We would be well advised to exert ourselves to slow the spread of this new venereal infection of our generation. We can do this without waiting for scientific miracles. I speak, of course, of education. There is a lesson in what smallpox did to the American Indians after 1492; a new disease can wreak vast damage. It happened in the past and can happen again, barring the intervention of scientists, supported by thoughtful public servants and an enlightened public.

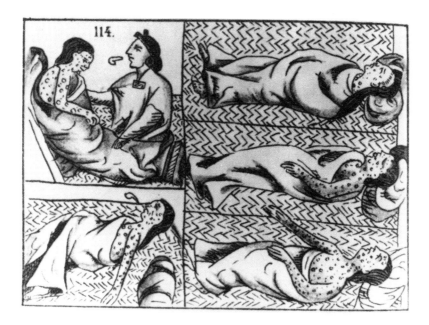

Aztec smallpox victims in the sixteenth century, from Fray
Bernardino de Sahagun, *Historia De Las Casas de Nueva
Espane*, vol. 4, book, 12, plate 114.

NOTES

1. Ulrich von Hutten, *Of the Wood Called Guaiacum*, trans. Thomas Paynel (London: Thomas Bertheletregü, 1540) as quoted in Alfred W. Crosby, *The Columbian Exchange: Biological and Cultural Consequences of 1492* (Westport: Greenwood Press, 1972): 122-64.

2. Russell Thornton, *American Indian Holocaust and Survival: A Population History since 1492* (Norman: University of Oaklahoma Press, 1987): 39-40.

3. Ibid., 44.

4. Alfred W. Crosby, *Ecological Imperialism: the Biological Expansion of Europe, 900-1900* (Cambridge: Cambridge University Press, 1986): 207-8.

5. Alfred W. Crosby, *Columbian Exchange*, 56.

6. Ibid., 55.

7. Ibid., 40-2.

8. Alfred W. Crosby, "Virgin Soil Epidemics as a Factor in the Aboriginal Depopulation in North America," *William and Mary Quarterly*, 3rd Series, (April 1976): 293-6.

9. *New York Times*, 24 December 1989, 6: 27 March 1990, 1; *Austin-American Statesman*, 9 December 1990, A16; Crosby, *Ecological Imperialism*, 197.

10. Crosby, *Columbian Exchange*, 58.

An AIDS Chronicle

Norbert Gilmore

Future Uncertain

AIDS is as much an idea as a disease. It is an epidemic of concepts as well as of disease. Whether its concepts are considered "good" or "bad," "right" or "wrong," they are as important to understanding this epidemic as is understanding the disease and premature death it produces.[1] The history of this epidemic, the scientific achievements, and the successes and failures to control it and its consequences[2] cannot be understood without understanding these concepts.[3]

The AIDS epidemic has been a slow but relentless epidemic. Eighteen million people are expected to be infected with HIV and six million people will die from AIDS by the year 2,000.[4] No country, today, can claim to be free of AIDS; it has become a medical and social calamity. But, there have been some successes. A putative but disputed cause for AIDS has been found.[5] There is the promise of treatment. There is also an expectation that soon there will be a vaccine that will prevent any further spread of AIDS.

Now, the era of discovery is ending; efforts to control this epidemic are shifting from knowing to doing. The next decade will see conceptual shifts and programme development designed to reduce exposure to HIV, to deliver care and treatment to those who need it, to minimize its harmful impact, and to sustain these efforts.[6] Such changes will bring increasing bureaucratization, competition and professionalism[7] as efforts to control this epidemic are fitted into the systems and structures, whether good or bad, designed to prevent disease, care for the sick and protect those made vulnerable by it.[8]

Beginnings: From Disease to Epidemic to Calamity

AIDS, it might be claimed, started in the Garden of Eden but AIDS the disease and its epidemic spread appear to be new. HIV may be 600 to 1,200 years old.[9]

16

Sporadic cases of AIDS-like disease and evidence of HIV infection have been found as early as the 1950s[10] but inexplicably, the widespread dissemination of HIV and AIDS appears not to have begun until the 1970s.[11] It spread invisibly, unrecognized until 1980 when a small number of men in the United States developed unusual diseases suggesting their immune systems had been destroyed. As more and more men developed these diseases, it became apparent this immune destruction was a new disease and an epidemic one.

Before 1981, immunodeficiency in adults was rare.[12] It was only seen in someone whose immune system had been profoundly but recognizably damaged such as recipients of kidney transplants who were treated with drugs that prevented rejection of their kidney grafts. This changed in 1980 when a small number of men in Los Angeles, San Francisco and New York developed unusual infections or malignancies which only developed in adults who were immunodeficient.[13] These men had been healthy but, inexplicably, they had become immunodeficient. Each had a history of sex with men and was a member of the gay community. That appeared to be their only feature in common. By the spring of 1981, with more and more men found to have these unusual diseases, it became clear that a distinctive but nameless disease had erupted out of the gay community in North America.

First Reports

In June 1981, the Centers for Disease Control, responsible for surveillance and control of epidemics in the USA, published a brief report describing the disease[14] of five of these men, alerting public health agencies, and the health care system in general, about this new disease. A month later, disease in an additional twenty-six men was reported.[15] Meanwhile, the first public report of this disease was published in the New York Times.[16] It had little impact at the time.

The number of cases reported to the Centers for Disease Control steadily increased. Twelve weeks after the first alert, the Centers for Disease Control reported 106 people in the USA were known to have developed this still unnamed disease.[17] They included six men who had not had sex with men, and one woman, each of whom had a history of non-medical injection drug use.

AIDS was a baffling disease[18] and often misunderstood.[19] However, many of its features were recognized early on. The growth of this epidemic was less explosive than earlier ones. Not until much later would its incubation time be known, that it took years after infection began for serious disease to appear.[20] AIDS was always associated with irreversible destruction of the immune system—the body's defense against a hostile, microbial world. It explained why people with AIDS developed rare, opportunistic diseases such as Pneumocystis carinii pneumonia (PCP) or Kaposi's sarcoma (KS). Its cardinal feature was the loss of cells that normally protected people from these diseases.[21] So profound was this loss that it was incompatible with prolonged survival. AIDS killed more than half of the men who developed it.[22]

Most people thought this sickness was confined to homosexual men[23] although within three months it was known that homosexual and heterosexual men, women, and injection drug users had developed it.[24] They included black, hispanic and white Americans. Many people also considered this sickness was an "American" one even though it was known that a small number of Europeans had developed it.[25]

No one knew if AIDS might be an infectious disease, or due to some toxin in the environment such as inhaled nitrites ("poppers")[26] or to the life-styles of those who developed it, such as from exposure to semen or the consequence of accumulated infections in particular sexually transmitted ones so prevalent but in no way exclusive to the gay community.[27] The first clue to unravelling this mystery was the discovery of a cluster of immunodeficient men in California that suggested this disease might be sexually transmissible.[28] In the midst of this cluster was one man, labelled "Patient Zero," whom some people erroneously thought started the epidemic.[29]

By the summer of 1982, the disease had been christened with the name AIDS.[30] Despite reports that 12 percent of cases in men and 4 percent of cases in women in the USA had a history of injection drug use,[31] that it could be spread by blood transfusions and blood products,[32] that babies of mothers who had AIDS had also developed it,[33] and that people from Haiti residing in the USA had developed it,[34] the association of AIDS with homosexuality persisted.

Haiti was the poorest country in the Caribbean, and the discovery of AIDS there confounded understanding of how it spread. Heterosexual transmission seemed unlikely, since surveillance begun in 1982 in most industrialized countries showed the incidence of AIDS was almost entirely among men having sex with men. Some Haitian men who had developed AIDS did have a history of sex with men but they were too few to explain the spread of AIDS there. Voodoo, scarification, inadequate cleansing of injection equipment and possibly blood transfusions rescued a faltering disbelief that AIDS was not spread by heterosexual activity. At the same time but without appreciable impact, rumours were spreading in Europe that AIDS had also been found in Africa.[35] Not until 1985 would the glacier-like dimensions of AIDS in Africa, the Caribbean and South America as a relentlessly moving heterosexual pandemic be fully appreciated.[36]

Early on, injection drug users were known to have developed AIDS but neither the speed with which AIDS could be spread by sharing uncleansed injection equipment nor the massive numbers of people infected by this mode of spread would be fully appreciated[37] until 1985. The epidemic in this population was dwarfed by the spread of AIDS among homosexual men and its impact on the gay community.[38] Meanwhile, AIDS continued to spread rapidly among injection drug users in many parts of the world, including the United States, Eastern and Western Europe, and Thailand.[39]

In January 1983, the Centers for Disease Control reported that women in the United States who were the heterosexual partners of men with AIDS had developed this disease.[40] It was now clear that AIDS could be spread by sexual intercourse, by exposure to blood and, when pregnant, from a mother who is infected to her child.[41] With the recognition of heterosexual transmission and that many of these women were partners of injection drug users,[42] the ominous implications of the AIDS epidemic were no longer escapable.[43]

In May 1983, the United States declared AIDS to be its "No. 1 health priority." At the same time, the New York Times ran its first front page story on AIDS, two weeks short of two years from the time AIDS had been discovered.[44] Nevertheless, the full impact of AIDS in the United States and in many other parts of the world would not come until 1985 when the world discovered that Rock Hudson had AIDS and was dying.[45] Meanwhile, AIDS was becoming a "hot" news item and media reports on AIDS became more frequent;[46] the gay community was mobilizing itself to meet its steadily increasing morbidity, mortality and the injustices AIDS produced; and the scientific community was mobilizing to search for a cause and treatment of AIDS.

HIV: The Sacred and Profane

The search for the cause of AIDS began before the discovery of AIDS when the first virus to cause cancer in humans was found in the 1970s.[47] The cells which this virus infected and then transformed into cancerous ones were the same as those destroyed in AIDS.[48] Scientists began searching for evidence that this virus, or a variant of it, was the cause of AIDS. Two years after AIDS was discovered, the first evidence that such a virus might be the cause of AIDS was found.

In May 1983, a research team from Harvard University in Boston reported they had found evidence that adults with AIDS were infected with HTLV-I.[49] In June, a research team from the National Cancer Institute in Washington reported they had found further evidence that adults with AIDS were infected with this virus.[50] However, researchers from the Institut Pasteur in Paris reported different findings. They had found a new virus, similar to but distinct from HTLV-I. They named this virus lymphadenopathy-associated virus or LAV.[51] The world seemed unimpressed with this report, until almost a year later when the research team from Washington announced they too had found a variant of HTLV-I. They named it human T-lymphotropic virus type III (HTLV-III).[52] They had also discovered a way to grow it in the laboratory in "industrial" quantities, and had developed a simple test by which infection with it could be detected.[53] Suddenly, the world reacted. A cause of AIDS had been discovered.

The virus discovered in Washington (HTLV-III) was soon found to be indistinguishable from that discovered in Paris (LAV) almost one year earlier.[54] Controversy erupted about who had "discovered" this virus, and this became a prime-time drama. The major players were Professors Montagnier in France and Gallo in Washington and their governments. At risk were reputations of scientists, royalties from their discoveries, and national pride. In 1987, a compromise was reached when French and American governments signed an entente, assigning the discovery of HIV to both Montagnier and Gallo, forming an international foundation to promote and fund research on AIDS, and agreeing that most of the royalties from this discovery would be given to this foundation.[55] During all of this, the scientific community renamed these viruses. They were given a single name: human immunodeficiency virus (HIV).[56]

Despite this entente, controversy persisted and it erupted again in 1989 when the research team in Washington was accused of fraud.[57] It was alleged that the virus which they claimed to have discovered was not discovered by them but it was a sample, purloined from the Institut Pasteur, of the virus discovered by French investigators. The investigation of these allegations of scientific misconduct continues today.[58]

Behind this controversy was another that went to the very heart of science, namely the nature of scientific evidence and of causation. Once it was recognized that HIV might be the cause of AIDS, data rapidly accumulated associating HIV with AIDS.[59] None of the data refuted HIV as a cause of AIDS but it failed to convince everyone.[60] Some scientists claimed HIV was unproven as a cause of AIDS. They contend HIV is an innocuous virus and HIV infection only indicates a person has been exposed to whatever might be the cause of AIDS.[61] Most scientists believe HIV has a causal role in AIDS; for some, HIV is a necessary but insufficient cause of AIDS and some as yet unidentified co-factor is necessary to explain why not everyone, who has been infected with HIV for a very long time, develops AIDS and why some people develop it rapidly whereas others do so slowly. With improved research methods and the efficacy of treatments such as AZT, concern that HIV is unproven as a cause of AIDS is abating.

The discovery of HIV triggered a frenzy of research. It became possible to grow the virus, study its characteristics, its spread and the damage it produced in the body. More importantly, it became possible to search for a treatment that might cure HIV infection and a vaccine that could prevent infection by making people resistant to HIV.[62]

By 1985, many industrialized countries had moved to screen blood donations. The availability of methods to improve the safety of blood again showed the massive gap between the rich and poor. Many non-industrialized countries could not afford to screen blood donations. Even now, unscreened blood continues to be used in many parts of the world, including some where the prevalence of infection exceeds 20 percent of the urban population![63]

Testing was rapidly made available in many countries to determine if people were infected and to assist in the diagnosis of AIDS. As with the development of testing for hepatitis B virus, HIV testing created frustrating problems and controversy.[64] The foremost of which was the abuse of the information which resulted. Confidentiality of information became a paramount concern.[65]

Research quickly showed HIV infection was very widespread among the gay community, among non-medical injection drug users, and in some parts of Africa. It was clear that HIV could spread rapidly. Over half of the gay men studied in San Francisco, two-thirds of injection drug users in New York city, and over 20 percent of people in some African cities were found to be infected with HIV.[66] Studies also showed not everyone who was infected with HIV developed AIDS, but among those that did, this was a slow infection, taking as long as a decade for AIDS to develop.[67] AIDS had already been declared the number one health priority in the USA, and now it was clear that it had become a medical calamity. It had also become a social calamity.

In July 1985, the study of the safety and efficacy of a potential anti-viral drug (azidothymidine or AZT) began. By August 1986, it was obvious that AZT could prolong life and decrease some of the consequences of immunodeficiency in adults with AIDS.[68] This lead to a change in the approach to HIV antibody testing and treatment. There now were benefits to early detection and aggressive treatment of HIV infection and its consequences.[69] However, controversy quickly followed the announcement of this success. The cost of AZT, its limited availability, and the restricted access to it quickly lead to anger and frustration.[70] In the midst of this controversy, AZT remained (and still remains) unavailable in most non-industrialized countries. It simply cannot be afforded in countries which cannot afford to screen blood donors or adequately diagnose and treat those who had developed AIDS.[71]

There is, as yet, no vaccine against HIV infection. Intensive efforts are underway to develop one, including the testing of several vaccine prototypes.[72] However, success seems distant. Avoiding exposure, or reducing the risk of infection when exposed, has been and is likely to remain for most people the only possibility to control this epidemic during the remainder of this century.[73]

Africa: The Heart of Sadness

If there is one image that will wrench tears from the public, it is that of an orphaned child dying from AIDS.[74] During the 1990s, over five million children under fifteen years of age will lose their mothers to AIDS. Worldwide, at least three million child-bearing women are believed to be infected with HIV and 700,000 of their children are also infected.[75] In some African cities, up to 30 percent of women are infected[76] and 23 percent of pregnant women are infected.[77]

The first awareness that AIDS had entrenched itself in Africa came in 1983-1984 with reports of AIDS in sub-Saharan Africa. Prior to this, there had been reports of Africans being treated for AIDS in Europe.[78] In Uganda, it had its own name "Slim" disease, characterizing the wasting this infection can produce.[79] By 1985, it was apparent that AIDS in Africa was a staggering problem.[80] Many Africans and their governments were angry that the origin of AIDS was attributed to sub-Saharan Africa, and many denied it was present there or, if they admitted to its presence, that its size and impact were minimized.[81] Since then, there has been report upon report of the massive infiltration of HIV in many cities in sub-Saharan Africa, along trade routes, and now is spreading into rural areas.[82] Prostitutes are a major source of its spread in some areas, with over 60 percent of them infected with HIV.[83] HIV is spread primarily by heterosexual sexual activity in a region where access to and use of condoms and HIV testing, and health care, are almost non-existent.[84] A similar situation has been reported from Central and South America.[85] The toll of suffering, morbidity and mortality wrought by AIDS, compounded by tropical and sexually-transmitted diseases, malnutrition and poverty, is unimaginable in industrialized countries.[86]

In 1985, researchers at the Institut Pasteur and in Portugal discovered a variant of HIV, named HIV-2, in western Africa.[87] It was subsequently found to produce the same disease as the original strain of HIV (named HIV-1) and to spread the same way. While its discovery was not unexpected, it was a set-back, making the search for a simple test for and a vaccine against HIV infection more difficult.

Telling It All: Teaching the Public about AIDS

June Osborn likened the world with AIDS to the day after Hiroshima,[88] and for many people, the bomb detonated in the spring of 1985: Rock Hudson had AIDS! In July 1985, the cover of *Life* magazine stated "Now No One is Free from AIDS"; Australia was stunned when its government aired its "Grim Reaper" public education advertisement; the United Kingdom launched a massive public education campaign in November 1986;[89] and in October 1986, the United States Surgeon General's report shocked the US with its sweeping call for people to use condoms to reduce the risk of HIV transmission and for schools to provide sex education.[90] The public was frightened, and their fears and confusion were amplified by the sensationalism and scrutiny of the media. However, governments had finally begun to respond.

Internationally, the World Health Organization responded by developing its Special Programme on AIDS, and its Director General declared AIDS to be "the world's chief public health problem."[91] It called for every government to develop a national plan to combat this epidemic. In Atlanta, the first annual international conference on AIDS was held in the spring of 1985. The United Nations debated the issue;[92] the World Health Assembly passed a resolution calling for an end to discrimination based on HIV infection and on AIDS;[93] and in 1988, the World Health Organization and the government of the United Kingdom convened an meeting of Ministers of Health.[94] Its London Declaration emphasized the importance of prevention, education, and respect for persons. By 1988, the United States, Canada, and Australia each produced strategic reports on the epidemic.[95]

Activism: AIDS and the Body Politic

As much as AIDS has been an epidemic of disease and death, it has also been an epidemic of metaphors and symbols that separate people. AIDS is not a "nice" sickness; seldom do the uninfected people want someone with AIDS near them. Afraid, ignorant or bigoted, they have stereotyped, stigmatized and "cast out" the people with AIDS and carriers of HIV. At the same time, with the accumulating toll of disease and death, the most affected communities grew and strengthened. These communities, in particular the gay community, educated their members how to avoid exposing themselves and others to HIV, cared for those who were infected or ill, promoted, recruited and participated in research efforts to understand and control this epidemic and treat those infected, and learned how to be advocates for their members and others made vulnerable, or more vulnerable, because of AIDS.[96] They have been the "unsung heroes" of this epidemic.[97] Among the better known of these community responses are Gay Men's Health Crisis in New York, AIDES in Paris and the Terrence Higgins Trust in London.[98] In many industrialized countries, philanthropic organizations were started such as the American Foundation for AIDS Research (AmFAR) and National AIDS Trusts in Australia and in the UK.

These communities united in the common purpose of demanding respect for those who are ill, infected or exposed to HIV. Often they were angry and impatient with the slowness of bureaucracy to respond to their needs and for access to treatment. This lead to the founding of coalitions of people living with AIDS. One of the best known and most effective groups is ACT UP. It was founded in New York in March 1987, to improve services of government and health care systems and access to them.[99]

Community development and activism in non-industrialized countries is only beginning. Development programmes promoting community development are, perhaps, the most visible.[100] Often, efforts to educate, care for and protect people in such countries is part of a wider effort to secure access to human rights.[101]

Reactions of some governments have, at times, been arbitrary, irrational, discriminatory, and aggravated the suffering and harms produced by AIDS. This is exemplified by repressive laws and policies that restrict the entry to these countries of people who are infected with HIV or who have AIDS and who would otherwise be admissible to them.[102] In contrast to its leadership in the area of research on this epidemic, the United States had the most restrictive law, until it was recently rescinded.[103] Perhaps the most repressive reaction has been by Cuba which indefinitely isolates its citizens who are infected.[104] Repression has also directly obstructed efforts to educate people and to change behaviour with legislatures invoking censorship to threaten or limit educational efforts.[105]

The Hidden Epidemic: The Junk Virus

HIV has steadily and sometimes rapidly penetrated into injection drug user communities. This is a calamity making the epidemic among the gay community seem simple. In 1959, William Burroughs described drug dependence as a "junk virus,"[106] and substance abuse has many features of an epidemic. There are the health and social consequences of injected drugs themselves, social structuring among injection drug users is often very primitive, and the growing use of cocaine facilitates repetitive injecting behaviour, more than do the opiates, expediting the spread of HIV. Perhaps most importantly is the stereotyping that injection drug use elicits. Non-medical injection drug use is generally illicit.[107] The association of injection drug use with what many consider unlawful behaviour, the impact of the drugs themselves and the poor socioeconomic status of most drug users antagonizes efforts to erase stereotyping and stigmatization. In addition, some injection drug users engage in prostitution to pay for their drugs.[108] Until drug misuse is seen to be a sickness (the "medicalization" of drug misuse), rather than predominantly a criminal activity (its "criminalization"), marginalization will continue to facilitate the spread of AIDS.

Some efforts to halt HIV transmission by the sharing of uncleaned injection equipment have been successful. These outreach programmes usually distribute free injection equipment and condoms to those using these services. While inaccessibility to injecting equipment appears to facilitate HIV transmission, access to equipment without effective programmes to educate drug users has not stemmed the spread of HIV.[109]

Conclusions: Future Imperfect

Analysis of the AIDS epidemic eventually arrives at the question of how this epidemic should be judged now, and how it will be judged by historians. Among these criteria are: first, what was done to control its spread; second, what was done to control the harms it produced including but not restricted to disease and death; and third, what improvements in society did it produce.[110] There has been success in preventing infection in some communities, and failure in others; diagnosis and treatment are now available but are accessible to only a minority of people infected; beneficial spin-offs and cultural development seem overwhelmed by events that have turned science into a commodity, and by the "double jeopardy" of dying and being persecuted, stigmatized or discriminated against because one is infected with HIV or has AIDS. These are not conclusions but challenges for an imperfect future.

NOTES

1. For a discussion of the terms "disease," "illness" and "sickness," as used in this paper see B.S. Turner, *Medical Power and Social Knowledge* (London: Sage, 1987), 1-17.

2. For scientific achievements, see R.C. Gallo, L. Montagner L, "The Chronology of AIDS Research," *Nature* (1987: 326): 435-436; for achievements in diagnosis, care and treatment, see R.E. Chaisson, "Living with AIDS," *Journal of the American Medical Association* (1090: 263): 434-435 and G.H. Friedland, "Early treatment for HIV: the time has come," *New England Journal of Medicine* (1990: 322): 1000-1002; and for social impact, see J.E. Osborn, "AIDS and Public Policy," *AIDS* (1989:3 (suppl 1)): S297-S300 and M.D. Grmek, *History of AIDS: Emergence and Origins of a Modern Pandemic* (Princeton N.J.: Princeton University Press, 1990), 156-70. For shortcomings in science, see B.J. Culliton, "Inside the Gallo probe," *Science* (1990: 248): 1494-98; E. Rubinstein, "The untold story of HUT78," *Science* (1990: 248): 1499-1507; and H.G. Miller, C.F. Turner and L.E. Moses, eds., *AIDS: The Second Decade* (Washington: The National Research Council/National Academy Press, 1990); for shortcomings in diagnosis, care and treatment, see D. Baltimore, S.M. Wolff, eds., *Confronting AIDS*. (Washington: National Academy of Sciences Institute of Medicine/National Academy Press, 1986) and T. Cooper, ed., *Confronting AIDS: Update 1988* (Washington: National Academy of Sciences Institutes of Medicine/National Academy Press, 1988). For shortcomings in social development see C. Pierce, D. Vandeveer, *AIDS: Ethics and Public Policy* (Belmont, CA:, Wadsworth, 1988); D. Crimp, ed., *AIDS: Cultural Analysis/Cultural Activism* (Cambridge, MA: The MIT Press, 1988); and R. Cohen, L.S. Wiseberg, "Editorial," *Double Jeopardy — Threat to Life and Human Rights. Discrimination against Persons with AIDS* (Cambridge, MA: Human Rights Internet, March 1990), 3.

3. R. Dubos, *Mirage of Health* (Garden City, N.Y.: Anchor Books, 1959) and A.M. Brandt, "The syphilis epidemic and its relation to AIDS," *Science* (1988: 239): 375-80.

4. J. Chin, P.A. Sato and J. Mann, "Projections of HIV infections and AIDS cases to the year 2000," *Bulletin of the World Health Organization* (1990: 68): 1-11.

5. In this paper, AIDS is presumed to be a consequence of HIV infection, regardless of whether it is a direct or indirect consequence of this infection. While there is uncertainty about the mechanism by which HIV infection might lead to, or result in AIDS (sufficient or necessary causation; whether or not co-factors determine progression to disease or modulate the progression of its manifestations; or that HIV might only be a marker for another cause of AIDS), there is consensus that HIV is associated with, or defines the process of AIDS from exposure to disease. Attributing causation of AIDS to HIV as used in this paper neither confirms nor denies causation, but only implies the utility of HIV as a marker for this process.

6. N. Gilmore, "Human immunodeficiency virus infection and AIDS: concepts and constructs," *Proceedings of the Third European Community Workshop on Quantitative Analysis of AIDS, Modelling and Scenario-analysis.* J.C. Jäger, ed. (Bilthoven, Netherlands: RIVM, 18 December, 1989) (forthcoming) and B.S. Blumberg and R.C. Fox, "The Daedalus Effect: changes in ethical questions relating to hepatitis-B virus," *Annals of Internal Medicine* (1985: 102): 390-94.

7. S. Panem, *The AIDS Bureaucracy* (Cambridge, MA: Harvard University Press, 1988), 136-49.

8. For a discussion of the origins and evolution of community responses to HIV/AIDS, see C. Patton, *Inventing AIDS* (London, Routledge, 1990), 5-23.

9. M. Eigen and K. Nieselt-Struwe, "How old is the immunodeficiency virus?" *AIDS* (1990: 4 (Suppl 1)): S85-S93.

10. M.D. Grmek, op. cit. (fn. 2), 119-37.

11. J.M. Mann, "Global AIDS: epidemiology, impact, projections, global strategy," *AIDS Prevention and Control* (Oxford: Pergammon Press, 1988), 3-13.

12. Certain infections such as Pneumocystis carinii pneumonia (PCP), mucocutaneous

candidiasis and chronic, ulcerative Herpes simplex infection rarely occur in adults unless they are immunodeficient. Similarly, Kaposi's sarcoma (KS) is a rare malignancy in industrialized countries. Other than in elderly men, KS only rarely develops in otherwise healthy people. That is, these infections (often termed opportunistic since they need the opportunity of immunodeficiency to develop) and malignancies such as KS or non-Hodgkin's lymphomas never develop in people whose immune systems function normally. The development of these diseases, therefore, indicates the immune system has been severely damaged, that is the person is immunodeficient.

13. M.D. Grmek, op. cit., 3-12.

14. Centres for Disease Control, "Pneumocystis pneumonia: Los Angeles," *Morbidity Mortality Weekly Report* (1981: 30): 250-52.

15. ___, "Kaposi's sarcoma and Pneumocystis pneumonia among homosexual men: New York city and California," *Morbidity Mortality Weekly Report* (1981: 30): 305-8.

16. L.K. Altman, "Rare cancer seen in forty-one homosexuals," *New York Times* (3 July 1981): 20.

17. Centers for Disease Control, "Follow-up on Kaposis sarcoma and Pneumocystis pneumonia," *Morbidity Mortality Weekly Report* (1981: 30): 409-10.

18. J. Marx, "New disease baffles medical community," *Science* (1982: 217): 618-22.

19. A.G. Fettner and W.A. Check, *The Truth about AIDS* (New York: Holt, Rinehart and Winston, 1985).

20. R.M. Anderson, "Mathematical and statistical studies of the epidemiology of HIV," *AIDS* (1989: 3): 333-46.

21. These cells are named T-helper, T4 or CD4 lymphocytes. They coordinate the functions of the immune system. In AIDS, they are progressively depleted. They are easily enumerated in blood specimens, providing quantification of immune damage.

22. M.S. Gottlieb, R. Schroff, H.M. Schanker, et al., "Pneumocystis carinii pneumonia and mucosal candidiasis in previously healthy homosexual men: evidence of a new acquired cellular immunodeficiency," *New England Journal of Medicine* (1981:305): 1425-31; H. Masur, M.A. Michelis, J.B. Greene, et al., "An outbreak of community-acquired Pnuemocystis carinii pneumonia: initial manifestation of cellular immune dysfunction," *New England Journal of Medicine* (1981: 305): 1431-38; F.P. Siegel, C. Lopez, G. Hammer et al., "Severe acquired immunodeficiency in male homosexuals, manifested by chronic perianal ulcerative herpes simplex lesions," *New England Journal of Medicine* (1981: 305): 1439-44.

23. D. Altman, *AIDS in the Mind of America* (Garden City, N.J.: Anchor Press, 1986).

24. J. Kinsella, *Covering the Plague: AIDS and the American Media* (New Brunswick, N.J.: Rutgers University Press, 1989), 75.

25. K.B. Hymes, J.B. Greene, A. Marcus, et al., "Kaposi's sarcoma in homosexual men: a report of eight cases," *Lancet* (1981: 2): 598-600, and H.K. Thomsen, M. Jacobsen and A. Malchow-Moller, "Kaposi's sarcoma among homosexual men in Europe," *Lancet* (1981: 2): 688.

26. M. Marmor, A.E. Friedman-Kien, L. Laubenstein, et al., "Risk factors for Kaposi's sarcoma in homosexual men," *Lancet* (1982: 1): 1083-87.

27. J. Leibowitch, *A Strange Virus of Unknown Origin* (New York: Ballantine, 1985).

28. Centers for Disease Control, "A cluster of Kaposi's sarcoma and Pneumocystis carinii pneumonia among homosexual male residents of Los Angeles and Orange counties, California," *Morbidity Mortality Weekly Report* (1982: 31): 305-7.

29. R. Shilts, *And the Band Played On: Politics, People and the AIDS Epidemic* (New York: St Martin's Press, 1987), 157-8. Such labelling misunderstood the difference between transmission of infection and susceptibility to develop disease once infected. Patient Zero may have been one of the earliest people to develop AIDS but whether or not he was earliest to be infected or to spread this infection is unknown.

30. The name "acquired immune deficiency syndrome" (soon changed to acquired immunodeficiency syndrome) and its acronym "AIDS" were first used in a publication dated 4 April 1982 (Centers for Disease Control, "Diffuse undifferentiated non-Hodgkin's lymphoma among homosexual males: United States," *Morbidity Mortality Weekly Report* (1982: 31): 277-79). Also, see M.D. Grmek, op. cit. (fn.2), 32.

31. Centers for Disease Control, "Update on Kaposi's sarcoma and opportunistic infections in previously healthy persons: United States," *Morbidity Mortality Weekly Report* (1982: 31): 294-301.

32. ___, "Pneumocystis carinii pneumonia among persons with hemophilia A," *Morbidity Mortality Weekly Report* (1982: 31): 365-7; and Centers for Disease Control, "Possible transfusion-associated acquired immune deficiency syndrome (AIDS): California," *Morbidity Mortality Weekly Report* (1982: 31): 652-4.

33. ___, "Unexplained immunodeficiency and opportunistic infections in infants: New York, New Jersey, California," *Morbidity Mortality Weekly Report* (1982: 31): 665-7.

34. ___, "Opportunistic infections and Kaposi's sarcoma among Haitians in the United States," *Morbidity Mortality Weekly Report* (1982: 31): 353-4. This report was soon followed by others which confirmed AIDS inside and outside of Haiti (J. Vieiria, E. Franck, T. Spira, et al., "Acquired immune deficiency syndrome in Haitians," *New England Journal of Medicine* (1983: 308): 125-9; A.E. Pitchenik, M.A. Fischl, G.M. Dickinson, et al., "Opportunistic infections and Kaposi's sarcoma among Haitians: evidence of a new acquired immunodeficiency state," *Annals of Internal Medicine* (1983:98):277-84; T. Andreani, R. Modigliani, Y. Le Charpentier, et al., "Acquired immunodeficiency with intestinal cryptosporidiosis: possible transmission by Haitian whole blood," *Lancet* (1983: 1): 1187-90; and J.W. Pape, B. Liautaud, F. Thomas, et al., "Characteristics of the acquired immunodeficiency syndrome in Haiti," *New England Journal of Medicine* (1983: 309): 945-50).

35. The earliest publication of AIDS in Africa originated in Zaïre (B. Lamey and N. Malemeka, "Aspects cliniques et épidémiologiques de la cryptococcose à Kinshasha. A propos de quinze cas personnels," *Médicine Tropicale* (1982: 42): 507-14). Subsequent publications included: N. Clumeck, F. Mascart-Lemone, J. De Maubege, et al., "Acquired immunodeficiency syndrome in black Africans," *Lancet* (1983: 1): 642; J.B. Brunet, E. Bouvet, J. Leibowitch, et al., "Acquired immunodeficiency syndrome in France," *Lancet* (1983: 1): 700-1; I.C. Bygbjerg, "AIDS in a Danish surgeon (Zaïre 1976)," *Lancet* (1983: 1): 925; J. Vandepitte, R. Verwilghen and P. Zachee, "AIDS and cryptococcosis (Zaïre 1977)," Lancet (1983: 1): p. 925; and G. Offenstadt, P. Pinta, P. Hericard, et al., "Multiple opportunistic infections due to AIDS in a previously healthy black woman from Zaïre," *New England Journal of Medicine* (1983: 308): 775.

36. Despite publications about AIDS in Africa, appreciation of the full extent of the problem was slow and clouded in political misunderstanding and denial. At the first International Symposium on AIDS in Africa (Brussels, 22 November 1985) some African governments denied AIDS was a problem in their countries, prohibited delegates from speaking about it, and were upset by accusations that HIV originated in Africa, leading to confusion and controversy about the dimensions of the problem in Africa (C. Norman, "Politics and science clash on African AIDS," *Science* (1985: 230): 1140-2).

37. D.C. Desjarlais and S.R. Friedman, "The epidemic of HIV infection among injecting drug users in New York city: the first decade and possible future directions," *AIDS and Drug Misuse*, J. Strang and G.V. Stimson, eds. (London: Routledge, 1990), 86-94.

38. A.R. Moss, "Control of HIV infection in injecting drug users in San Francisco," ibid., 77-85.

39. A. Wodak and A. Moss, "HIV infection and injection drug users: from epidemiology to public health," *AIDS* (1990: 4 (Suppl 1)): S105-S109.

40. Centers for Disease Control, "Immunodeficiency among female sex partners of males with acquired immune deficiency syndrome (AIDS): New York," *Morbidity Mortality Weekly Report* (1983: 31): 697-8.

41.___, "Prevention of acquired immune deficiency syndrome (AIDS): Report of Inter-agency Recommendations," *Morbidity Mortality Weekly Report* (1983: 32): 101-3.

42. H. Masur, M.A. Michelis, G.P. Wormser, et al., "Opportunistic infection in previously healthy women: initial manifestations of a community acquired immunodeficiency," *Annals of Internal Medicine* (1982: 97): 533-9.

43. A.S. Fauci, "The acquired immune deficiency syndrome. The ever-broadening clinical spectrum," *Annals of Internal Medicine* (1983: 249): 2375-6.

44. J. Kinsella, op. cit. (fn. 24), 71.

45. Ibid., 142-5.

46. Media responses in the United States did not peak until 1987 but there was a large increase at the time of the announcement that AIDS had become the number-one health priority in the USA (ibid., fig. 11, p. 156).

47. This was a retrovirus, named human T-leukemia virus type I or HTLV-I. It was renamed human T-lymphotropic virus type I, and the distinct virus associated with AIDS was named human T-lymphotropic virus type III (HTLV-III).

48. HIV preferentially infects cells expressing the CD4 molecule, and so preferentially infects T-helper lymphocytes.

49. M. Essex, M.F. McLane, T.H. Lee, et al., "Antibodies to cell membrane antigens associated with human T-cell leukemia virus in patients with AIDS," *Science* (1983: 220): 859-62.

50. R.C. Gallo, P.S. Sarin, E.P. Gelmann, et al., "Isolation of a human T-cell leukemia virus in acquired immunodeficiency virus," *Science* (1983: 220): 865-8.

51. F. Barré-Sinoussi, J.-C. Chermann and F. Rey, "Isolation of a T-lymphotropic retrovirus from a patient at risk for acquired immune deficiency syndrome (AIDS)," *Science* (1983: 220): 868-71.

52. R.C. Gallo, S.Z. Salahuddin, M. Popovic et al., "Frequent detection and isolation of cytopathic retrovirus (HTLV-III) from patients with AIDS and at risk for AIDS," *Science* (1984: 224): 500-503 and M.G. Sarngadharan, M. Popovic, L. Bruch et al., "Antibodies reactive with human T-lymphotropic retroviruses (HTLV-III) in the serum of patients with AIDS," *Science* (1984: 224): 506-8.

53. M. Popovic, M.G. Sarngadharan, E. Read and R.C. Gallo, "A method for detection, isolation and continuous production of cytopathic retroviruses (HTLV-III) from patients with AIDS and pre-AIDS," *Science* (1984: 224): 497-500.

54. See R.C. Gallo and L. Montagner, op. cit. (fn. 2).

55. H.L. Singer, "Institut Pasteur v. United States: The AIDS patent dispute, the Contract Disputes Act and the international exchange of scientific data," *American Journal of Law and Medicine* (1989: 15): 439-59; L.K. Altman, "U.S. and France end rift on AIDS," *New York Times* (1 April 1987): A1; and M.D. Grmek, op. cit. (fn. 2), 76-7.

56. J. Coffin, A. Haase, J. Levy, et al., "Human immunodeficiency viruses," *Science* (1986: 232): 697.

57. J. Crewdson, "The great AIDS quest," *Chicago Tribune* (19 November 1989: Sec. 5 (Special Report)).

58. B.J. Culliton, op. cit.; and E. Rubinstein, op. cit.

59. H. Rubin, "Is HIV the causative factor in AIDS?" *Nature* (1988: 334): 201.

60. W. Blattner, R.C. Gallo, H.M. Temin, "HIV causes AIDS," *Science* (1988: 241): 514-7.

61. P.H. Duesberg, "Retroviruses as carcinogens and pathogens: expectations and reality," *Cancer Research* (1987: 47): 1199-220; and P.H. Duesberg, "HIV is not the cause of AIDS," *Science* (1988: 241): 514-7; and J. Kinsella, op. cit. (fn. 24), 45-7.

62. M.P. Girard, J.W. Eichberg, "Progress in the development of HIV vaccines," *AIDS* (1990: 4 (Suppl 1)): S143-S150.

63. E.A. Preble, "Impact of HIV/AIDS on African children," *Social Science and Medicine* (1990: 31): 671-80; and *Global Program on AIDS: Progress Report No. 6* (Geneva: World Health Organization, May 1990), 27.

64. B.S. Blumberg and R.C. Fox, loc. cit. (fn. 6).

65. M. Gunderson, D.J. Mayo, F.S. Rhame, "AIDS: Testing and Privacy," *Ethics in a Changing World*, M.P. Battin and L.P. Francis, eds. (1989: 2): 1-240, and B.M. Dickens, "Legal limits of AIDS confidentiality," *Journal of the American Medical Association* (1988: 259): 3449-51.

66. G. Slutkin, J. Chin, D. Tarantola, J. Mann, "Sentinel surveillance for HIV infection: a method to monitor HIV infection trends in population groups," (Geneva: World Health Organization, 1988), (WHO/GPA/DIR/88.8).

67. R.M. Anderson, op. cit.

68. M.A. Fischl, D.D. Richman, M.H. Grieco, et al., "The efficacy of azidothymidine (AZT) in the treatment of patients with AIDS and AIDS-related complex," *New England Journal of Medicine* (1987: 317): 185-91.

69. F.S. Rhame, D.G. Maki, "The case for wider use of testing for HIV infection," *New England Journal of Medicine* (1989: 320): 1248-54.

70. D. Crimp, A. Rolston, *AIDS DemoGraphics* (Seattle: Bay Press, 1990), 13.

71. J. Mann, op. cit. (fn. 11).

72. M.P. Girard, op. cit. (fn. 62)

73. J.E. Osborn, "AIDS and public policy," *AIDS* (1989: 3 (Suppl 1)): S297-S300.

74. M. Black, "Children and AIDS: An Impending Calamity," (New York: UNICEF, 1990), 13; and S. Hunter, "Orphans as a window on the AIDS epidemic in sub-Saharan Africa: initial results and implications of a study in Uganda," *Social Science and Medicine* (1990: 3): 681-90.

75. J. Chin, "Global estimates of AIDS cases and HIV infections: 1990," *AIDS* (1990: 4 (Suppl 1)): S277-S283.

76. M. Black, op. cit., 10.

77. M.-L. Newell, C.S. Peckham and P. Lepage, "HIV-1 infection in pregnancy: implications for women and children," *AIDS* (1990: 4 (Suppl 1)): S111-S117.

78. See fn. 35.

79. D. Serawadda, R.D. Mugerwa, N.K. Sewankambo et al., "Slim disease: a new disease in Uganda and its association with HTLV-III/LAV infection," *Lancet* (2): 849-52.

80. T.C. Quinn, J.M. Mann, J.W. Curran and P. Piot, "AIDS in Africa: an epidemiologic paradigm," *Science* (1986: 234): 955-963.

81. See fn. 35.

82. J.W. Carswell, G. Lloyd, J. Howells, "Prevalence of HIV-1 in east African lorry drivers," *AIDS* (1989: 3): 759-61; Editorial: "AIDS: prevention, policies, and prostitutes," *Lancet* (1989; 1): 1111-1113; E.R. Koenig, "International prostitutes and transmission of HIV," *Lancet* (1989: 1): 782-3; and *AIDS and the Third World* (London: Panos Institute/New Society Publishers, 1989).

83. J.K. Kreiss, D. Koech, F.A. Plummer et al., "AIDS virus infection in Nairobi prostitutes. Spread of the epidemic to East Africa," *New England Journal of Medicine* (1986: 314): 414-18.

84. J. Mann, "Global AIDS: revolution, paradigm and solidarity," *AIDS* (1990: 4 (Suppl 1)): S247-S250.

85. T.C. Quinn, F.R.K. Zacharias, R.K. St John, "AIDS in the Americas: an emerging public health crisis," *New England Journal of Medicine* (1989; 320): 1005-7.

86. R.H. Morrow, R.L. Colebunders, J. Chin J, "Interactions of HIV infection with endemic tropical diseases," *AIDS* (1989: 3 (Suppl 1)): S70-S87; and D.W. Cameron and N.S. Padian, "Sexual transmission of HIV and the epidemiology of other sexually transmitted diseases," *AIDS* (1990: 4 (Suppl 1)): S99-S103.

87. F. Clavel, D. Guétard, F. Brun-Vézinet et al., "Isolation of a new human retrovirus from West

African patients," *Science* (1986: 233): 343-6.

88. J. Osborn, op. cit. (fn. 73).

89. Office for Information Reference Services, AIDS Control in Britain. (London: Foreign and Commonwealth Office, December 1987) (Document 290/87).

90. C.E. Koop, "Surgeon General's report on acquired immunodeficiency syndrome," *Journal of the American Medical Association* (1986: 256): 2783-9.

91. This programme was subsequently renamed the Global Program on AIDS mandated to prevent further transmission of AIDS, decrease the impact of this epidemic on individuals, groups and societies, and coordinate efforts between and among countries to stop this epidemic (see M.D. Grmek, op.cit. (fn. 2), 182-3.

92. World Health Organization, Global Programme on AIDS, op. cit. (fn. 63), appendices 4 and 5, 53-7.

93. World Health Assembly, "Avoidance of discrimination in relation to HIV-infected people and people with AIDS," (Geneva: World Health Association, 1988) (WHO Doc. WHO/GPA/INF/88.2).

94. J. Mann, op. cit. (fn. 84).

95. J.D. Watkins, Chairman, "Report of the Presidential Commission on Human Immunodeficiency Virus Epidemic," (Washington: US Government Printing Office, 1988) (Doc. O-214-701: QL3, 1988); M. Chrétien, E.A. McCulloch, "AIDS: A Perspective for Canadians," (Ottawa: Royal Society of Canada, 1988).

96. C. Patton, op. cit. (fn. 8); D. Altman, op. cit. (fn. 23).

97. C. Norman, "The epidemic's unsung heroes," *Science* (1985: 230): 1020.

98. J.F. McGuire, "AIDS: the community-based response," *AIDS* (1989: 3 (Suppl 1)): S279-S282.

99. D. Crimp, op. cit. (fn. 2); and D. Crimp and A. Rolston, op. cit. (fn 70).

100. D. Nabarro and C. McConnell, "The impact of AIDS on socioeconomic development," *AIDS* (1990: 4 (Suppl 1)): S265-S272.

101. U.N. Centre for Human Rights, Report of an International Consultation on AIDS and Human Rights. (New York: United Nations, 1991).

102. N. Gilmore, A.J. Orkin, M. Duckett and S.A. Grover, "International travel and AIDS," *AIDS* (1989: 3 (Suppl 1)): S225-S230; and M. Duckett and A.J. Orkin, "AIDS-related migration and travel policies and restrictions: a global survey," *AIDS* (1989; 3 (Suppl 1)): S231-S252.

103. L.O. Gostin, P.D. Cleary, K.H. Mayer, A.M. Brandt and E.H. Chittenden, "Screening immigrants and international travellers for the human immunodeficiency virus," *New England Journal of Medicine* (1990: 322): 1743-6.

104. R. Bayer and C. Healton, "Controlling AIDS in Cuba. The logic of quarantine," *New England Journal of Medicine* (1989: 320): 1022-4.

105. C. Patton, op. cit. (fn. 8), 52-7.

106. W.S. Burroughs, *Naked Lunch* (New York: Grove Press, 1959), vi.

107. C. O'Neill, "Intravenous drug abusers," *AIDS and the Law: A Guide for the Public*, H.L. Dalton, S. Burris, Yale AIDS Law Project, eds. (New Haven, CT: Yale University Press, 1987), 253-80.

108. C.B. Wofsy, "AIDS and prostitution," *AIDS in Children, Adolescents and Heterosexual Adults*, R.F. Schinazi and A.J. Nahmias, eds. (New York: Elsevier, 1988), 168-9.

109. E. Tempesta and M. Di Giannantonio, "The Italian epidemic: a case study," Strang and Stimson, eds., op. cit (fn. 35), 108-17.

110. N. Gilmore, "Sex, AIDS and cultural change," *Sieccan Journal* (1988: 3): 1-13.

AIDS and the Reconceptualization of Homosexuality

Dennis Altman

Dedicated to the memory of James Baldwin, whose writings helped many of us to understand that it was society, not us, which was the problem.

It was an historic accident that AIDS appeared as a new disease, first diagnosed among male homosexuals, at a time of rapid change in social and cultural attitudes to homosexuality in most Western countries. There has already been considerable discussion on the way the gay connection affected the conceptualization of AIDS. Equally important is the way the link with AIDS has affected the social construction of homosexuality.

AIDS has not altered the fundamental reality of homosexuality (although it may have meant some people are less willing to adopt a gay identity; evidence on this point remains scanty). On balance it seems that AIDS has strengthened the growth of gay identity and community already evident before its onset in most Western countries. Indeed, it seems likely that the response to AIDS by both the gay community and the larger society is primarily a function of the extent to which gays had carved out some degree of political legitimacy for ourselves in the 1970s. Where a gay movement had succeeded in establishing some official recognition, (for example the Netherlands, Scandinavia, California, and parts of Australia), this affected the response of governments in the fight against AIDS. Where there had been less success in establishing a gay movement this was also reflected in official attitudes towards AIDS (as in almost every authoritarian society and not a few allegedly democratic ones).

The most dramatic impact of AIDS on concepts of gay identity is in the area of sexuality; the epidemic has severely strained the mores of sexual adventure and experimentation that seemed an integral part of gay male life until the early 1980s. In so doing, it has made clear that the gay community is based on more than a shared set of sexual arrangements; indeed, AIDS itself has become part of the common experience of gay men, which may further isolate us from both lesbians and non-gays, while strengthening our own communal organizations.

In writing this article I have drawn heavily on my own experience, first while I was researching my book, *AIDS in the Mind of America*[1] on both coasts of the United States in 1984-85, and subsequently back in Australia, where I have been both a government advisor and vice-president of the Victorian AIDS Council (a juxtaposition that already says something about the approach adopted by the Australian government, in contrast to the United States federal government). Over the past few years I have briefly visited Canada, Sweden, France, Britain, and New Zealand, but any references I make to the situation outside my immediate experience need be tentative and exploratory. What is clear, however, is that wherever there exists a self-conscious gay community and identity, AIDS has become an overwhelming preoccupation that hangs over all of us.

My own career suggests to me that the distinction between "academic" and "activist" is a false one. But it is striking how little work on politics has gone on under the rubric of gay/lesbian studies. We badly need comparative studies of the gay movement and of specific campaigns, many (like the two major referenda in California on gay-related topics) have virtually been ignored by gay scholars.[2] My own ignorance was sharply brought home to me in the discussion following the presentation of this paper at an international conference, particularly in light of comments from participants from Mexico and Brazil.

AIDS and the Question of Gay Identity

Early in the epidemic I speculated whether the fear and stigma associated with AIDS would lead to a decline in the number of men who chose to identify themselves as gay, or at least adopt homosexual behaviour as an integral part of their lives. That I can pose this in terms of choice suggests that I still adhere to a constructionist view of homosexuality, despite the strength of some of the recently made criticisms of this theory.[3]

At this point it seems to me that there exists no evidence to suggest that such a decline has occurred, although it is true that I am working almost entirely on the basis of impressionistic data. My feeling is that at least as many teenagers are adopting a gay identity and/or homosexual behaviour pattern as was true ten years ago, and that in most Western countries of which I have first hand knowledge they are able to integrate an awareness of AIDS into this identity or behaviour. (This feeling is reinforced by one New Zealand study that claimed: "The personal psychological awareness of sexual orientation reported by young people now is quite consistent with what was reported by the previous generation. But the social experience of these people, and their patterns of sexual activity, have changed quite radically.")[4] It may also be true that some men are seeking to change their sexual identity in response to AIDS — as Brendan Lemon wrote in a recent short story: "Somewhere toward the end of the AIDS decade, Paul decided to go straight."[5] I doubt if this is the experience of significant numbers of men.

Thus, on one level, the title of this paper is somewhat misleading, for AIDS has not apparently affected the incidence, nor the fundamental meaning of homosexuality in Western societies. It has, however, meant very real changes in the ways we experience homosexual identity, both at an individual and a collective level.

Some observers have claimed that since the onset of AIDS gay men have been less likely to define themselves in sexual terms. Certainly it is true that not inconsiderable numbers of men are remaining celibate for long periods of time, without this affecting their sense of gay identity. But it seems to me that any concept of gay identity becomes quite meaningless if we try to deny it is an identity clearly based upon sexual preference, even if this preference is not always acted upon.

It is true that a particular style of gay life, closely linked to a constant search for sexual adventure and excitement, a world depicted in novels such as *Faggots, Tricks, or Dancer for the Dance*, has declined, at least in the major centres of gay America. Bath-houses and backroom clubs have been closed down due to the epidemic in both New York and San Francisco, and have lost clients in those cities where they have been permitted to stay open. There is some evidence that gay businesses have declined in at least those cities most affected by the epidemic.

Even allowing for this it is my impression that the sort of gay world created by the twin engines of cultural change and commercialization during the 1970s has been largely untouched by AIDS. Indeed, outside the United States, new saunas have opened in the past two years in Melbourne, Montréal and Paris, and in the United States the title of Randy Shilts's book on AIDS, *And the Band Played On*, is still an appropriate description of much of gay life. On my last trip to the United States. I was struck by the sheer size and verve of gay life in cities such as Dallas and Boston.

Growth of Community Organizations

In many countries, the AIDS epidemic has seen the development of large gay community organizations concerned with providing education, support services, and counselling to both those with AIDS and to the much larger group who are threatened by it. Almost everywhere AIDS organizations arose out of, and remain closely linked to, the gay community, although the first and the largest, New York City's Gay Men's Health Crisis remains one of the few to declare itself as such. Indeed, a number of AIDS organizations have quite specifically sought to include

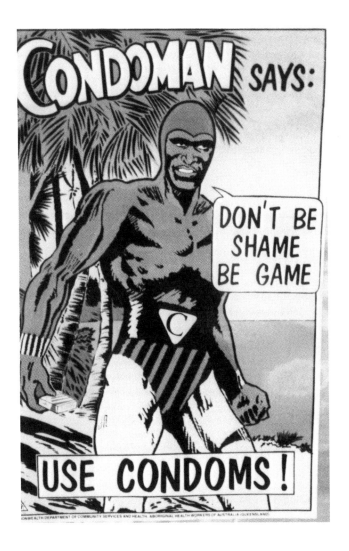

Condoman Campaign, Aboriginal Health Workers of Australia, Queensland. Poster.

and represent other groups than gay men, both as a reflection of medical realities and political desirability.

In some cases it may be that AIDS organizations have developed to a point where it is no longer accurate to think of them as gay community organizations. Indeed, AIDS makes the definition of the gay community problematic in a new way. Now it is not merely the traditional division between homosexual identity and behaviour, and the argument as to whether lesbians and gay men constitute one or two communities, that are involved. There are numbers of people who, without being homosexual in any sense, have committed themselves to working with gay community organizations, just as there are men who regard themselves as feminists. I don't know what term to use for them, but I do know that they are more a part of my community than those homosexual men and women who support politicians such as Reagan and Thatcher whose policies oppress us.

AIDS has undoubtedly created a strong sense among many gay men and women that we have a responsibility to do something about this disease, not just on an individual level, but also as members of a community. "We have to look after other gay men, because nobody else gives a damn," was a feeling encountered very often, at least in the United States, in the early years of the epidemic. This feeling was evident in the outpouring of hundreds of thousands of gay women and men, and their supporters, at the recent march on Washington, where anger at federal inaction on AIDS was clearly a major driving force.[6]

My own experience with the Victorian AIDS Council suggests that voluntary AIDS organizations become important community resources, through which people, in addition to the work they are directly involved with, also develop very deep ties of friendship and support. In Melbourne we have had the luxury of a low case-load and considerable government support — the state government responded to the epidemic by financing the establishment of a Gay Men's Community Health Crisis Centre — and our situation is a much easier one than in American cities of similar size such as Houston or Miami-Fort Lauderdale. Our experience suggests, however, that with proper resources the gay community can generate impressive organizational responses to the epidemic.

In addition to such straightforward arguments about the ways AIDS has strengthened gay community, we need consider two other areas: the paradox that more overt homophobia based on AIDS has also served to strengthen gay identity/community, and the ways in which the gay community has produced a large body of cultural reflection upon the meaning of the epidemic, thus unintentionally reinforcing the perception of AIDS as a specifically gay disease.

While it is true that AIDS is not in any intrinsic sense a gay disease, it is the gay communities of the Western world who have produced cultural images and reflections on the meaning of the epidemic, through films, novels, theatre, art works — think of the 800-square-foot quilt memorializing those dead from AIDS that was part of the Washington protests. (The quilt disproved Edmund White's suggestion that AIDS has "tilted energies away from the popular arts . . . and redirected them towards the 'solitary' high arts").[7] It is hardly accidental that theatre, far more immediate an artform than either the novel or the cinema, has proven a particularly appropriate forum to canvass the emotions and issues raised by AIDS, as other papers have demonstrated; Larry Kramer's *The Normal Heart* was as important a commentary for the politics of its time and place as earlier *cris du coeur* such as Arthur Miller's *The Crucible* were.

There is little doubt that AIDS has given new energy to our opponents, which in turn has led to a marked increase in anti-gay violence and attempts to repeal legislative gains of the past two decades. *Newsweek* considered these developments so striking, at least in Britain, that it ran one story headed "An Ugly Anti-Gay Backlash," and in the United States there have been Congressional hearings that have demonstrated the recent rise in homophobic violence. As AIDS has provided a new pretext for right-wing fundamentalists, whether of the religious kind like Jerry Falwell or secular like Jean Le Pen and the British Tories, to attack homosexuals, the response, at least in the United States, has been to mobilize gays to fight back. Large-scale political action by the gay community on AIDS-related issues began with the campaign waged in late 1986 to defeat the LaRouche-initiated referendum in California, which would have introduced quarantine for anyone testing HIV positive. A strong campaign, and support from many politicians and health authorities, defeated the measure by almost two-to-one.[8] Since then there has been a marked increase in direct gay political action, as in the rise of groups like ACT UP (New York) or ACTING OUT (San Francisco) and in the civil disobedience actions that accompanied the March on Washington and subsequent events in the U.S.

Examples from elsewhere are harder to find. In the spring of 1987 a rally of 10,000 Germans protested proposals for harsh measures by the Bavarian Land government, and in both Sydney and Melbourne antibody-positive activists have organized rallies in protest of the expense and limited availability of AZT.

This discussion has been largely restricted to gay men, although in some countries lesbians have played an important part in AIDS movements. In my own city of Melbourne the great majority of women who participate in AIDS work have been straight, and I suspect that one consequence of AIDS has been to increase separateness between gay women and men, not least because the official perception of "the gay community" as male reinforces the already male-centredness of that movement. This is emphatically not the case in the United States, where AIDS has quickly moved from being perceived as a gay male issue to one that has provided new unity between lesbians and gay men. In the United States lesbians have provided considerable leadership in the AIDS battles, from early on in the epidemic (think, for example, of the role of the "Blood Sisters" in offering support to gay men) to the March on Washington where a majority of those arrested for direct action were women.[9] I would hope this renewed sense of community between gay women and men extends to other countries.

I do not want to offer too rosy a view of gay community and support as the response to AIDS. The other side of this is the considerable fear, paranoia, and unfocused anger that is also evident in some of the gay world. For some the reaction to the epidemic has been irrational anger or apathy — irrational not in the sense that it is not understandable, or in the case of anger, unjustified, but irrational because it does little to meet the challenge. (A good example of this sort of anger is the way in which a once great paper, the New York Native has denounced some of the most hard-working supporters of the gay community, such as Mathilde Krim and Jeff Levi, when they in any way disagreed with the increasingly eccentric line taken by that paper). While many of us have found a way of coping with fear and loss by our participation in community and support organizations, others have retreated to a sort of emotional autism, so scared — and scarred — by the prospect of the disease that they avoid any form of emotional contact. As Paul Reed recently wrote: "It would seem that our community is becoming increasingly fractured and useless, that there is no reason for self-improvement, for spiritual nourishment, for emotional maturity."[10]

AIDS and Gay Legitimacy

One of the paradoxes of AIDS is that it has forced governments to deal with gay movements and openly gay individuals to an unprecedented extent. Whereas the response of all but a handful of governments has been to demand greater surveillance and repression of homosexuality, a demand not unheard in even the most progressive of societies, most liberal democracies have seen the necessity to establish contact with their gay communities to better respond to AIDS. On a global scale, the countries in which a meaningful gay community/movement exists form a minority; one can only fear the worst as fear of AIDS adds to official homophobia and authoritarianism in the countries of Eastern Europe and much of the Third World, and applaud the efforts of the World Health Organization to persuade governments of the need to recognize their gay populations.

I can best illustrate the progress of gay legitimation through AIDS by referring to Australia, possibly the first country to accord official recognition of the gay movement's stake in determining AIDS policy. In late 1984 the Federal government established the National Advisory Committee on AIDS, chaired by Australia's best known woman journalist, and appointed two gay leaders to its membership. Since then the Federal government has facilitated the establishment of a Federation of AIDS Organizations, made up of the predominantly gay state

AIDS Councils; and it recently funded a conference of educators and researchers into gay/bisexual behavioural change. The opening session of that conference, where a woman psychologist lectured an audience including government officials on fisting, water sports, and other "exotic sex practices," was a vivid mark of how AIDS has made the previously "unmentionable" the subject of official discourse, and helped legitimize (and, let it be acknowledged, control) gay sex, as well as the gay movement.

In a number of Western European countries there has been some consultation with gay groups, though in very few has it been as institutionalized and publicly recognized as it has in Australia. The United States is a special case, because of the importance of local governments; while San Francisco included gay representatives in city policy-making from very early on in the epidemic — the City already had an Office of Gay and Lesbian Health when AIDS hit — elsewhere, gay AIDS organizations have been totally ignored. When President Reagan finally established a Presidential Commission on AIDS in mid-1987 he reluctantly included one openly gay man, but one who was there for his medical expertise, rather than his links to the gay movement. Even this degree of recognition seems unlikely in countries such as Mexico, Brazil, the Philippines, or Japan, where there are gay organizations that are almost totally unacknowledged by the authorities.

Nonetheless, it is undoubtedly the case that in almost every Western country — though least so, as far as I know, in southern Europe — AIDS has meant a new visibility for gays, and increased access to governments. One of the consequences of this is the creation of a new class of gay leaders, people who sit on government committees, hold government-financed jobs, and travel at government expense to international conferences. As one of these people, I know only too well the risks of becoming alienated from the people we seek to represent.

AIDS and the Construction of Sexuality

There are few examples in history to match the dramatic changes in sexual behaviour which have occurred among homosexual men since the onset of widespread safer sex advice. (There are, of course, few comparable times when sexual behaviour has been so closely scrutinized and monitored, which itself raises some real questions: Is gay behaviour, even identity, changed by the enormous attention that has been paid to it by both professionals and the media as a consequence of AIDS? When does legitimacy and representation become control and co-option?).

Considerable numbers of epidemiological surveys and reports from sexually transmitted disease clinics in a number of countries all point to a sharp decrease in unprotected anal intercourse in the homosexual population. It is not merely that tens of thousands of men have incorporated condoms into the act of intercourse; there is considerable anecdotal evidence that anal intercourse itself has been abandoned by very many gay men (which makes the terms "sodomite" even less appropriate as a synonym for homosexual).

At the same time, AIDS has led to the creation of new forms of sexual expression, of which the American "jack-off clubs" are the most obvious. The ability of many thousands of men to eroticize forms of behaviour once thought of as mere preludes to "real" sex — most obviously mutual masturbation — is a strong indication of the elasticity of sexual desire. It is important to note, however, a point which reinforces my earlier arguments, that what is involved is a change in specific *behaviour* but not in the object of *desire*.

For some, AIDS has become a reason to argue against sexual adventure and erotic experimentation: AIDS is being used by many prominent forces in our society to argue for a return to "traditional values," by which they seem to mean heterosexual monogamy and homosexual celibacy. Within the gay world, debate about what sort of sexual behaviour is appropriate since AIDS is often marred by bitter and irrational arguments, in which wild accusations of either puritanism or irresponsibility are thrown back and forth. Thus Randy Shilts's otherwise excellent book is marred by his total inability to accept that not everyone who thought it wrong to close the bath-houses in San Francisco was irresponsible and unconcerned by the spread of AIDS (just as those on the other side of the debate saw everyone who believed in closure as homophobic and probably fascist).[11]

Outside several cities in the United States, government-enforced closures of sex venues has, in fact, occurred much less than one might have predicted several years ago. In a number of Western countries there has been a recognition of the value of such venues as places where men can be encouraged to change risky behaviour; and in Australia, after some initial decline, it is my observation that sex venues are once again flourishing — but with new practices, above all the almost automatic acceptance by most patrons of the use of condoms for anal sex.

The most interesting changes are, however, not in sexual behaviour but in patterns of interaction and intimacy, where we can only venture guesses based necessarily on very limited personal experience. More gay men are, I think, developing close friendships and affectionate relationships in which genital sexuality plays a lesser role, and affection and shared commitment to community a greater. Writing before the onset of AIDS, Edmund White suggested that: "The current notion of hot sex in New York [may] be a mere transition, a new recuperation of old oppression, and we would expect this period to be followed by a sweeter, calmer one in which romance and intimacy and sustained partnership between lovers would emerge again."[12] There are those who would argue that this is now happening because of AIDS.

AIDS and the Return to Gay Liberation

Over the past year it has struck me that AIDS is leading gay men and our organizations towards some of the practices associated with the gay liberation movements of fifteen years ago. Consciousness-raising is now referred to as workshopping, and gay pride as self-esteem, but the basic premise that internalized self-hatred can only be overcome by empowering people to overcome social stigma is being rediscovered as a central plank of attempts to alter sexual behaviour patterns. (Research evidence at this point is rather inconclusive, but it does seem that gay men who have low self-image and little contact with a "gay community" find behavioral change more difficult than others.)[13]

During the late 1970s and early 1980s it became fashionable to dismiss earlier gay liberation ideals and structures as unrealistic and utopian. The gay movement sought a new respectability, summed up in the establishment of groups like the American National Gay Task Force and Gay Business Associations, and their counterparts elsewhere.[14] To some extent AIDS has meant a strengthening of this tendency, in the already discussed entry into advisory groups and government bureaucracies. But it has also meant a new militancy and a new stress on grassroots organizing. In the United States the new gay bureaucrats were among those arrested (by police wearing yellow gloves) in protests against government inactivity in Washington, D.C., and calls for civil disobedience have come from formerly mainstream leaders such as Los Angeles' Duke Comegys, co-chair of the Human Rights Campaign Fund.[15] In Australia, where we have far less reason to protest government response, AIDS has brought a new population into gay organizations, where newcomers are re-learning some of the basic precepts of the gay liberation movement of fifteen years ago.

It is difficult for those of us who have not lived in the major centres of the epidemic to recognize the extent to which it has devastated our community. A friend of mine in New York tells of going to the funeral of someone who had died of AIDS, and commenting on how small the attendance was. That's because, he was told, most of those who would have come are already dead. In New York, San Francisco, Los Angeles, and a growing number of other cities anyone — gay or straight, woman or man — with ties to the gay community is experiencing the sort of devastation that Andrew Holleran catches in this interchange in his wonderful story *Friends at Evening*:

> "So you think nothing will ever, ever be the same?" said Ned.
> "Nothing," said Mister Lark, screwing the cap on his jar of face cream.
> "We're all going in sequence at different times. And will the last person please turn out the lights?"[16]

The long-term implications of this amount of death and suffering for those who survive AIDS are as yet hard to determine. We know something of the psychological costs in the short term; we have yet to come to grips with the full extent of the longer-terms effects. Large numbers of gay men in their thirties and forties are dealing with the constant presence of death several decades before they would otherwise expect it. Even if medicine finds ways of curing and preventing this disease, a whole generation of gay men will bear its scars for the rest of our lives.

When AIDS first hit there was an understandable reaction that claimed it invalidated the sexual liberationist struggles of the previous decade. Some went further and prophesied that it meant the end of gay life as we had come to understand it in the past two decades. This, after all, was not an impossible scenario — gay life in Germany, which had seemed fairly well established in the 1920s, was very quickly wiped out by Hitler. But six years into the epidemic I think we can be fairly sure that while the losses have been enormous, and the grief of those of us who survive will stay with us for the rest of our lives, gay life, gay identity, and gay community will not disappear. As Paul Berman wrote in the *Village Voice*:

> The sexual revolution of the last twenty years can be reined in, it can be redirected, but it can't be repealed . . . Naturally the plague will cause changes in sexual behaviour and imagination, both in the immediate present as emergency measures and in the post-emergency long run. But those long-run changes will be an evolution towards something new, not a return to something old. Neither utopia nor conservation will be the future.[17]

However horrible the devastation caused to our people by AIDS, the gay communities constructed in the last two decades will survive and grow.

NOTES

1. Published in Britain under the title, *AIDS and the New Puritanism* (London: Pluto, 1986).

2. One of the few exceptions is Barry Adam, *The Rise of a Gay and Lesbian Movement* (Boston: Twayne Publishers, 1987).

3. Frederick Whitam and Robin W. Mathy, *Male Homosexuality in Four Societies* (New York: Praeger, 1986); S. Epstein, "Gay Politics, Ethnic Identity: The Limits of Social Constructionism," *Socialist Review* 93/94 (1987).

4. Phil Parkinson, "Stigma and Risk," unpublished, presented in Wellington, 18 September 1987.

5. Brendon Lemon, "Female Trouble," *Christopher Street* (L16): 48.

6. "The March on Washington," *The Advocate* (10 November 1987): 11-35; L. Cagan, "More than a March," *Zeta Magazine* (January 1988): 35-6.

7. Edmund White, "Esthetics and Loss," *Artforum* (January 1987).

8. "LaRouche Initiate Stopped Dead," *New York Native* (7 November 1986).

9. Cindy Patton, "No Turning Back," *Zeta Magazine* (January 1988): 67-73.

10. Paul Reed, *Serenity*, (Berkeley: Celestial Arts, 1987): 17.

11. Randy Shilts, *And the Band Played On* (New York: St. Martin's Press, 1987).

12. Edmund White, *States of Desire* (New York: Penguin Books, 1980): 279.

13. The Macquarie University AIDS Research Project (Sydney) is producing evidence which strongly supports this conclusion.

14. I develop this argument in my *The Homosexualization of America* (Boston: Beacon Press, 1986).

15. Mark Vandervelden, "Civil Disobedience," *The Advocate* 29 (September 1987).

16. Andrew Holleran, "Friends at Evening," *Men on Men: Best New Gay Fiction*, George Stambolian, ed. (New York: Penguin Books, 1986): 95.

17. Paul Berman, "Culture Shock," *The Village Voice* (23 June 1987).

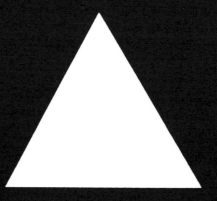

SILENCE = DEATH

AIDS, AESTHETICS AND ACTIVISM

AIDS Demo Graphics

Douglas Crimp

A simple graphic emblem — SILENCE=DEATH printed in white Gill sanserif type underneath a pink triangle on a black ground — has come to signify AIDS activism to an entire community of people confronting the epidemic.

This in itself tells us something about the styles and strategies of the AIDS activist movement's graphics. For SILENCE=DEATH does its work with a metaphorical subtlety that is unique, among political symbols and slogans, to AIDS activism. Our emblem's significance depends on foreknowledge of the use of the pink triangle as the marker of gay men in Nazi concentration camps, its appropriation by the gay movement to remember a suppressed history of our oppression, and now, an inversion of its positioning (men in the death camps wore triangles that pointed down; SILENCE=DEATH's points up). SILENCE=DEATH declares that silence about the oppression and annihilation of gay people, then and now, must be broken as a matter of our survival. As historically problematic as an analogy of AIDS and the death camps is, it is also deeply resonant for gay men and lesbians, especially insofar as the analogy is already mediated by the gay movement's adoption of the pink triangle.[1] But it is not merely what SILENCE=DEATH says, but also how it looks, that gives it its particular force. The power of this equation under a triangle is the compression of its connotation into a logo, a logo so striking that you ultimately have to ask, if you don't already know, "What does that mean?" And it is the answers we are constantly called upon to give to others — small everyday direct actions — that make SILENCE=DEATH significant beyond a community of lesbian and gay cognoscenti.

Although identified with ACT UP (AIDS Coalition to Unleash Power), SILENCE=DEATH precedes the formation of the activist group by several months. The emblem was created in the winter of 1986/87 by six gay men calling themselves the Silence=Death Project, who printed the emblem on posters and had them "sniped" at their own expense.[2] The members of the Silence=Death Project were present at the formation of ACT UP in March 1987, and they lent

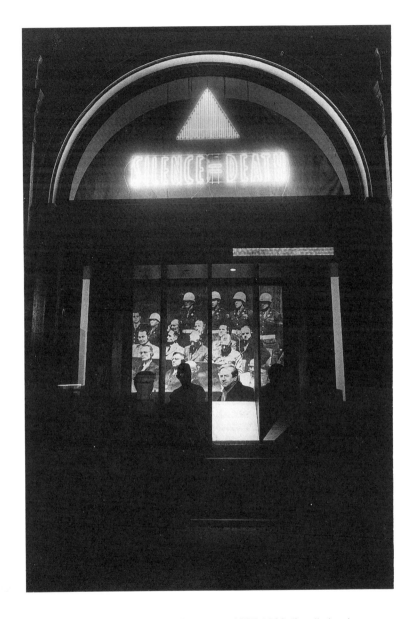

ACT UP. *Let the Record Show . . .* , 1987-1988. Installation in the Window on Broadway of the New Museum of Contemporary Art, New York. Photo: Robin Holland.

the organization their graphic design for placards used in its second demonstration at New York City's main post office on April 15, 1987. Soon thereafter SILENCE=DEATH T-shirts, buttons, and stickers were produced, the sale of which was one of ACT UP's first means of fundraising.

Nearly a year after SILENCE=DEATH posters first appeared on the streets of lower Manhattan, the logo showed up there again, this time in a neon version as part of a window installation in the New Museum of Contemporary Art on lower Broadway. New Museum curator Bill Olander, a person with AIDS and a member of ACT UP, had offered the organization the window space for a work about AIDS. An ad hoc committee was formed by artists, designers, and others with various skills, and within a few short months *Let the Record Show*, a powerful installation work, was produced. Expanding SILENCE=DEATH's analogy of AIDS and Nazi crimes through a photomural of the Nuremburg trials, *Let the Record Show* indicted a number of individuals for their persecutory, violent, homophobic statements about AIDS — statements cast in concrete for the installation — and, in the case of then president Ronald Reagan, for his six-year-long failure to make any statement at all about the United States' number-one health emergency. The installation also included a light-emitting diode (LED) sign programmed with ten minutes of running text about the government's abysmal failure to confront the crisis.[3]

Let the Record Show demonstrated not only the ACT UP committee's wide knowledge of facts and figures detailing government inaction and mendacity, but also its sophistication about artistic techniques for distilling and presenting the information. If an art world audience might have detected the working methods of such artists as Hans Haacke and Jenny Holzer in ACT UP's installation, so much the better to get them to pay attention to it. And after taking in its messages, who would have worried that the work might be too aesthetically derivative, nor original enough? The aesthetic values of the traditional art world are of little consequence to AIDS activists. What counts in activist art is it propaganda effect; stealing the procedures of other artists is part of the plan — if it works, we use it.

ACT UP's ad hoc New Museum art project committee regrouped after finishing *Let the Record Show* and resolved to continue as an autonomous collective — "a band of individuals united in anger and dedicated to exploiting the power of art to end the AIDS crisis." Calling themselves Gran Fury, after the Plymouth model used by the New York City police as undercover cars, they became, for a time, ACT UP's unofficial propaganda ministry and guerrilla graphic designers. Counterfeit money for ACT UP's first-anniversary demonstration, WALL STREET II; a series of broadsides for New York ACT UP's participation in ACT NOW's spring 1988 offensive, NINE DAYS OF PROTEST; placards to carry and T-shirts to wear to SEIZE CONTROL OF THE FDA (Federal Drug Admin-

istration); a militant *New York Crimes* to wrap around the *New York Times* for
TARGET CITY HALL — these are some of the ways Gran Fury contributed to
the distinctive style of ACT UP. Their brilliant use of word and image has also
won Gran Fury a degree of acceptance in the art world, where they are now
given funding for public artworks and invited to participate in museum exhibitions and to contribute "artist's pages" to *Artforum*. [4]

Like the [American] government's response to the AIDS activist agenda, the
art world's embrace of AIDS activist art was long delayed. [5] Early in 1988,
members of the three ACT UP groups, Gran Fury, Little Elvis, and Wave Three
protested at the Museum of Modern Art (MOMA) for its exclusion of AIDS
activist graphics. The occasion was an exhibition organized by curator Deborah
Wye called *Committed to Print: Social and Political Themes in Recent American Printed
Art*. Work in the show was divided into broad categories: gender, govern-
ments/leaders, race/culture, nuclear power/ecology, war/revolution, econom-
ics/class struggles/the American dream. The singleness of "gender" on this list, the
failure to couple it with, say, "sexuality," already reveals the bias. Although spanning
the period from the 1960s to the present, *Committed to Print* included no work
about either gay liberation or the AIDS crisis. When asked by a critic at the *Village
Voice* why there was nothing about AIDS, the curator blithely replied that she
knew of no graphic work of artistic merit dealing with the epidemic. AIDS activists
responded with a handout for museum visitors explaining the reasons for
demonstrating:

- We are here to protest the blatant omission from *Committed to Print* of any
  mention of the lesbian and gay rights movement and of the AIDS crisis.
- By ignoring the epidemic, MOMA panders to the ignorance and indifference
  that prolong the suffering needlessly.
- By marginalizing twenty years of lesbian and gay rights struggles, MOMA
  makes invisible the most numerous victims of today's epidemic.
- Cultural blindness is the accomplice of societal indifference. We challenge the
  cultural workers at MOMA and the viewers of *Committed to Print* to take
  political activism off the museum walls and into the realm of everyday life.

The distance between "downtown" and "uptown" New York City — and
between its constituent art institutions — was rarely so sharply delineated as it
was with MOMA's blindness to SILENCE=DEATH, for it was only a few months
earlier that Bill Olander had decided to ask ACT UP to design *Let the Record Show*,
after having seen the ubiquitous SILENCE=DEATH poster the previous year:
"To me," he wrote, "it was among the most significant works of art that had yet
been inspired and produced within the arms of the crisis." [6] For more traditional
museum officials, however, a current crisis is perhaps less easy to recognize, since

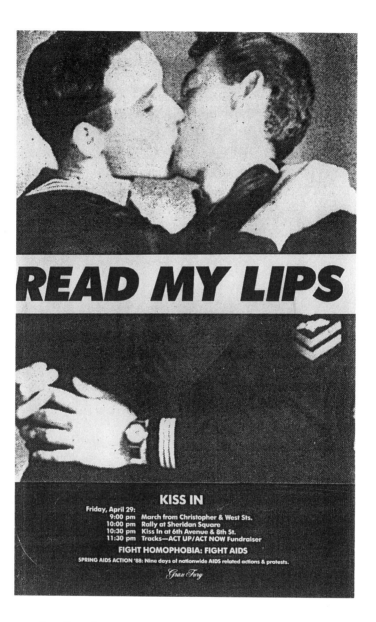

Gran Fury, *Read My Lips (boys)*, 1988. Poster, also used as a T-Shirt.

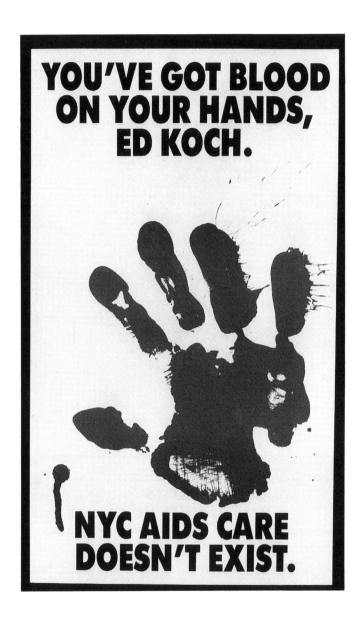

Gran Fury, *You've Got Blood on Your Hands*, 1988. Poster.

they "see" only what has become distant enough to take on the aura of universality. The concluding lines of MOMA curator Wye's catalogue essay betray this prejudice: "In the final analysis it is not the specific issues or events that stand out. What we come away with is a shared sense of the human condition: rather than feeling set apart, we feel connected."[7] The inability of others to "feel connected" to the tragedy of AIDS is, of course, the very reason we in the AIDS activist movement have had to fight — to fight even to be thought of as sharing in what those who ignore us nevertheless presume to universalize as "the human condition."

There is perhaps a simpler explanation for MOMA's inability to see SILENCE=DEATH. The political graphics in *Committed to Print* were, it is true, addressed to the pressing issues of their time, but they were made by "bona fide" artists — Robert Rauschenberg and Frank Stella, Leon Golub and Nancy Spero, Hans Haacke and Barbara Kruger. A few collectives were included — Group Material and Collaborative Projects — and even a few ad hoc groups — Black Emergency Cultural Coalition and Artists and Writers Protest Against the War in Vietnam. But these were either well-established artists' organizations or groups that had been burnished by the passage of time, making the museum hospitable to them. The SILENCE=DEATH Project (whose AIDSGATE poster had been printed in the summer of 1987) and Gran Fury (who by the time of the MOMA show had completed their first poster, AIDS: 1 IN 61) were undoubtedly too rooted in movement politics for MOMA's curator to see their work within her constricted aesthetic perspective. They had, as yet, no artistic credentials that she knew of.

The distance between "downtown" and "uptown" has thus figured in more ways than one. For throughout the past decade postmodernist art has deliberately complicated the notion of "the artist" so tenaciously clung to be MOMA's curator. Questions of identity, authorship, and audience — and the ways in which all three are constructed through representation — have been central to postmodernist art, theory and criticism. The significance of so-called appropriation art, in which the artist forgoes the claim to original creation by appropriating already-existing images and objects, has been to show that the "unique individual" is a kind of a fiction, that our very selves are socially and historically determined through pre-existing images, discourses, and events.

Young artists finding their place within the AIDS activist movement rather than the conventional art world had reason to take these issues very seriously. Identity is understood by them to be, among other things, coercively imposed by perceived sexual orientation or HIV status; it is, at the same time, wilfully taken on, in defiant declaration of affinity with the "others" of AIDS: queers, women, Blacks, Latinos, drug users and sex workers.[8] Moreover, authorship is collectively and discursively named: the SILENCE=DEATH project, Gran Fury, Little Elvis,

53

Testing the Limits (an AIDS activist video production group), DIVA-TV (Damned Interfering Video Activist Television, a coalition of ACT UP videomakers), and LAPIT (Lesbian Activists Producing Interesting Television, a lesbian task group within DIVA). Authorship also constantly shifts: collectives' memberships and individual members' contributions vary from project to project.

Techniques of postmodernist appropriation are employed by these groups with a sly nod to art world precursors. In a number of early posters, for example, Gran Fury adopted Barbara Kruger's seductive graphic style, which was subsequently, and perhaps less knowingly, taken up by other ACT UP graphic producers. In the meantime, Gran Fury turned to other sources. Their best known appropriation is undoubtedly the public service announcement on San Francisco (and later New York) city buses produced for Art Against AIDS' On the Road, under the auspices of the American Foundation for AIDS Research. Imitating the look of the United Colors of Benetton advertising campaign, Gran Fury photographed three stylish young interracial couples kissing and topped their images with the caption KISSING DOESN'T KILL: GREED AND INDIFFERENCE DO. The punch of the message, its implicit reference to the risk of HIV transmission, and its difference from a Benetton ad derive from a simple fact: of the three kissing couples, only one pairs boy with girl. If their sophisticated postmodern style has gained art world attention and much-needed funding for Gran Fury, the collective has accepted if only hesitantly, often biting the hand that feeds. Their first poster commission from an art institution was discharged with a message about art world complacency: WITH 42,000 DEAD, ART IS NOT ENOUGH. Familiar with the fate of most critical art practices — that is, with the art world's capacity to co-opt and neutralize them — Gran Fury has remained wary of their own success. Such success can ensure visibility, but visibility to *whom?*

For AIDS activist artists, rethinking the identity and role of the artists also entails new considerations of audience. Postmodernist art advanced a political critique of art institutions — and art itself as an institution — for the ways they constructed social relations through specific modes of address, representations of history, and obfuscations of power. The limits of this aesthetic critique, however, have been apparent in its own institutionalization: critical postmodernism has become a sanctioned, if still highly contested, art world product, the subject of standard exhibitions, catalogues and reviews. The implicit promise of breaking out of the museum and marketplace to take on new issues and find new audiences has gone largely unfulfilled. AIDS activist art is one exception, and the difference is fairly easy to locate.

The constituency of much politically engaged art is the art world itself. Generally, artists ponder society from within the confines of their studios; there they apply their putatively unique visions to aesthetic analyses of social conditions. Mainstream artistic responses to the AIDS crisis often suffer from just such

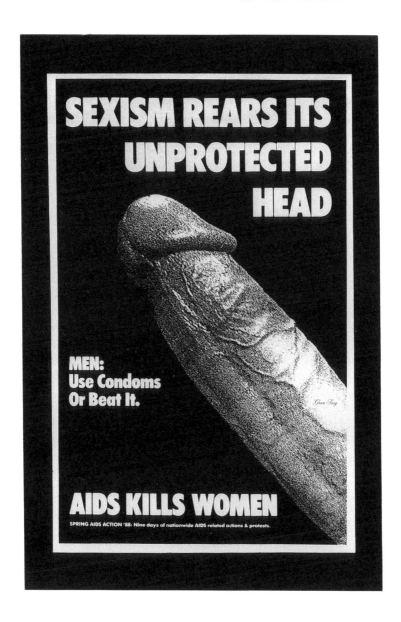

Gran Fury, *Sexism Rears Its Unprotected Head*, 1988. Poster.

isolation, with the result that the art speaks only of the artist's private sense of rage, or loss, or helplessness. Such expressions are often genuine and moving, but their very hermeticism ensures that the audience that finds them so will be the traditional art audience.[9]

AIDS activist artists work from a very different base. The point of departure of AIDS activist graphics is neither the studio nor the artist's private vision, but AIDS activism. Social conditions are viewed from the perspective of the movement working to change them. AIDS activist art is grounded in the accumulated knowledge and political analysis of the AIDS crisis, produced collectively by the entire movement. The graphics not only reflect that knowledge, but actively contribute to its articulation as well. They codify concrete, specific issues of importance to the movement as a whole, or to particular interests within it. They function as an organizing tool, by conveying, in compressed form, information and political positions to others affected by the epidemic, to onlookers at demonstrations, and to the dominant media. But their primary audience is the movement itself. AIDS activist graphics enunciate AIDS politics to, and for, all of us in the movement. They suggest slogans (SILENCE=DEATH becomes "We'll never be silent again"), target opponents (the *New York Times*, President Reagan, Cardinal O'Connor), define positions ("All people with AIDS are innocent"), propose actions ("Boycott Burroughs Wellcome"). Graphic designs are often devised in ACT UP committees and presented to the floor at the group's weekly meetings for discussion and approval. Contested positions are debated, and sometimes proposed graphic ideas are altered or vetoed by the membership. In the end, when the final product is wheatpasted around the city, carried on protest placards, and worn on T-shirts, our politics, and our cohesion around those politics, become visible to us, and to those who will potentially join with us.

NOTES

1. Although factions within the AIDS activist movement have used holocaust metaphors indiscriminately — "genocide," for example, is a term that often appears in early ACT UP fact sheets — it should be remembered that forced, punitive quarantine has been both a constant threat, and in some places and for some groups, a reality for people with HIV infection. For a detailed consideration of the gay and AIDS activist movements' adoption of the pink triangle, see Stuart Marshall, "The Contemporary Political Use of Gay History: The Third Reich," paper presented at *How Do I Look? A Queer Film and Video Conference*, Anthology Film Archives, New York, October 21-22, 1989 (conference papers forthcoming).

2. "Sniping" is a means of ensuring that posters pasted on boardings will remain there for a specific time period, without being covered over by anyone else's posters. In New York City, "snipers" are usually paid by promoters to put up rock concert advertisements and to replace them if they are torn down or pasted over.

3. For a more complete description of *Let the Record Show* see the introduction to *AIDS: Cultural Analysis/Cultural Activism*, Douglas Crimp, ed. (Cambridge: MIT Press, 1988): 7-12.

4. Gran Fury, "Control," *Artforum* 28 (October 1989): 129-30, 167-8.

5. Long, that is, in relation to how time is and must be figured in the AIDS crisis. I do not mean to imply that the agenda of AIDS activist artists includes any special interest in art world acceptance — far from it. The art world is only one of many sites of the struggle. My point is that, whatever the position of AIDS activist artists, art institutions should recognize all vital forms of aesthetic production.

6. Bill Olander, "The Window on Broadway by ACT UP," in *On View* [handout] (New York: New Museum of Contemporary Art, 987): 1.

7. Deborah Wye, *Committed to Print: Social and Political Themes in Recent American Printed Art* (New York: Museum of Modern Art, 1988): 10.

8. "I am a member of the gay community and a member of the AIDS community. Furthermore, I am a gay member of the AIDS community, a community that some would establish by force, for no other end but containment, toward no other end but repression, with no other end but our deaths — a community that must, instead, establish itself in the face of this containment and repression. We must proudly identify ourselves as a coalition" (Gregg Bordowitz, writing about the Testing the Limits Video Collective, in "Picture a Coalition," *AIDS: Cultural Analysis/Cultural Activism*, 195).

9. Individual artists' aesthetic responses to AIDS have not always been genuine or moving; sometimes they are exploitative and damaging. To take a notorious example, Nicholas Nixon's serial photographic portraits of people with AIDS (PWAs) reinforce mainstream media stereotypes of PWAs as isolated, despairing victims. When the photographs were shown at the Museum of Modern Art in the fall of 1988, ACT UP members protested, demanding NO MORE PICTURES WITHOUT CONTEXT. Part of the context excluded from Nixon's pictures, of course, is everything that kills people with AIDS besides a virus — everything that AIDS activists, PWAs among us, are fighting.

Public Art on AIDS:
On the Road with Art Against AIDS

Jan Zita Grover

W ell, the 1980s in the U.S. are over, thank God . . . Though the next two decades don't look as if they're going to be appreciably better: the kinder, gentler cold warrior has waged war in the Gulf, and Jesse Helms is still attempting to establish policy in the arts and public health. Amid this curious and poisonous atmosphere, public art is being heralded as an example of artists "fighting back": a new or renewed "commitment" to political engagement on the part of artists. Never mind that most of the engagement has been around intra-artworld concerns, the straw-grasping still serves as consolation for those of us shell-shocked by the precipitous fall-back from the early days of women's, black, and gay liberation in the late 1960s and early 1970s. Artists may have used public art to deal with a narrow range of public issues, but at least they were offering something to those of us who were not buying paintings at $40,000 a crack on 57th Street. Public art: in most cases not enough, but better than nothing.

Most public art projects have been artist-generated and produced with public funds as one-shots or small series of events. Though many artists have been drawn to the use of billboards, LED displays, and public transportation as places to take their messages, the money and political clout needed to use these media on a wide scale have been conspicuously missing. This article is about a public art project that had a conspicuous amount of both at its disposal. Art Against AIDS' public-art project, *On the Road,* although now over two years old, remains an interesting case-in-point of the problems and achievements possible in a political arts project conceived nationally rather than locally. Like AIDS policy itself, the lack of a "critical regionalism"[1] in public art condemns much of what gets organized and produced to realtime irrelevance. What was this corporate-sponsored public art project able to accomplish?

In May, 1989, 100 artists' billboards, bus-shelter posters, and busboards appeared in San Francisco as part of AmFAR's (American Foundation for AIDS Research) ongoing Art Against AIDS project to raise money for AIDS research. Twenty-two artists, selected by Ann Philbin of Livet Richard Company (the New York publicity firm that produces Art Against AIDS' events), participated in *On the Road*, named for its sitting on and alongside transit routes and for the plans to tour it across the United States.[2]

What did this massive public-art project accomplish in San Francisco? What was it designed to accomplish? And how did it fare when the project went "on the road" to Washington D.C., Atlanta, and other North American cities? To answer these questions, we need to look at how *On the Road* originated.

In January 1989, AmFAR's fundraisers visited Lynne Sowder and Nathan Braulick of First Bank Systems (FBS) to try to set up an art-auction in Minneapolis similar to its successful New York sale. Sowder and Braulick felt strongly that AmFAR's New York model wouldn't work "because there were too few galleries and private collectors in the Twin Cities to raise the kind of money that AmFAR's New York auction had."[3] Such a model "wouldn't be useful in most U.S. cities." Moreover, "elegant grand dinners and all these rich people" left little room for participation by artists with only local fame or no fame at all.[4]

The New York (and eventually Los Angeles and San Francisco) auction, as *On the Road* curator Anne Philbin and AmFAR publicist Marissa Cardenal described it, was a very "upscale event." The work solicited came from nationally known artists; the auction catalogues were glossy and four-coloured; expensive cocktail parties and dinners surrounded the auctions like glittering nets, socialites and entertainment celebrities.

Instead of taking this model into Minneapolis and other cities, Sowder and Braulick proposed "mainstreaming the issue of AIDS" by putting it in "a different information flow on streets and public transit." This part of the "package" was based on *Artside Out*, a public-art project they had produced in summer 1985 for FBS in Minneapolis. Their model had another important component: it would draw local artists who were not invited to participate in the upscale auctions into AmFAR's activities.

Another part of the *On the Road* model tapped local corporate support. According to Art Against AIDS publicist Susan Martin, AmFAR needed a way to draw corporations into its donor base. The auctions had not succeeded in doing this because most corporate art collections had "specific agendas" (i.e., collecting "areas") for purchasing, while the donated artwork auctioned by Art Against AIDS consisted of whatever the solicited artists chose to give.[5] From a fundraising viewpoint, *On the Road* offered regionally based corporations sponsorship of a stable project that ensured publicity for their role as well as patronage of local artists. But not only local artists: most of the artists chosen for *On the Road* were ones that corporate sponsors or their curatorial staffs would be familiar with: artists with national reputations who could draw corporations into sponsorship.

In San Francisco, AmFAR fundraisers took this "package" directly to corporate CEOs after researching corporations for "their record of AIDS donations." (Some of the San Francisco sponsors had been active in funding AIDS projects before;

some had done nothing.) Corporations that made a "substantial" (i.e., $10-$15,000 minimum) donations to the project were offered "site acknowledgements": billboards linking their names with the Art Against AIDS/*On the Road* project (Esprit, the "lifestyle" clothing manufacturer, and Chevron of California both received site acknowledgement billboards).[6] Sponsorship was a blank check; corporations were not given a chance to veto the work that would be exhibited.

Using additional in-kind contributions from billboard, busboard, shelter-poster, and poster-production companies, curator Philbin was able to keep space-rental and production costs low, so three sets of *On the Road* posters were produced for a costs of roughly 20 percent of the funds raised. (The other two sets of posters were planned for use in other cities, further reducing cost-to-profit ratios there.) The net after-production costs in each city were to be divided between AmFAR's national operations and local AIDS service organizations.

Although the money *On the Road* raised in San Francisco is negligible compared with AmFAR's other Art Against AIDS projects,[7] its organizers suggest that it accomplished several things that the "New York model" did not: it "increased public awareness of AIDS and gave artists an opportunity to reach people who might never set foot in a gallery or otherwise think about AIDS."[8]

On the Road's achievements in these respects are ambiguous and difficult to assess, but its claims should interest anyone concerned with artists as producers of meaning and the cultural (in-)specificity of public art.

Artists as Savants

On the Road commissioned artists as producers of meanings about AIDS rather than merely as producers of commodities that could be sold to raise money for AIDS. The project's originators, Lynne Sowder and Nathan Braulick, and its AmFAR organizers and curator were all unanimous in stating that artists with "a political attitude toward art-making," with "social consciousness,"[9] would have something worth saying to a diverse public about AIDS.

The basis for this belief lay in a widely-shared construct of the artist as guru, shaman, social priest/ess, seer who scouts out the territory lying ahead and brings back messages from the future to the rest of us. In most of its contours, this is a distinctly twentieth-century, Western, urban and, above all, middle-class idea of the artist's role. In the case of AIDS, it is not particularly borne out by evidence. Except for gay artists (who are widely viewed as having an "inevitable" or "personal" stake in addressing AIDS), few artists have worked on the subject. But plenty of them dismiss AIDS as a non-issue to the "general [art] public," as just so much coddling of homosexuals.[10]

While gay artists as individuals and communities (e.g., the New York video collective Testing the Limits; the Los Angeles activist-designer's group Stiff Sheets)

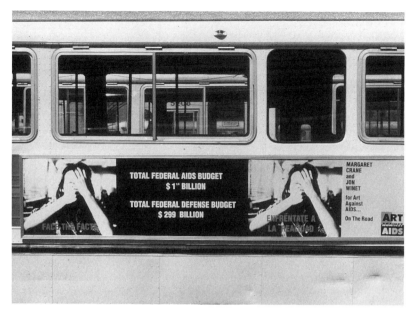

TOTAL FEDERAL AIDS BUDGET
$ 1" BILLION

TOTAL FEDERAL DEFENSE BUDGET
$ 299 BILLION

FACE THE FACTS

ENFRENTATE A
LA REALIDAD

MARGARET
CRANE
and
JON
WINET

for Art
Against
AIDS...

On The Road

ART
AGAINST
AIDS

Margaret Crane and Jon Winet, project for *Art Against AIDS*,
San Francisco, 1989.

have produced an abundance of extraordinary work on AIDS,[11] most of the
artists who participated in *On the Road* had not addressed AIDS in their work
before they were solicited for this project.[12] On the face of it, this made them
odd choices for a public art project about AIDS — unless, as Lynne Sowder
phrased it, it is true that "artists as a community are more aware than other
people."

This supposes that once presented with a problem or issue, artists' insights
are more incisive than other people's. Can artists' insights substitute for other
kinds of experience such as, for example, direct action on AIDS — political
organizing, demonstrating, buddying? Can artists' insight/intuition substitute for
what feminist critics in the 1970s termed "the authenticity of experience"?

In the case of *On the Road*, the unspecificity of most of the participants'
experience was doubled by curator Philbin's decision to encourage work that
could be shown wherever the project went. While Philbin didn't impose any
restrictions on what the artists could do with their poster space, by commis-
sioning mostly New York-based artists who had not worked on AIDS before, she
weighted the project towards what I would describe as an imperial localism —
New York's — that has very little to do with how AIDS is perceived elsewhere
in the country. For example, a didactic piece like Gran Fury's *Kissing Doesn't Kill:*

61

Greed and Indifference Do makes more sense as a comment on prejudice and government inaction in New York City (if one reads government inaction into it at all) than it does in San Francisco, where local government foots seventy percent of the cost of providing AIDS care. Truisms like Keith Haring's *AIDS: Get the Facts . . . Understand It. Prevent It* and Barbara Kruger's *Fund Health Care Not Warfare* look bland and unspecific in a city where the AIDS Foundation's Bleachman and use-a-condom billboards already blanket public space.

Meaning is Cultural

But my point here is not to use my own reactions to *On the Road*'s public art as a gauge of its success — in fact, I think any individual's attempt to do so is both hopeless and invalid. If anything is clear from my interviews and conversations with a wide variety of people who saw *On the Road* in San Francisco, it is that public art's meanings are a multiple and immanent as its viewers. But the cultural codes in some of the pieces are sufficiently stable and consensual to produce broadly-based meanings. These in turn suggest both the strengths and limitations of work produced by artists with limited exposure to the issues they are commissioned to "explore":

- AIDS is viewed as a dark, catastrophic reality, something that we flee from (Barbara Ess's wordless image of a women screaming in front of a city backdrop).
- AIDS presupposes death/time-running-out (Mark Durant's image of a running child, the text reading, *I promise you a warm embrace from my shadow*; Laurie Simmons' *Walking Hourglass*).
- AIDS is an overpowering force, something that people are powerless against (Enrique Chagoya's gigantic Mickey Mouse hand flicking people like mosquitoes).
- AIDS is sadness and loss (William Wegman's *'Purple Netted' Fay Wray* — the dog head down, buckling under the weight of a heavy purple net).

Several pieces are almost entirely open to viewers' projections:

- Nayland Blake's black poster with its Victorian tracery of flowers and the legend, *Don't Leave Me This Way*.
- Cindy Sherman's woman (coded by dress as middle-aged and middle-class) standing in a hallway, gazing into an off-frame light source.
- Mark Tansey's Veil — nude and semi-nude figures in an off-stage dark, staring through an open curtain into a highly lit area.

Several of the pieces are relatively unambiguous — chiefly because they depend on didactic texts:

- Group Material and John Lindell's *All People With AIDS are Innocent*, a message on a white background bracketed by the symbol of medicine, Aesculapius's staff, snakes, and olive branches, and the Seal of the Presidency.
- Barbara Kruger's *Fund Health Care Not Warfare*.
- Keith Harings's *AIDS: Get the Facts . . . Understand It. Prevent It.*
- Erika Rothenberg's *Teenagers Don't Die of AIDS. It's usually a time bomb that goes off in your 20s. USE A CONDOM.*
- Jos Stances's *Adam and Eve, AIDS touches Everyone.*

As public art, then, *On the Road* offers vague advice to the public; expresses fear, grief, loss; functions in an almost entirely projective way. How do these messages raise "public awareness of AIDS," how (or do they) extend already existing public discourses on AIDS?

The answers to this question lies less in the work itself than in the complex interactions taking place between the work, its site, the viewer's expectations for public art, and the viewer's prior experience of AIDS.

Sites of Meaning

The cultural codes embedded in artwork are never its sole determinants of meaning, even when those codes are as widely shared as most of those in *On the Road*. Probably anywhere in the U.S., viewers could look at the sumptuous catalogue illustrations of the project's art pieces and "get" the connotations I've attributed to them. But such meanings probably dominate only in the pages of a catalogue, where other determinants of meaning are absent, where we lack other ways to make sense of what we see. In the case of public art, we bring local and specific expectations to our viewing: our sense of how this billboard reads on the site of this individual corner of this local street in this particular town.[13] To see how this works, let's look at *On the Road* on its first stop.

On the Road had its debut in San Francisco, a city whose experience with AIDS is unlike any other's.[14] The city is very concentrated in size and population — less than six miles wide and eight miles long, only 731,000 residents. More than 7,000 San Franciscans have been diagnosed with AIDS since 1982; the city's cumulative incidence rate is 102 (i.e., 102 cases per 100,000 population averaged over the reporting period 1982-1989), the highest in North America. Up until last year, more than half the people diagnosed with AIDS lived in the Eureka Valley (the Castro) and Duboce Triangle, two old neighbourhoods off upper Market Street. For residents and shoppers in the area, living on close terms with AIDS has been common since 1983, when people began being diagnosed in great numbers.

In San Francisco's gay and lesbian communities, AIDS has become a central focus of political action and community activity, with fundraising projects and volunteer service new constants in many people's lives. And of course there have been many deaths — about 8,000 to date. The streets are deep in loss and anger.

But while this is particularly true of the Castro, public-health surveys indicated that it is also generally true of San Francisco: most of its citizens are aware of AIDS and are better informed about it than citizens of other cities. The city government has responded with great generosity to the crises; almost three-quarters of the funding for AIDS-related services in San Francisco come from the city budget (only 30 percent of the costs are reimbursed from state and federal funds). Most of the indirect costs of helping people with AIDS [PWAs] stay independent and at home (housecleaning, shopping, transportation, peer counselling, pet care, etc.) are borne by city volunteers. In short, San Francisco's many communities have responded to the crises — individually, collectively, institutionally — with generosity and resourcefulness.

This is the city and a bit of the history into which *On the Road* inserted itself. Most of the work was shown south of Market Street in an area occupied chiefly by light industry, galleries, lofts, nightclubs, and leather bars. Except on weekend nights, when the clubs and bars attract huge crowds, most of this area has little foot traffic, so relatively few people saw all or most of the work except from cars or buses. A similar number of sites were used north of Market Street in business districts with heavier foot-traffic. *On the Road* also rented sites in predominantly blue-collar Oakland and university-town Berkeley across the Bay.

Culturally Specific Meanings

I talked with a variety of people about their reactions to *On the Road*: AIDS activists, AIDS healthcare workers, people I met on the street who were looking at the work or waiting for buses, artists, people I know who have HIV infection. The range of response was wide and appeared to be most heavily influenced by viewers' prior experience with AIDS, except in the case of artists, who seemed most affected by the extent of the project as a work of public art.

The most consistent reaction was that no one I spoke to liked the Laurie Simmons or Barbara Ess pieces — "Oh, that's horrible," "Not more doom and gloom," "It makes me feel written off." *All People with AIDS are Innocent* got many positive reactions from these same viewers. (Although not from all activists: Anne Philbin reported that a prominent AIDS activist in San Francisco told her that the slogan was passe is San Francisco because "everybody already knows that"— an example of the cultural myopia that made *All People with AIDS are Innocent* useful in the first place.) Erika Rothenberg's *Teenagers Don't Die of AIDS. It's Usually a Time Bomb That Goes Off in Your 20s. USE A CONDOM* got many votes of approval from people on the street and from a friend with HIV infection, but thumbs down

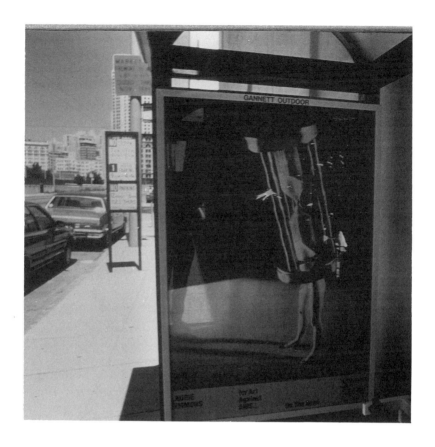

Laurie Simmons, project for *Art Against AIDS*, San Francisco, 1989.

from AIDS health-educators, who pointed out that "fear tactics" have never worked in a public-health campaign, whether against teen pregnancy, smoking, or sexually transmitted diseases. Jos Stances' *AIDS Touches Everyone* billboard offended a number of gay viewers, who saw its Adam-and-Eve illustration as either inscribing them within heterosexuality, or excluding them, as usual. William Wegman's *Purple Netted* drew a wide range of reactions: "Is this supposed to mean dogs can die of AIDS?" from a sophisticated AIDS physician; a positive reaction from an artist with HIV infection who read the image projectively and found it "so sad, so touching." Most of the people I spoke with found the didactic posters (Kruger's, Haring's, Stances', Crane-Winet's) unremarkable because they "didn't say anything" — in other words, they didn't say anything these San Franciscans didn't already know from personal or media (newspaper, radio, television) experience.

On the Road clearly worked differently for its random viewers. For San Franciscans, much of the didactic work was "old news," ineffective in light of the far more hard-hitting poster campaigns of the Stop AIDS Project, Mobilization Against AIDS, the SF AIDS Foundation, and the Shanti Project. Significantly, these viewers' experience of AIDS was deeper and more complex than that of most of the artists commissioned to "raise public awareness." On the other hand, many of these same viewers found the most ambiguous work, like William Wegman's dog buckling beneath the weight of a dark heavy net or Nayland Blake's *Please Don't Leave Me This Way* very affecting. Here again, the local and the specific may have played a part in their reactions: for all the deaths San Franciscans have experienced, there have been few public, collective expressions of grief. These ambiguous works of mourning may have offered viewers such a site.

On the Road's next stop was Washington, D.C., in March 1990. AIDS in Washington looks much different than AIDS in San Francisco. Since the first of this year, the District of Columbia has reported the highest incidence of new AIDS cases in the U.S. Most of these are intravenous drug-users and their sexual partners; most of them are also black and poor.[15] D.C. is also one of the most racially segregated cities in the U.S.; work like Gran Fury's aroused more fury there over its interracial couples than over its elliptical indictment of government inaction. Though I cannot comment from direct experience about Washington, I think it probable that projective pieces like Wegman's and Blake's may "read" obscurely in a city whose AIDS problem is obscured by crack, violence, and imperial politics. Sitting *On the Road's* billboards and bus shelters in a city so divided produced meanings for the work wholly unlike those generated in San Francisco. Corporate sponsors were less willing to underwrite positions that, while commonplace in San Francisco (*All People with AIDS are Innocent, Fund Health Care Not Warfare*), remained controversial in a conservative Southern city. *On the Road's* meanings continued to change as it arrived on its other stops.

The Possibility of Public Art

During a Dia Foundation-sponsored discussion on The *Cultural Public Sphere* (1987),[16] Martha Rosler commented that,

> apparently the artists' billboards perceived to be the most successful are those with the least specificity in relation to their physical locales and, I suspect, those closest to the familiar forms of advertising . . . Their viewers may constitute their audience but not their publics.[17]

For Rosler, the promises of public art have not panned out. Beguiled as artists may be with public space, they have not sufficiently thought through how to select and address audiences out of publics: "the out-of-doors neither symbolizes nor necessitates collectivity."[18]

On the Road did not set out to build a collectivity. Its billboards and posters were not unified in what they attempted to do or say; instead, they constituted a catalogue of twenty-two artists' individual solutions to producing public statements on AIDS. Only the multi-coloured Art Against AIDS logo tied their work together.

San Franciscans' responses to *On the Road* supports Rosler's argument. Massive and impressive as the project was from an organizational point-of-view, it advanced no collective position on artists' stake in AIDS, called for no particular actions on that part of its viewers, challenged no media stereotypes about PWAs. Because the project did not make a coherent statement, viewers' reactions depended more on their personal and community experiences of AIDS than on what the artists presented.

Its organizers believed that the unspecificity of *On the Road*'s public art was no impediment to its power; it would simply play differently in different cities. Where AIDS is not discussed much publicly (for example, in Washington), Philbin believed that any public statements about AIDS was likely to attract attention. This is the time-honoured (and untestable) premise of advertising and public relations: any publicity is better than no publicity. It is a premise regularly invoked with corporate clients — in this case, clients-as-patrons — for after San Francisco, *On the Road* needed to win corporate support for public art that now had a track history and a viewable "portfolio," some of which could be expected to seem controversial to makers of widgets and weapons.

The fact that *On the Road*'s artists made work that stressed mourning, loss, and truisms over tough issues may be an inevitability, given that most of them were largely inexperienced with AIDS and that the project was answerable to corporate sponsorship — the only way that such a massive project has yet been produced. No alternative models for public art of the scale of *On the Road* and on a subject still widely (and marvellously) viewed as "controversial" exist. The

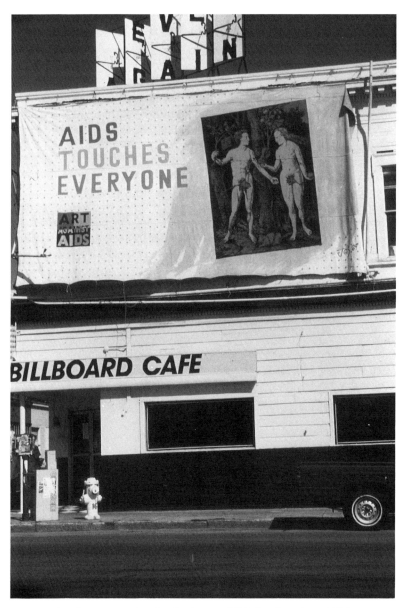

Jos Stances, project for *Art Against AIDS*, San Francisco, 1989.

project confronts us with the organizational and conceptual problems that have been there all along in public art: who are its audiences? what can be effectively said in public space? what is the message? and who will sponsor it?

NOTES

1. Kenneth Frampton, "Toward a Critical Regionalism: Six Points for an Architecture of Resistance," The Anti-Aesthetic Essays on Postmodern Culture, Hal Foster, ed. (Seattle: Bay Press, 1986).

2. The artists were Terry Allen, John Baldessari, Nayland Blake, Enrique Chagoya, Mark Durant, Barbara Ess, Gran Fury, Group Material, Keith Haring, Jerry Kearns, Barbara Kruger, Robert Mapplethorpe, Erika Rothenberg, Cindy Sherman, Laurie Simmons, Lorna Simpson, Jos Stances, Mark Tansey, William Wegman, Brian Weil, and Margaret Crane/John Winet.

3. Conversation with Nathan Braulick, 20 July 1989. All subsequent quotations from sources are from telephone conversations held in July 1989.

4. Conversation with Lynne Sowder, 26 July 1989.

5. Conversation with Susan Martin, 20 July 1989.

6. The locally-based sponsors lined up by AmFAR in San Francisco included Esprit, Chevron ("The People at Chevron"), Bank of America, TransAmerica (insurance), the Werner Erhard Foundation (Erhard was the founder of 'E.S.T.'), Black, Starr & Frost (jewellers), Morgan Stanley & Co. and Deloitte Haskins + Sells (investments) and Kenneth Cole Productions (fashion). On the Road raised $100,000 from these Bay Area sponsors.

7. For example, its 1987-88 New York auction and benefits raised $2.5 million; its Los Angeles activities ("[which] follow[ed] the New York City format") raised over $1.3 million (The Art Against AIDS Campaign [press release, AA/106.d]).

8. Marissa Cardenal, op. cit., Nathan Braulick, Susan Martin, Anne Philbin, and Lynne Sowder all cited these same goals/effects, as did Bruce W. Ferguson's "Statement" for On the Road in the catalogue, Art Against AIDS [San Francisco] (New York: AmFAR, 1989), 208-9.

9. Anne Philbin and Lynne Sowder's comments, respectively.

10. See my "AIDS: Keywords," AIDS: Cultural Analysis/Cultural Activism, Douglas Crimp, ed. (Cambridge: MIT Press, 1988), 17-30.

11. An introduction and overview of this community-generated art on AIDS can be found in my catalogue, AIDS: The Artists' Response (Columbus: Ohio State University, 1989), available for $2.50 plus postage from Wexner Center for the Arts, 1440 N. Main Street, Columbus, OH 43201-1226, U.S.A.

12. Exceptions to this are Nayland Blake, Gran Fury, Group Material-John Lindell, Keith Haring, and Brian Weil.

13. This is not to say that individual galleries and museums aren't also highly specific sites in the sense of having their own history, their own politics. But since museums claim universality and timelessness for the work they show, the grounds are at least laid for viewers to regard anything seen there as unrelated to culturally specific issues, whether of the artists' time/place or their own.

14. I take it as axiomatic that no city's experience of AIDS is like any other's, but San Francisco's is more different from other cities' than, for instance, Montréal's is from Minneapolis's.

15. In contrast, 94 percent of San Francisco's reported AIDS cases are gay and bisexual men.

16. Martha Rosler, "The Birth and Death of the Viewer: On the Public Function of Art," Discussions in Contemporary Culture, Number 1, Hal Foster, ed. (Seattle: Bay Press, 1987).

17. Ibid., 14.

18. Loc. cit.

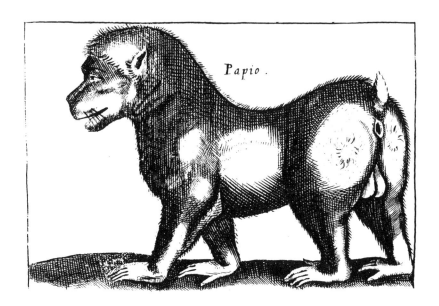

Papio.

PROLOGUE

Ten minutes covers a very infinitesimal part of all our shared concerns and lived experiences in the world context of AIDS. This was the time period in which we made a performance presentation in the framework of the SIDART panel on visual arts at the Fifth International Conference on AIDS, June 1989 in Montreal. Three art critics showed slides, and three artists showed videotapes. Ours was the only performance, a style no more mannerist than the panel conference style which dominated the event. It seemed appropriate in order to remind people that they were not at school.

Privileging the importance of fragmentation in our work, the performance was as much integral to, as descriptive of, our artistic practice. We felt that a more lucid and less didactic presentation would open avenues of interest and approach for non-arts or non-academically oriented people in the audience. With this adaptation of the performance to a book format, we hope to respect equally the particular medium involved — one can spend more time with a book, which has an increased capacity to convey visual information as well as the written word.

The work of art around which we structured our performance, entitled *Miasme/Hyène et la valve* (Miasma/The Hyena and the Valve), was also part of *Eat Me/Drink Me/Love Me* (New York, 1989/90), our installation conceived at the invitation of the late Bill Olander of The New Museum of Contemporary Art. The performance itself involved the assumption of several personas including that of a doctor and a carnival presenter, the reading of both a reworked Aesop's fable set in a hammam and a section of Christina Rossetti's *Goblin Market*, as well as a sound track of a scratched version of *Peter and*

70

Animal Love:
Miasme/Hyène et la valve

Martha Fleming & Lyne Lapointe

for John Fletcher, died August 1989
whom I had known since the age of thirteen,
and who said to me in our last telephone conversation:
"There's more than one way to skin a cat."

the Wolf. We performed with our friends and colleagues Petunia Alves and Diane Obomsawin.

Animal Love includes primary research material uncovered through our long-term examination of science and sexuality begun in 1983 for the Musée des Sciences, and continuing through to *Eat Me/Drink Me/Love Me.* Among related issues, we were interested in how certain animal life has become associated with sexual fear and is then represented to us as fearful. For example, the false construction of the will of insects to enter our bodily orifices. What is really signified therein is a sense of one's own orifices as somehow dark, inaccessible places one doesn't want to go to, and that one would prefer nobody else went to either. A colonization of one's orifices themselves by a social status quo is effected by one's fear of their being transgressed and penetrated. Though we did a great deal of reading and research about the issues presented that evening under the heading of *Animal Love*, we acknowledge a particular debt to John Boswell's book, *Christianity, Social Tolerance and Homosexuality*, a section of which touches on the development of cultural elisions between gayness and animalness. Boswell says that "the earliest and most influential of all arguments used by Christian theologians opposed to homosexual behaviour were those derived from animal behaviour."

We make no apology for the apparent simplicity of our presentation, for its humour, for its ecological and animal rights approach, nor do we think it naive or reductive to discuss AIDS in this light. Here then are some connected ideas of interest to us as lesbian artists working with the vortex of the representation of sexuality and of health, as well as their relationship to the actual practice of two ostensibly divergent disciplines: art and science, rent apart in a period ineptly called the Enlightenment.

The hyena's hair is of a dirty, greyish colour, marked with black, disposed in waves down its body. Its tail is short, with pretty long hair,

and immediately under it, above the anus, there is an opening into a kind of glandular pouch, which separates a substance of the consistence but not of the odour of civet. This opening might have given rise to the error of the ancients, who asserted that this animal was every year alternately male and female. It is an obscure and solitary animal, to be found chiefly in the most desolate and uncultivated parts of the torrid zone, of which it is a native. It resides in the caverns of mountains, in the clefts of rocks, or in dens that it has formed for itself under the earth. Its eyes shine by night, and it is asserted, not without the greatest appearance of truth, that it sees better by night than by day. Some have said that this animal changes the colour of its hair at will, and some, that the shadow of the hyena kept dogs from barking.
— Goldsmith's *Natural History*, first published in 1773.

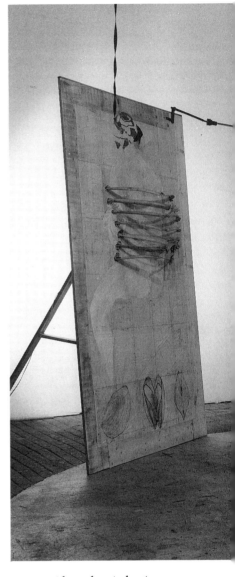

Nor can it be believed that the hyena ever changes its nature or that the same animal has at the same time both types of genitalia, those of the male and the female, as some have thought, telling of marvellous hermaphrodites and creating a whole new type — a third sex, the androgyne, in between a male and a female. They are certainly wrong not to take into account how devoted nature is to children, being the mother and begetter of all things. Since this animal [the hyena] is extremely lewd, it has grown under its tail in front of the passage for excrement a certain fleshy appendage, in form very like the female genitalia. This design of the flesh has no passage leading

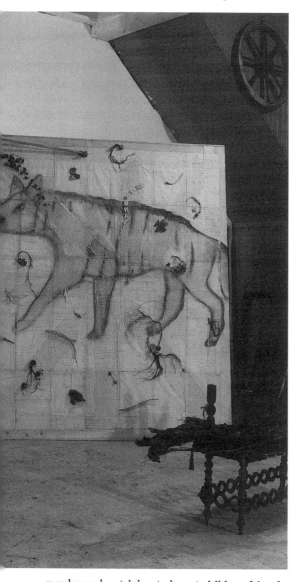

to any useful part, I say, either to the womb or to the rectum. It has, rather, only a great cavity, whence it derives its fruitless lust, since the passages intended for the procreation of the fetus are inverted. This same thing occurs in the case of both the male hyena and the female, because of their exceptional passivity. The males mount each other, so it is extremely rare for them to seek a female. Nor is conception frequent for this animal, since unnatural insemination is so common among them. It seems to me on this account that Plato in the Phaedrus deprecates pederasty, calling it 'bestial' because those who give themselves up to [this] pleasure 'take the bit' and copulate in the manner of quadrupeds, striving to beget children [thus].

— Clement of Alexandria (d. ca. 215): Paedagogus 2.10, from Boswell: *Christianity, Social Tolerance and Homosexuality, 1980.*

All the bivalve tribe are hermaph-
rodite, but they require no assistance from each other towards
impregnation. The muscle, as is
well know, consists of two equal
shells, joined at the back by a
strong muscular ligament that
answers all the purposes of a
hinge. By the elastic contraction
of these, the animal can open her
shell at pleasure. The muscles are
moored by what is vulgarly called
the beard of the fish. It consists of
a bundle of blackish, horny, fibres
or threads which are formed of a
glutinous matter, secreted by a
conglomerate gland placed at the
base of the 'foot,' a tongue-shaped
organ lying at the base of the
byssus, distinguished by its dark
violet colour, and capable of considerable extension and retrac-
tion. There is a furrow drawn
along its middle, gathering to a
fleshy sheath, which does surround the base.

— Goldsmith's *Natural History*.

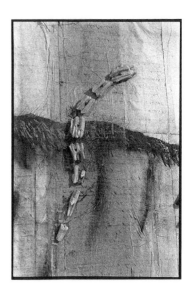

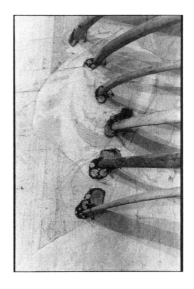

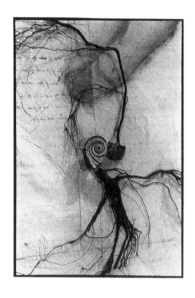

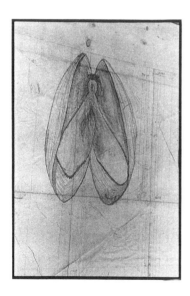

It has long been familiar to physicians that there was produced by marshes and swamps a poisonous and aeriform substance, the cause, not only of ordinary fevers, but of intermittents, and to this unknown agent of disease, the term marsh miasma has been applied. — McCollough's *Malaria*, published in 1827.

Le microbe est un paresseux, contemplatif du vide. Il n'est pas dangereux, il vit ou en terrain faible, ou en terrain fort. Il est animé par la société et la société en a peur. Elle le chasse mais il ne se sauve pas. Il est relativement heureux, et n'a aucune conscience de son pouvoir. Il se déplace dans les courants d'air. La seule limite du microbe, et il en est très conscient, c'est qu'il vit dans la matière. C'est sa seule dépense. Quand il rêve, il se voit flottant, heureux dans le vide. Il existe une croyance populaire qui dit qu'on attraie les microbes. Sans le microbe, nous ne pourrions pas vivre. Il porte une quantité de paradoxes infinis sur ses épaules, sans se plaindre.
— Written and read by Diane Obomsawin, 1989.

If we are together truly to beat this illness, we must be multi-disciplinary in our approach, and radical in our critique of a *scientific* methodology which produces diagnosis, prognosis and prescription, because this empiricism is also a root of the origin and perpetuation of the epidemic itself. Similarly, in the visual arts, we practitioners who rattle an *artistic* methodological cage being habitually ravished of the authority of our

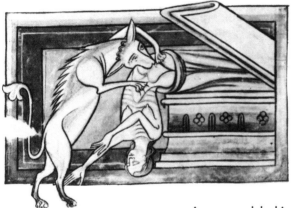

voice by a solid, socially established hierarchy based on the primacy of the written word, must stand the ground of our knowledge of the manipulation of imagery, a knowledge more profound than that to which the academy gives lip service.

As gay and lesbian artists looking at this illness and making things to look at about this illness, we must de-medicalize the image of AIDS by firmly grounding our work in the reality of the social, economic, political, psychic *and* ecological realities which have produced AIDS and continue to support it. There is a terrain of discussion to be opened between scientific and cultural researchers which could productively realign representations and realities in both domains.

In light of the historical, cultural bestialization of same-sex love, in which model both gay lesbian sex and animals are constructed as savage, what is to be made of AIDS research on animals in laboratory conditions? And what can we expect of this methodology in terms of a "cure"?

Somewhere between The Bearded Lady and The Elephant Man, between Batman and Catwoman, between the monkey lab and the urban jungle, there is a conceptual problem whose undoing might help us truly to see AIDS and homophobia in a cultural/ ecological context.

Without wishing to point a special finger at animal researchers — for our attitudes to animals are shared cultural property, and we are all experts in the lack of respect for our environment and the consequent denigration of the self — nor

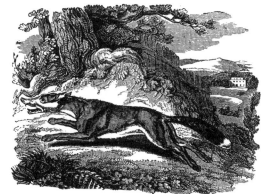

wishing to imply that reckless testing and interventionist experimentation on human beings is either the sole or even a desirable alternative, we feel that animal laboratory research is in part the product of a cultural complex from which same root springs homophobia. We as lesbians have come to understand the deep structure of this complex through our long-term analysis of the construction of our sexuality and that of our brothers as bestial, and through the socio-cultural production of AIDS and AIDS sciences. We as cultural producers can therefore help to rectify the problem through our practice in the same visual field.

These kinds of understandings are related directly to the crisis in representation which some cultural theorists have justly linked with AIDS. Surely this crisis in methodology has parallels within the medical and scientific discourses, given the reliance of pathology on visible evidence, however microscopic. The circulation of scientific "information" privileges the visual too.

Why have we rendered the flora and fauna of our world into a representational construct mirroring the arbitrary gradations of our heavily interested sexual belief systems? The Linnean system of the classification of plants was the botanical rule for centuries, and was based on dividing plants into male and female worlds, whose interactions were analogised to fit the social mores of the seventeenth century. How does this cultural construct key into science's project of predicting and dominating nature? As gays and lesbians knowing only too well what is meant socially by words such as "natural" and "un-natural," how can we allow a life-and-death issue such as AIDS to be analyzed according to a scientific methodology which is based in these alienating precepts? It is preposterous but true, for example, that the current human HIV test is based on an animal virus developed in laboratory conditions.

On a continuous line of questioning, what is the rapport between social mechanisms of marginalization which segregates us as unwanted and non-productive elements of society, and the obligation of scientific methodology to isolate chemical and physical cause and effect relationships within the restricted confines of the laboratory? How does the stress of a lab animal affect the findings of the scientist? How does their stress relate to the social stress we experience as gay men and lesbians in a heterosexist society?

Further, how does the methodological obligation to isolate draw medical attention away from the actual circumstances in which AIDS is produced and experienced by real people, gay or straight, in any one of the many Worlds which we choose

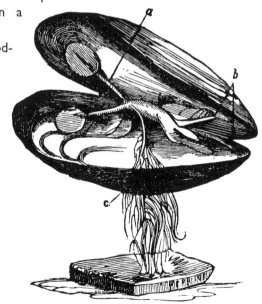

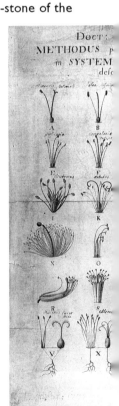

hierarchically to divide? How is it preferable to render animals ill in order to observe them, to the detriment of the quality and the quantity of attention afforded to people already suffering, a practice which at the same time ignores the actual social, economic and psychic conditions in which the illness is spread?

The notion of evolution is one of the foundation-stones of modern science. Instead of viewing humanity as one organic element of a complex ecology at one with other animals great and small, evolutionary theory insists that humanity is the summum of a selective, *procreative* progression. To this extent, it is also a foundation-stone of the reduction of (non-procreative) homosexuality to a "lower order" of "animal desire." The homosexuality/bestiality model has structural similarities to the rapport between misogyny and homophobia. According to this model, women are weak, and gay men, in willingly casting the mantle of power off at least one shoulder, are equated with women, and are gone to join . . . "a lower order." Lesbians, in turn, "aspire un-naturally."

Miasme/Hyène et La Valve is a work of art which proposes gay/lesbian friendship in the AIDS crisis, underlining the importance of recognizing both our similar and our differing experiences as an asset in terms of dialectical tools with which to resolve the crisis in spite

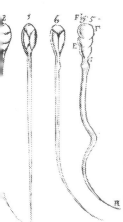

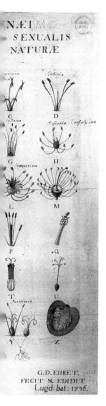

of science's excision of women's experience from its methodology.

For all women, in our formative (read obligatorily heterosexual) years at least, the sex act always contains the immediate possibility of the world-changing consequence of pregnancy. The legacy of this is that even the most pleasurable sex is early on twined with deep physical fears. These feelings are also tied in with fear of abuse and abandonment, fear of rejection, and, from our oppressed position, fear of the revolutionary power of our own desire and pleasure. For women with AIDS, the virus is therefore an intolerable manifest destiny. Those of us who are lesbians live also with the fear of discovery and social isolation. Some of this will sound familiar to our gay brothers, but some of it may also be new in their experience with AIDS. Gay men coming to grips with AIDS can learn a lot from women's analysis of the production of our fear of sex and fear of pleasure and of who is served by the maintenance of this fear, as well as from a millennia of our reliance on alternative medicine and our political organizing around sexual health care issues. And, more darkly, from the history of the social rejection of the importance of these issues.

The Miasma is a cloud of invisible germs which carry an illness. The miasma was often associated with bubonic plague. It is a vague term which precedes microscopy and germ theory, but which persisted through to the end of the nineteenth century with the discovery of mosquitos as carriers of malaria. In passing, the mosquito's function of penetration to the blood vessel is a staple of the kind of bestial iconography of homophobic AIDS ideologists.

Miasma, then, is a form of flora, the flora of infectious or noxious exhalations from putrescent organic matter. It is the home of the germ. The miasma in our work is a veil of meaning, of prejudice, through which we are trained to discern the much-maligned hyena. As for the Bather, the

mere site of her bath is one of the few places in the history of the world to which men are barred from entry, and is consequently a staple of Western male heterosexual fantasy. The bather is fettered, even in her place of refuge, by the spectre of the whalebone corset, and all that it means. Social constraint is again elided with the animal. Both the rigidity of the bones and the clinical, instrumental brass arm which links the two panels refer to apparati invented in early portrait photography and later refined and adapted for criminological and judicial photography: a restrainer which kept the portrait subject still for the long exposure required by the camera. Its lens is similar to that of the microscope which brought us germ theory out of Leeuwenhoek's "animalcules." Interestingly enough, in terms of the masculinist, procreative agenda of science, among the first substances observed by "men of science" under the new glass of the seventeenth century was semen.

The valve, or mussel, or oyster, isolated and clinically presented at the bottom of the panel, makes reference to the veiled pornographic function of the original painting by Ingres, as well as the divisive effect of the gaze on female identity, sexual and otherwise. But the body is also a psychic terrain, and not merely a group of organs — the mussel itself is a 'bearded lady,' anchoring her oyster to the shifting sea floor with the tendrils of her tuft. And what of "unwanted" hair, what of the bestial meanings of "excessive," pelt-like hair as somehow gender-transgressive, what of the *bambina pelosa?*

In this work, the hyena and the bather turn to each other for the first time with the eagerness of recognition and the freshness of intuited friendship: their eyes are about to meet. It is a work about prejudice and stigma, but it is also a work about solidarity and friendship between gay men and lesbians.

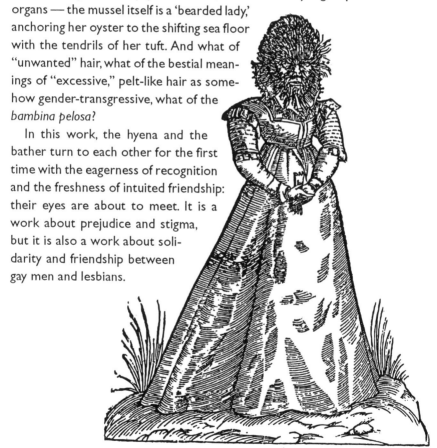

At the Fifth International Conference on AIDS (subtitled The Scientific and Social Challenge) which took place in June 1989 in Montréal, Section C was called Basic Research (Biomedical). That "basic research" be equivalent to "biomedical" research is indicative of the laboratization of an analysis of AIDS. Here are titles of some of the presentations involving animals by researchers in this field:

Genetic Analysis of SIV Derived from Mandrill

Experience with Eight HIV-Vaccine Trials in Chimpanzees

Cross Reactivity of Goat Sera Generated against Five HIV-Derived gp120 Recombinants and Synthetic Peptides

Comparison of Immune Responses in Mice Immunized with Native HIV-2 Envelope Glycoprotein or Corresponding Immunosome

Mapping of T and B Cell Epitope of HIV-1 NEF Protein in Immunized Chimpanzees

Rhesus Monkeys Immunized with Recombinant Vaccinia Viruses Containing HIV-1 Envelope Genes Develop Antibodies Reactive with Envelope of Divergent HIV-1 Strains

Immune Responses of Rabbits and Chimpanzees to Inactivated Whole Virus Concentrates of HIV-1

Phosphonoformate Inhibits Feline Retrovirus Infections in Cats

Pharmacokinetics, Toxicity and Prophylactic Antiviral Activity of Pmea in Feline Retrovirus Infected Cats

The Role of the VPX and VPR Genes in Simian Immunodeficiency Virus Life Cycle

Serological and Molecular Analysis of the Immunodominant Loop from Neutralization Resistant Variants Derived from HIV Inoculated Chimpanzees

Transgenic Constructs involving HIV-1 Genes

Relationship Among Primate Retroviruses

Primates for the Study of AIDS-Related Disorders

Prevention of Simian AIDS by Passive Protection

Characteristics of SIV AGM Isolated from Wild Caught Animals in Central African Republic

Prophylactic Effects of AZT Following Exposure of Macaques to an Accutely Lethal Variant of SIV

SIV from Sooty Mangabey Monkeys: An African Primate Lentivirus Closely Related to HIV-2

HIV-1 Infection of Human PBL-Reconstituted SCID Mice

Transmission of SIVmnd in a Semi-Free Range Breeding Colony of Mandrills in Gabon

Localisation of a Domain of Human CD4 Required for HIV-Mediated Synctytium Formation by Comparison with CD4 cDNAs Isolated from The Chimpanzee and Rhesus Monkey

Infection of Rhesus Macaques with a Moledularly Cloned Simian Immunodeficiency Virus

Feline Immunodeficiency Virus: Genetic Organization and Regulation

Evaluation by PCR of HIV-1 Status of Chimpanzees Challenged with HIV after Receiving Human HIVIG

Molecular Cloning and Sequence Analysis of Feline Immunodeficiency Virus

Infection of The New Zealand White Laboratory Rabbit

Neuropathological Study of SIV infected Macaques

Clinical, Immunological and Virological Follow-Up of HIV-2 Infected Rhesus Monkeys

Monkeys with Simian AIDS Produce an Anti-body Directed against a Histone-like Protein on CD4+ T-Cells

Vaccine Protection against Simian Immunodeficiency Virus Infection

Evidence for Progression to Diseases in Chimpanzees Chronically Infected with HIV-1?

Genetic Variation of SIV in Experimentally Infected Macaques: Tissue Versus Tissue Culture

Aerosol Delivery of Pentamidine to the Deep Lung: A Model of Isotopic Quantitation in Baboons

Persistent HIV-2 Infections of Rhesus, Macaques, Baboons and Mangabeys

A Rabbit Model of HTLV-1 Infection

CD8+ and CD4+ Responses to HIV-1 Antigens in Mice Immunized with VV

Macrophages from 1 P-BM5 Infected Mice Induced Murine AIDS

Intercomparisons of Different SIV Isolates in Rhesus and Cynomolgus Macaques

Strain Specificity of Lymphocyte Proliferative Responses in Experimental Animals Immunized with Recombinant HIV-1 gp120 Antigens

FIV-AIDS Model for Testing Novel Vaccine Approaches for Human AIDS

Isolation and Preliminary Characterisation of a Neurotropic Stain of Feline Leukemia Virus

In Situ Immunoassaying Suggests Central Neuroendocrine Involvement in Infant Feline AIDS (FAIDS)

In Vivo Analysis of the Minimal Infectious Dose of an Acutely Lethal Pool of Simian IV

HIV-1 Infection in a Continuous Rabbit Macrophage Line

Infection with Simmian Immunodeficiency Virus Via Conjunctival and Oral Mucosae in a Newborn Rhesus Macaque

Therapy of Mouse AIDS with Diethyldithiocarbamate

Pathology of Feline Immonodeficiency Virus Infection

Un modèle expérimental du SIDA chez la souris, qui élicite des infections et des angiosarcomes

Adaptation of Human Immunodeficiency Virus Serologic Tests to the Simian IV Model

Enhancement of Anti-viral Therapy in HIV Infection using BBB Modification with Insulin: Animal Data and Clinical Considerations

Experimental HIV-2 Infection of Old World Monkeys

Culture Requirements for HIV-1 Isolation from Infected Chimpanzees

HIV-1 Antigenemia in Athymic "Nude" Mice

Langerhans Cells in Rhesus Monkey Oral Mucosa Before and After Infection with Simian Retreovirus Serotype-1

Innoculation of Baboons and Macaques with Virus Produced from SIV

Infection of Rhesus Macaques with Molecularly-Cloned HIV-2

Clinical and Immunological Staging of Feline Immunodeficiency Virus Infection

Establishment of FEV-Producing Cell Lines From FIV Seropositive Cats

Human Recombinant IL-2 Induces Cytotoxic LGL from FeLV Infected IL-2 Immunosuppressed Cats

Isolation and Partial Characterization of an HIV-1 Related Virus Occurring Naturally in Chimpanzees in Gabon

HIV-1 Infection in the Rabbit

Experimental Infection of Cynomolgus Monkeys with HIV-2

Effects of Whole Body Hyperthermia on Cats Infected with Feline Leukemia Virus

Experimental Infection of Specific Pathogen-Free Cats with UK Isolates of Feline Immunodeficiency Virus

A Mouse Model for Investigating HIV-1 Replication

Analysis of Guinea Pig Dermal Hypersensitivity to HIV Whole Virus Immunogen

Growth Characteristics of Simian Kaposi's Sarcoma in Nude Mice

Development of a Study Set on the Pathology of Simian Retroviral Diseases

Immunization of Rhesus Macaques with Inactivated SIV Fails to Protect against Mucosal or IV Challenge

HIV Immunization and Challenge of HIV Seropositive and Seronegative Chimpanzees

Immunogenicity of Potential HIV Vaccines in Chimpanzees

Simian Immunity to HIV-1 Candidate Vaccines

Still Searching

John Greyson

There's a drawing I made, a mother letting her dead son slide into her arms. I could do a hundred similar drawings but still can't seem to come any closer to him. I'm still searching for him, as if it were in the very work itself that I had to find him.
— Käthe Kollwitz, 1916

The tapes I've made addressing AIDS aren't autobiographical, yet they inevitably trace my changing responses to the epidemic, my search for the stories that the *Globe and Mail* won't print, the stories of my friends, of our communities, of what we're all going through, the things that haven't been seen and said. It is impossible to imagine an end to the search: there are still hundreds of tapes begging to be made.

Moscow Does Not Believe in Queers (1986), simply references AIDS as part of an exploration of East/West sexual politics. The tape is an eccentric, dramatized diary of my experiences as an out gay delegate to a 1985 international youth conference in Moscow, during the first year of glasnost. Central to the project is an interrogation of tourist journalism, foregrounding in particular the impossibility of overcoming cold war discourses, the impossibility for me, as a Westerner, to adequately represent what Moscow's gay underground might actually look like. As part of my strategy, I chose two cultural references from the West (both unavailable in Moscow), that summed up the contradictory extremes of the culture I was coming from. On the one hand, hysterical tabloid headlines about Rock Hudson, the first Hollywood celebrity with AIDS, whose diagnosis was being trumpeted from every airport newsstand during the flight to Moscow; on the other hand, unsafe bum-fucking images from a best-selling gay porn tape.

The contradictions of each image interested me. Rock represented a break-through in the previous deafening media silence about AIDS, yet the coverage of his diagnosis and eventual death was homophobic and AIDS-phobic to the extreme. At the same time, on the porn front, Toronto's gay community was very aware of censorship issues, joining with artists and feminists to fight repressive film/tape censorship laws. The Ontario Censor Board had gained notoriety by

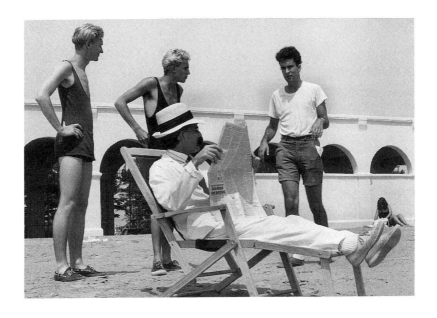

John Greyson, *The ADS Epidemic*, 1987. Still from the shoot.
Photo: Leena Randvee.

banning the feminist anti-porn film *Not a Love Story*, as well as such gay classics as Jean Genet's *Un Chant d'Amour* and Frank Riploh's *Taxi Zum Klo*. Canada Customs had become notorious for its regular seizures of books and magazines being shipped to Glad Day Books, Toronto's only gay bookstore, including porn and explicit safer sex materials. Within the gay community, many of the same people who were fighting the censorship of unsafe-sex porn, were also fighting for the representation of explicit safer sex images in AIDS education campaigns, since the official state education campaigns were predictably anti-sex and anti-gay.

These two counterpoints (Rock and porn), butt-cut together (as it were), served to construct an ambient cultural commentary about the day-to-day construction of AIDS representations within the Western mass media and the Western subculture. These in turn were contrasted with conversations and monologues about AIDS paranoia in Moscow, both at the conference and in the city's gay subculture. AIDS was integrated in the tape not as the central subject, but rather, as an inevitable aspect of the parameters of gay mens identities in both the East and the West that summer.

A year later, given the opportunity to make a commissioned work for a public shopping mall setting, I decided to make an AIDS awareness tape that targeted gay youth. *The ADS Epidemic*, a five-minute music video remake of Visconti's *Death In Venice* was the result. It tells of a new plague, Acquired Dread of Sex, that is sweeping the nation. In this remake, Aschenbach is a raging homophobe who eventually succumbs to an ADS attack, while Tadzio overcomes his fear of ADS to discover that condoms are his very favourite thing to wear. While stressing safer sex, the tape is equally concerned with combatting the "promiscuity equals death" ideology of most straight safer sex campaigns.

The upbeat pop song and humorous images ensured that audiences unfamiliar with either Visconti or Mann would still get the affirmative message. For *Death in Venice* fans, I hoped the tape might encourage a rethinking of European literature's most famous novella. The original parlayed its message of plague-as-metaphor-for-deviant-desire-and/or-fascism with disturbing ease. *The ADS Epidemic*, on the other hand, didactically identified homophobia and AIDS-paranoia as dangerous but treatable plagues in their own right.

With both *Moscow . . .* and *The ADS Epidemic*, I was concerned with exploring the psychological impact of AIDS on the gay community, especially in relation to the construction of AIDS in the mass media as a gay disease. The formation of AIDS Action Now in Toronto in January, 1988, inspired by the earlier formations of ACT UP groups in both New York and Los Angeles, served both to mobilize the community around a new conceptualization of what AIDS politics could mean, and also demonstrated a compelling need for another sort of tape — one that would capture the new militance of the AIDS activist movement, one that would explore the actual experience of HIV disease and AIDS within Toronto. An explosion of tapes from the U.S. and U.K., (including the work of Stuart Marshall, Stashu Kybartas, Isaac Julien, Tom Kalin, Andre Burke, Michael Balser, Andy Fabo, Testing the Limits, Pratibha Parmar, Gregg Bordowitz and Jean Carlomusto at Gay Men's Health Crisis in New York, and many others) offered a breathtaking spectrum of strategies in their various approaches to this urgent content. Inspired by such grassroots momentum, and involved in AIDS Action Now's plans for disrupting the Fifth International Conference on AIDS in Montreal in June 1989, I decided to make two low-budget tapes that summer, one documenting the conference, the other focusing on the activist agenda concerning treatment drugs.

Armed with a cheap Super-VHS camcorder and press passes, video artist Colin Campbell and I rushed willy-nilly through the four surreal days of the Fifth International. We went in with a loose set of priorities: document the four activist demonstrations that were planned; interview as many international grassroots AIDS educators and PWA activists as possible; and document the complacent opportunism of the 10,000 official "AIDS experts" in attendance, be they government leaders, multi-national mouthpieces or AIDS industry bureaucrats.

Given the hit-and-run nature of the conference, we grabbed what we could when we could, relying on luck and contacts for getting interviews and documenting interventions. The narrative structure, that of using a fictional conservative CBC reporter who would be kidnapped by AIDS activists, and eventually succumb to the Patty Hearst syndrome, occurred to me during the second day of shooting, and we made sure to shoot backdrop shots that an actor could be keyed into later. Similarly, the idea of getting pharmaceutical reps to talk about their AIDS profits only came to us while we were shooting in the trade fair. I had assumed that such business people would be smart enough to avoid the topic completely, especially since two such scruffy fag types with a pathetic little camcorder were the ones asking the questions. In fact, they were only too happy to talk growth forecasts, market shares and profit margins for their various products, seemingly unaware that the audience might not be the most sympathetic.

The song, What We Want Is, was written by composer Glenn Schellenberg and myself, taking its lyrics in part from the The World Is Sick poster campaign that AIDS Action Now had designed for the conference demos. (The tape's title, The World is Sick (sic), also comes from this campaign). We were interested in playing with the conventions of acid house, creating a danceable club song that also functioned as a call to arms, explicitly contradicting the traditional cynicism of sampled ironic quotation that provides the structure and frisson of much house music.

Interviews with international AIDS educators and PWA activists form the central core of the tape. Their eloquent testimonies emphasize the necessity of specificity, the necessity of creating AIDS education and service projects that originate within local cultural and community contexts (as opposed to being imposed from without). Their words are echoed in the speeches of the closing demonstration, with activists from around the world calling for international recognition that PWAs are not simply citizens demanding their full rights in society, but more, that PWAs are *the* leaders in fighting this epidemic.

In August, 1989, I also made *The Pink Pimpernel*, with several goals in mind. First and foremost, this tape was intended as a recruitment tape for AIDS Action Now (AAN). Secondly, it was intended to contribute to ongoing debates about different types or "styles" of activism within the gay community, fondly poking fun at the self-righteousness and seriousness of some self-styled AIDS politicos. Thirdly, it focuses on the politics of AIDS treatment drugs, using as a case-study the anti-viral AIDS treatment drug DDI.

The choice of DDI was an obvious one, since there was much excitement about it that summer as a potentially less toxic alternative to AZT. AIDS Action Now had targeted its manufacturer Bristol Myers for several demonstrations, and it was hoped that the tape could contribute to AAN's community education campaign. Because the situation was changing on a daily basis, however, the tape had to anticipate future changes in DDI's status. Thus in the interviews I conducted with AIDS activists and PWAs, we had to search for a way to ensure that their comments wouldn't become redundant based on an unknown future. We tried to make the interviews focus on DDI as an example of the general fight for getting promising treatment drugs released.

Two weeks after I finished editing, the situation did in fact change dramatically. Due to coordinated actions by AIDS Action Now and ACT UP New York against Bristol Myers, DDI was released on 'compassionate grounds' in Canada, but under an extremely limited definition of what these 'compassionate grounds' actually were. In practice, DDI was really only available in clinical trials comparing its efficacy with AZT. Similarly, the prognosis on DDI's value has ebbed and flowed, as new and sometimes contradictory evaluations of its toxicity, pricing and appropriate dosage levels continue to be made. Because *The Pink Pimpernel* chose not to engage in detailed specifics about such issues, focusing instead on the politics of getting the drug released, the tape hopefully remains a useful organizing tool.

The *Pink Pimpernel* consists of three intercut elements: documentary interviews with AIDS activists; the dramatic retelling of the classic 1940s melodrama *The Scarlet Pimpernel*; and four safer-sex ads by famous dead artists. Firstly, the documentary interviews, where AIDS activists and PWAs are constituted as the experts of the health crisis. Each interview subject is framed by Pink Panther cartoons. The intention was simple: every Pink Panther adventure consists of this feline dandy getting what he wants (food, clothes, a place to sleep) through sneaky and significantly non-violent (at least, compared to the Roadrunner) tricks against

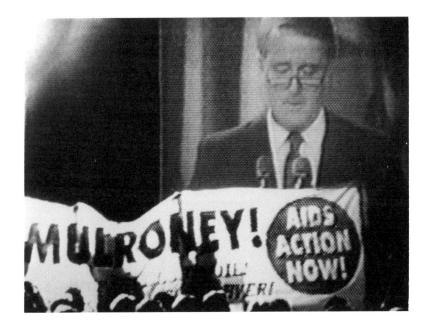

John Greyson, *The World is Sick (sic)* in which Canadian Prime Minister Brian Mulroney's speech is being booed by AIDS activists, 1989. Still from colour video.

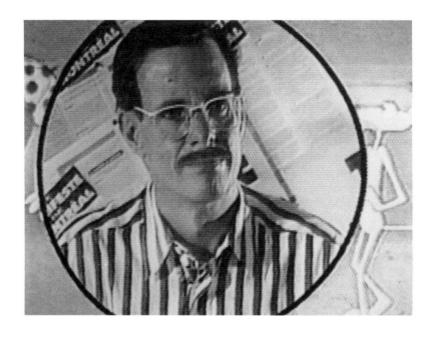

AIDS activist Michael Lynch in John Greyson's video *The Pink Pimpernel*, 1989. Still from colour video.

the stuffy rich old man. The Panther's subversive antics were a playful tribute to the imaginative strategies of the AIDS activist movement, where wit, style and irony are valued components in the preparation of demonstration banners and education campaigns.

The limited range of subjectivities represented by the six interview subjects in the tape (four white gay men, one white lesbian, one South Asian gay man) reflects a dilemma originating within AIDS Action Now, which despite concerted efforts remains overly representative of white clones with moustaches. In selecting the speakers, I had two choices: either do affirmative representation that would make the tape (and the organization) look more inclusive than it really is, or be honest about the tokenism and address it. I went for the latter strategy, but came up against a fundamental contradiction: propaganda tapes by definition aren't supposed to be self-critical. In the final edit, one speaker, Mary Louise Adams, addresses the issue by speaking about the evolving relationship between the women's self-health movement and the AIDS activist movement. She expresses optimism that gay men are finally acknowledging a debt to and learning from feminist critiques of the health-care system, and addresses how the organization is grappling with the racism and sexism, as well as the homophobia, of dominant AIDS agendas.

The Pink Pimpernel's title comes, of course, from the reactionary Alexander Korda classic *The Scarlet Pimpernel*, inspired by the romantic English novel of the same name. Starring Leslie Howard and Merle Oberon, it tells of an English dandy who was secretly helping the French aristocracy escape the Terror and the guillotine of revolutionary France. Cashing in on French bi-centennial fever, I updated the story to tell of two gay lovers, one a humourless AIDS activist, the other a frivolous fop named Percy. In reality, Percy is the Pink Pimpernel, who smuggles DDI across the border for people with AIDS in Toronto. Played in high melodramatic style, complete with a swooning kiss in the sunset under the closing credits, this slim narrative is an attempt to insert camp gay humour back into the sometimes too-earnest ranks of AIDS activism, and suggest, as PWA Michael Lynch notes in the tape, that a dandy can also be an activist. The goal was to recruit unpoliticized gay men into AIDS Action Now, attempting to seduce with tacky humour those who might otherwise run away from a more traditional serious documentary.

The smuggling narrative is no metaphor: at various times, and for various AIDS treatment drugs (including dextran sulphate, AZT and pentamidine), the AIDS activist and PWA self-empowerment movements on both sides of the Can-ada/U.S. border have adopted such semi-legal and illegal strategies, and will no doubt continue to do so in the future, while both governments continue to block the speedy and affordable release of most treatment drugs.

Four safer sex ads by famous dead gay artists punctuate the documentary and dramatic sequences. These one-minute remakes of Fassbinder's *Querelle*, Jean Genet's *Un Chant d'Amour*, and Warhol's *Blow Job* serve as mini-tributes to historic gay directors, and also act as mini-safer sex rewrites of the original unsafe plots, through the adroit insertion of condoms at key moments. The fourth, a remake of Claude Jutras' and Norman MacLaren's *A Chairy Tale*, was both a bit of token Canadian content and a fond reclaiming of the not-widely-known gay sexuality of these two revered directors.

These four safer sex ads were also an attempt to break with the constricting realist consensus that has developed among some AIDS educators concerning the production of safer sex materials. Granted, it is usually a battle-royale simply to be allowed to be sexually explicit in any campaign. However, a majority of the explicit posters and tapes that have been produced in Canada, the U.S. and Europe seem to believe that the simple illustration of a correct practice will automatically produce the same behaviour on the part of audiences. Too many educators seem to feel that target groups will respond in a monkey-see, monkey-do fashion, not taking into account the complex psychological ways different people respond to representations of sexuality. There is no automatic relation between the images that turn people on and the sort of sex they practice. Indeed, there are often profound differences between the pornographic fantasies people create/consume and the actual sex they engage in.

Through their humour, style, and coding within film history, these four mini-tapes announce at the outset that they don't pretend to be porn. Instead, their very distance from the aesthetics of porn invite viewers to watch with heightened awareness. Some educators have argued that the film history references make them elitist and inaccessible to the many viewers who don't know who Fassbinder is. I would counter this assertion with several arguments. First of all, such a statement constructs a mythic, monolithic "them," an uneducated uniform gay proletariat that must be condescended to if it is to be saved. This ignores the huge diversity of the community as well as the recent statistics which suggest that young, college-educated gay men who have been inundated with safer sex info for the past five years are nevertheless practicing unsafe sex, and are desperately in need of a different sort of safer sex education campaign that speaks to them. Secondly, the tapes offer multiple pleasures for those who do know the references, and a bit of on-the-spot cinema studies pedagogy for those who don't. It is exactly that sort of casual coded references that serve to extend our knowledge of the gay subculture and of gay history, contributing to a shared vocabulary. All five artists who are appropriated were arguably anti-elitist in their various practices and contexts, no matter how much art history has attempted to place them on a pedestal. Finally, the safer sex message and humour is still clear no matter how few film history courses you've taken.

Another tape, *The Great AZT Debate*, was made for a public access cable series

93

called *Toronto — Living With AIDS*, which Toronto artist Michael Balser and I initiated in 1990. Our project was inspired by the Gay Men's Health Crisis *Living With AIDS* show in New York, which has produced some of the most dynamic AIDS education tapes to date. The Toronto cable version commissions artists and community groups to produce half-hour low-budget works in any style on a specific AIDS subject. The funding is coming from guilty Federal and Provincial Health Ministries who are trying to curry favour with community AIDS activists outraged by the respective governments' years of indifference and neglect.

The Great AZT Debate is basically a round-table of PWAs talking about their personal pro and con experiences with AZT. Dressed up like an episode of *Wheel of Fortune*, complete with performance artists David MacLean as Vanna and Meryn Caddell as Pat Sajak, the format stresses the roll of the dice when it comes to getting accurate, up-to-date info about the drug. Our main purpose was to stress that there is no one answer, despite the attempts of some self-styled experts (be they doctors, activists, or PWA advocates) to say otherwise. Instead, each choice is contextual, and thus anyone considering taking the drug must weigh the considerable and ever-changing pros and cons in relation to their specific situation. The round-table format grew out of an AIDS Action Now educational speak-out, where it became clear that the variety of impromptu testimonials from people during the question and answer period were more memorable and powerful than the earlier, prepared presentations by two panelists. The tape is meant to fulfill a very specific need: offering audiences of PWAs a range of opinions from people in the same situation, focusing not just on the objective facts of dosage levels, complimentary therapies and side effects, but also on subjective experiential issues, like fear of not making the right choice, disempowerment at the hands of insensitive doctors, and anger at the lack of substantial answers and options.

Video as a technical information medium for treatment issues will never be able to substitute the clarity of a take-home-and-read brochure. What video can provide is the intimate sense of shared and often contradictory experience, of giving viewers in the same situation a sense of community, and hence vocabulary, and hence empowerment. AZT remains such a hotly contested issue that perhaps the most radical thing this tape accomplishes is simply that it enables people to listen respectfully to others who made different treatment decisions than they did.

The different ways I've used video to speak about AIDS since 1986 are a result of several interlocking factors. Most obviously, there is my own developing personal and political response to the epidemic, my search for a voice. Then, there is the impact of grassroots AIDS organizing, in Toronto and throughout the world, which has inspired the content. Perhaps most directly, there is the incredible groundswell of tapes by artists and activists, who continue to invent new ways to speak of and visualize the experiences of this appalling health crisis. This network of artists making video about AIDS is inspirational, not just because of the amazing tapes that result, but also, because of the spirit of unquestioning generosity that flourishes when it comes to sharing equipment, footage, and ideas, and the gleeful irreverence that ensues when it comes to debunking precious notions of authorship, copyright and artistic worth. Any cynical commentator who has lost faith in the efficacy of video as an agent of social change should plug into the AIDS video subculture. The tapes that have been made, and that continue to pour forth, constitute a collective search for empowerment. A search that offers audiences images and words that *The Globe and Mail* won't consider. A search that encourages audiences to create those images, and speak those words, for themselves.

The Spectacular Ruse

Monika Gagnon & Tom Folland

> Physical control and restraint are ideologically, strategically, and symboli-
> cally significant to the new right. Eras of rightists' ascendancy are marked
> by legislative shifts toward more stringent physical controls — law and
> order, capital punishment, punishment of sexuality, more stringent peda-
> gogical styles.
>
> — Cindy Patton, *Sex and Germs*[1]

The abjection of the body and of gay men is repeated throughout history under a variety of guises. Rosalind Miles in her *Women's History of the World* for instance, describes the burning of gay men at the stake of witches: ". . . [M]en accused of homosexuality were bound and mixed with the faggots of brushwood and kindling around her feet, 'to kindle a flame foul enough for a witch to burn in.' "[2] This union in adversity exemplifies our aim to trace the ideological underpinnings of seemingly disparate events in order to emphasize the signifi-cance of a political alliance between straight and lesbian women, and gay men. In temporarily suspending the specificities of these social groups, a common political affiliation might strategically be forged in order to identify points of contact, develop modes of critique and strategies of resistance. For historically, what is explicit in the destruction of sorceresses and gays is the threats they pose to so-called normal social and symbolic life, "the severe punishment of males who transgressed the restriction of sex to heterosexual coupling links them with women who similarly defied patriarchal definitions."[3]

While aware of the significance of historical specificity and the particular aims of different political struggles — the shared and separate agendas of lesbians and gays, for instance — we have sought to temporarily collapse such specificities to move toward a generality: to underline how control, subjection and abjection of particular social groups have a social and psychic functionality for the dominant order. Socially transgressive behaviour (any forms of "otherness" — social, sexual and cultural), can be understood as identified and isolated in order to reaffirm social definitions of sanctified norms; "correct" behaviour, in other words, must be defined in relation to what it is not. Equally important is how the historical tropes of subjugation have been revitalized, albeit in different forms, within the contemporary scenario of AIDS. The collapse of historical detail within our text has allowed for a context in which an historical continuity of domination might be traced.

The duality of sorceresses' and hysterics' social roles, two seemingly vastly different female types, has been examined at length by Catherine Clément. At once, escape and flight from the burdens of social constraint by these women — the witches' Sabbath, the hysteric's spectacle of femininity in crisis — are both recouped as an expulsion with a specific social functionality. Via Lévi-Strauss, Clément describes this simultaneous operation which expels whilst patrolling the effects of transgression:

> . . . like all subgroups that are unsituated in the complex of symbolic systems, women are threatened by the reverse of mobility, by symbolic repressions that are ready to limit the effects of symbolic disorder . . . The anthropoemic mode [of repression or integration], ours, consists in vomiting the abnormal ones into protected spaces — hospitals, asylums, prisons.[4]

The operation of protected and policed social spaces — hospitals, asylums, prisons — is to contain and survey those social groups deemed "dangerous." Once burnt at the stake, gays and women found themselves objects of medical scrutiny and examination in more insidious, if not as violent, forms of domination. "Homosexuality" was defined as a biologically-determined perversity, in interrelation with so-called normal sexual behaviours and practices that themselves fluctuated and varied at different historical moments and in different social contexts. Women's conjugal and parental role was naturalized to the extent that deviation from this sanctioned femininity was viewed as "abnormal."

The classificatory obsession with constructions of deviant subjectivities and sexualities was endemic to nineteenth century Europe, and coincided with the reorganization of the family, work and gender relationships under capitalism. Across a broad range of discursive practices as well as geographical areas, the insistence on increasing social controls can be compared, to signal a general impulse toward the surveillance and domination of so-called deviant behaviours by those who were deemed subversive to the white, heterosexual family unit under patriarchy: criminals, gays, immigrants, wayward women.

Instances of surveillance and control proliferate across the historical terrain of nineteenth century Europe. In the domain of policed sexualities, Alexandre Parent-Duchâtelet's highly influential demographic study of 12,000 registered Parisian prostitutes was published in 1836. His expertise as a specialist in sewers, drains and cesspools (perhaps inadvertently) linked his study of prostitution with "sewage, putrefecation and death," as Abigail Solomon-Godeau has written. She continues,

> If the public prostitute could be identified, registered and confined to certain areas; her activity limited to certain hours, her person segregated in a licensed brothel; if she could be monitored by the madame, the police, the gynecologist, then prostitution . . . could be managed and contained. The threat to the rationalized system lay in the growing ranks of clandestine, that is to say, nonregistered prostitutes.[5]

In the domain of other monitored sexualities, Michel Foucault marks the birth of the homosexual "as a species" in 1870, with an article on "contrary sexual sensations" by German psychiatrist Karl Westphal. Foucault writes,

> [T]he psychological, psychiatric, medical category of homosexuality was constituted from the moment it was characterized . . . less by a type of sexual relations than by a certain quality of sexual sensibility, a certain way of inverting the masculine and the feminine in oneself.[6]

Allan Sekula has emphasized the operation of photography within specific discourses of criminality and eugenics in the late nineteenth century, discourses in which "the photograph operated as the image of scientific truth."[7] Among other examples, Sekula cites Italian anatomist-craniometrician Cesare Lombroso's physical analysis and classification of criminals which contributed significantly to the development of criminal anthropology and the determination of a criminal "type" based on physical characteristics. In England, Francis Galton's photographic "composite images" underpinned conceptual bases for the "improvement" of the human species through selective breeding.

Although constructed for different purposes within differing historical contexts, these discursive operations that are called upon to construct categories of subversive subjectivity point toward a fluidity and interchangeability of certain disposable constituencies. In the contemporary context of AIDS discourse, Paula Treichler has underlined this fluidity. In relation to women's cultural association with illness and disease, she notes that up until recently, ". . . [there was] no need for female representation in the AIDS saga because gay men [were] already substituting for them as the Contaminated Other." [8]

French neurologist Jean-Martin Charcot's extensive work on hysteria in the late nineteenth century exemplifies the control of sexuality present in medicine's discursive constructions; these constructions were also reliant on the truth-value of photography, the belief in the reality of the image. Hysteria was called upon to define an expansive range of female symptoms and was historically, since the time of Hippocrates, attributed to a disorder of the womb. While the reduction of the woman to the spectre of her own body — both in Charcot's organicist explanations and in his use of photography — was acceptable, indeed preferable, insofar as her femininity was already defined by her bodily functions, her reproductive capacities, the identification of analogous hysterical behaviours in male patients and the crises of definition that ensued, acutely revealed the gender bias of so-called objective medicine.

Charcot first shifted emphasis away from the womb to the brain in order to transport his model of hysteria to the male. However, as Lynne Kirby has argued, "Male hysteria is not so much the coding of men as women, as the uncoding of men as men."[9] In other words, the implicit emasculation of the male hysteric within hysteria's discursive history produced telling ideological correctives that attempted to redefine what was, in effect, a rupture in strict conceptions of masculinity.[10]

Thus, while female hysteria was defined — like Lombroso's criminals, or Galton's racial typologies — by organic explanations and reaffirmed with an extensive photographic repertoire produced on the grounds of the Salpêtrière Hospital, the appearance of male hysteria necessitated a conceptual and methodological shift: social factors replaced organic explanations for the cause of hysteria in the male subject. As Elaine Showalter has radically suggested, the "shell-shock" diagnosed amongst World War I soldiers (one of the later euphemisms for hysterical behaviour among men), prompted a masculinity crisis precisely when masculine heroism was essential for the ideology of war, and thus catapulted organicist explanations toward the era of psychiatric modernism:

> The efficacy of the term 'shell-shock' lay in its power to provide a masculine-sounding substitute for the effeminate associations of hysteria and to disguise the troubling parallels between male war neurosis and the female nervous disorder epidemic before the war.[11]

This evidence of a masculinity in crisis and the desperate correctives called upon to mask its presence in social reality denoted the limits within which femininity and masculinity could be defined, within the patriarchal constrains of heterosexual reproduction.

■ ■ ■

> While gay men find their situation made problematic by a revived and newly legitimated climate of homophobia, women are also being subjected to a new set of gender-specific regulatory strategies designed to maximize their social utility as breeders while minimizing the social costs attached to sexual exchanges.[12]

What are the contemporary deployments of physical and symbolic control? Photography continues to be used today as a documentary tool within medical and scientific fields. The power of the medical image as an ideological mechanism of control and domination, however, has effectively shifted into the pervasive spectacles of popular tabloids, newspapers and television. And what, in the

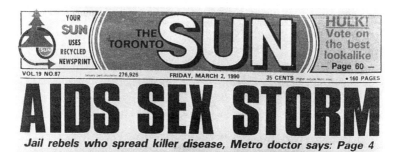

The Toronto Sun, Friday, March 2, 1990.

Renaissance, was a religiously sanctioned hatred of sorceresses and homosexuals, shifted, as their definition as transgressive behaviours became reinforced through the discursive constraints of law and medicine.

The practice of medicine must be understood, Bryan Turner writes in *The Body and Society*, as "essentially social medicine, because it is a practice which regulates social activities under the auspices of the state."[13] Thus public health, for example, one of the principle means of state-enforced health in the twentieth century is a political practice deeply implicated with the surveillance, policing, testing, regulation and accounting of, those considered to be its other: the poor, people of colour, immigrants, gays, straight and lesbian women. Formally expelled from the symbolic through ritual, these others are simply legislated to the margins of the social.

Two recent events and subsequent media spectacles that may at first seem unrelated, will serve to illuminate the broader social logic to which both belong: the controlled and punitive legal and medical framing of gay and female sexuality. When Chief Medical Officer of Ontario Richard Schabas recently attempted to reclassify AIDS and HIV infection as a "virulent" disease, he effectively framed those with AIDS and HIV infection (in Canada still predominantly gay men) as a legislated threat to "public health" by promoting a quarantine legislation. Had Schabas succeeded (fortunately this was voted down by the AIDS subcommittee of the Toronto Board of Health), this proposed legislation would have criminalized the sexual activity of persons with HIV infection and AIDS in Ontario. This might be considered in relation to Barbara Dodd's 1989 court case; a pregnant woman whose planned abortion was postponed by a court injunction procured by an ex-boyfriend. The injunction designated Dodd's fetus a ward of the state and she was prevented from having an abortion until the case went to trial. The subsequent appearance of a second boyfriend who also claimed to be the father had two effects: it cast doubt on the paternity of the first boyfriend and thus, on the viability of his legal claim to Dodd's fetus. It also had the effect of destabilizing Dodd's moral integrity with social connotations of promiscuity, given her transgression from monogamous behaviour. Dodd's personal history was promptly dragged before the courts in an attempt to portray her as manipulative and morally corrupt. Needless to say, had Dodd's boyfriend been successful in overriding Dodd's own rights over her body and her fetus (the injunction was overturned), the result would have been eerily prophetic of the state breeders in Margaret Atwood's futuristic novel *The Handmaid's Tale*, in which women's social function is reduced to their biological status as reproducers of the species.

Schabas, who in the past distinguished himself by advocating a mandatory list of names of people testing positive to HIV (referred to within the gay community as his "death list"), had also, with his recent attempt at reclassification, simply availed himself of the very familiar accusation of gay men with AIDS as sexual murderers. This construction of sexual murder is shared not only by Ontario public health officials (most of whom were in agreement with Schabas's quarantine proposal), but also promoted by popular tabloids: "AIDS SEX STORM" screamed one headline, "Jail rebels who spread killer disease." [14] In his letter to the editor of a Toronto newspaper defending his quarantine proposal (which is curious in its absence of any reference to gays considering that it is of course gay men that would be most affected), Schabas deploys another familiar image of sexual danger: the prostitute, in this case, one "who also shared needles with other addicts." [15] Leo Bersani has written that "Representations of AIDS have to be X-rayed for their fantasmatic logic; they document the comparative irrelevance of information in communication." [16] In this sense, it is not important whether or not these dramatic images are real. What is important is the extraordinarily slippery passage that is produced between AIDS, sex, drugs, prostitution and criminality: AIDS is conflated with crime in one terse headline; a prostitute shares needles with "other addicts." What these images of prisoners with AIDS and needle-sharing prostitutes do communicate is a deeply rooted fear and hatred of the Other, constructed as the "outside" of public health. And as with those media representations of Barbara Dodd, portrayed as irresponsible and promiscuous, the characterization of "immoral" behaviour depends on an idealized conservative moral righteousness.

These dangerous identities of sexuality are not fixed and immutable, and serve particular ideological and social needs. Paula Treichler, for example, discerns a shift in the victim/perpetrator construction of AIDS as it pertains to women in the climate of concern over the declining birthrate amongst middle class white women. Once categorized with babies and other so-called "innocent victims" of AIDS (non-drug-using/prostitute/gay/"racial" persons with AIDS), heterosexual women with AIDS are increasingly pictured as "carriers." As Treichler observes, "There is thus no intrinsic concern of women as *women*." [17] The pregnant mother with AIDS forfeits her status as a person with rights over her own body and takes on the position already occupied by gay men, criminals, prostitutes and drug users: morally responsible for her own condition and a threat to others.

Although Barbara Dodd was not infected with HIV, her trial was as equally marked by the complete disregard of any autonomous rights of person she might have claimed for her own body, as are PWAs. As a woman, Dodd was thus positioned as an absent term in this discourse of rights of possession or civil rights. Luce Irigaray writes that,

> just as, in commodities, natural utility is overridden by the exchange function, so the properties of a woman's body have to be suppressed and subordinated to the exigencies of its transformation into an object of circulation among men. [18]

While not in circulation among men, gays are equally excluded from this order in the same way that Irigaray characterizes women, as "ill-suited for the seriousness of symbolic rules."[19] Ill-suited for the seriousness of symbolic rules, gays and other disposable constituencies are equally unfit for inclusion within the symbolic terrain of "public health," thereby justifying state intervention into the use of their own bodies.

The reluctance to deal with AIDS by any means other than punitive, and the ingrained homophobia that accompanies any government action on the issue was signalled by [then] Canadian Federal Minister of Health Perrin Beatty's "Working Document for the Development of the National Strategy for AIDS," prepared in October 1989 for Health and Welfare Canada. The report was based on consultation with public health officials and community AIDS groups who are usually pitted against one another; one group thus represented the interests of the state, the other represented actual communities of people infected with, and/or working with people with HIV and AIDS. Despite this token representation of community AIDS service groups, the report, prepared by the independent group Sadinsky and Associates, vacillated in a state of anxious homophobia between affirming the rights of PWAs and oddly enough, posing those same people as a threat to public health. As a result, Beatty's "National Strategy for AIDS" (released June 28, 1990) contained nothing new, including no additional monies.[20]

The long-awaited release of Beatty's disappointing "National Strategy for AIDS" and the tortured logic of his earlier report, is only one of the many testimonials to the particular ideologic rupture AIDS has posed for notions of the social body and public health. AIDS and the social crises it has engendered must be viewed as part of the much longer history that we have attempted to sketch very briefly.

These examples demonstrate how rights to one's own body, and the rights to pleasure, are increasingly under attack. While this is particularly evident in the professional disciplines of law and medicine, the ways in which this ideology is carried through representations in popular media has also come to have an effect on contemporary visual art practices. Increasing examples of censorship in the visual arts must be understood within this volatile conservative climate in which the media is accused of being impartial and "too liberal." When political conservatism reaches into the traditionally "liberal" domain of the arts, it is paradoxically, the radical potential of images in art that becomes foregrounded. By insisting on intervening in the area of arts content, the conservative agenda unwittingly underlines the important and contradictory ideological work that the artwork can perform.

As we have suggested, the ideological work performed by images is central to defining subjectivity, particularly gender and sexuality. The nineteenth century deployment of medical and police photographs, or mass media's inflammatory "images" of AIDS, perform similar operations in naming illness and disease as deviant conditions. Those public health acts which deliberately ostracize and persecute both women and gay men similarly operate on highly socially constructed definitions of normalcy and deviance. Each instance demonstrates a position on the question of sexual and political liberation. Each instance demonstrates the profound stakes surrounding the image.

NOTES

Thanks to Mark Lewis for his comments on our manuscript.

1. Cindy Patton, *Sex and Germs: The Politics of AIDS* (Montréal: Black Rose Books, 1986): 83-84.

2. Rosalind Miles, *The Women's History of the World* (London: Paladin, 1989), 122.

3. Loc. cit.

4. Catherine Clément, "The Guilty One," *The Newly Born Woman* (Minneapolis: University of Minnesota Press, 1986): 8.

5. Abigail Solomon-Godeau, "The Legs of the Countess," *October* 39 (Winter 1986). Solomon-Godeau writes, "Parent-Duchâtelet's 'De la prostitution dans la ville de Paris' provided the model not only for fifty years of French reglementary systems, but also for British laws and investigations," 101.

6. Michel Foucault, *History of Sexuality*, Volume One: An Introduction (London: Penguin, 1979), 43.

7. See Allan Sekula, "The Body and the Archive," *October* 39 (Winter 1986): 40.

8. Paula Treichler, "AIDS, Gender and Biomedical Discourse: Current Contests for Meaning," *AIDS: The Burdens of History*, Elizabeth Fee and Daniel M. Fox, eds. (Berkeley: University of California Press, 1988), 217.

9. Lynne Kirby, "Male Hysteria and Early Cinema," *Camera Obscura* 17 (May 1988): 126.

10. See Monika Gagnon, "A Convergence of Stakes: Feminism and Representations of AIDS," forthcoming book anthology, James Miller, ed. (Toronto: University of Toronto Press, 1991), and "Territories of Convergence," *Territories of Difference*, Renee Baert, ed. (Banff: Walter Phillips Gallery, 1991), for a more extended discussion of male hysteria and its disruption of social conceptions of masculinity.

11. Elaine Showalter, *The Female Malady: Women, Madness and English Culture 1830-1980* (New York: Penguin Books, 1985), 164.

12. Linda Singer "Bodies — Pleasures — Powers," *Differences* 1 (Winter 1989): 46.

13. Bryan S. Turner, *The Body and Society* (New York: Basil Blackwell, 1984), 226.

14. "AIDS SEX STORM: Jail rebels who spread killer disease," *Toronto Sun*, 2 March 1990.

15. "AIDS lockup proposal endorsed," *Toronto Star*, 16 February 1990.

16. Leo Bersani, "Is the Rectum a Grave?" *October* 43 (Winter 1987): 210.

17. Treichler, 214.

18. Luce Irigaray, *This Sex Which is Not One*, Catherine Porter, tr. (Ithaca: Cornell University Press, 1985), 187.

19. Ibid., 193.

20. It is interesting to note that the amount of federal money for AIDS is just two million dollars more than the $110 million that [then] Minister of Culture and Communications Marcel Masse was allocated for postal subsidies for Canadian periodicals.

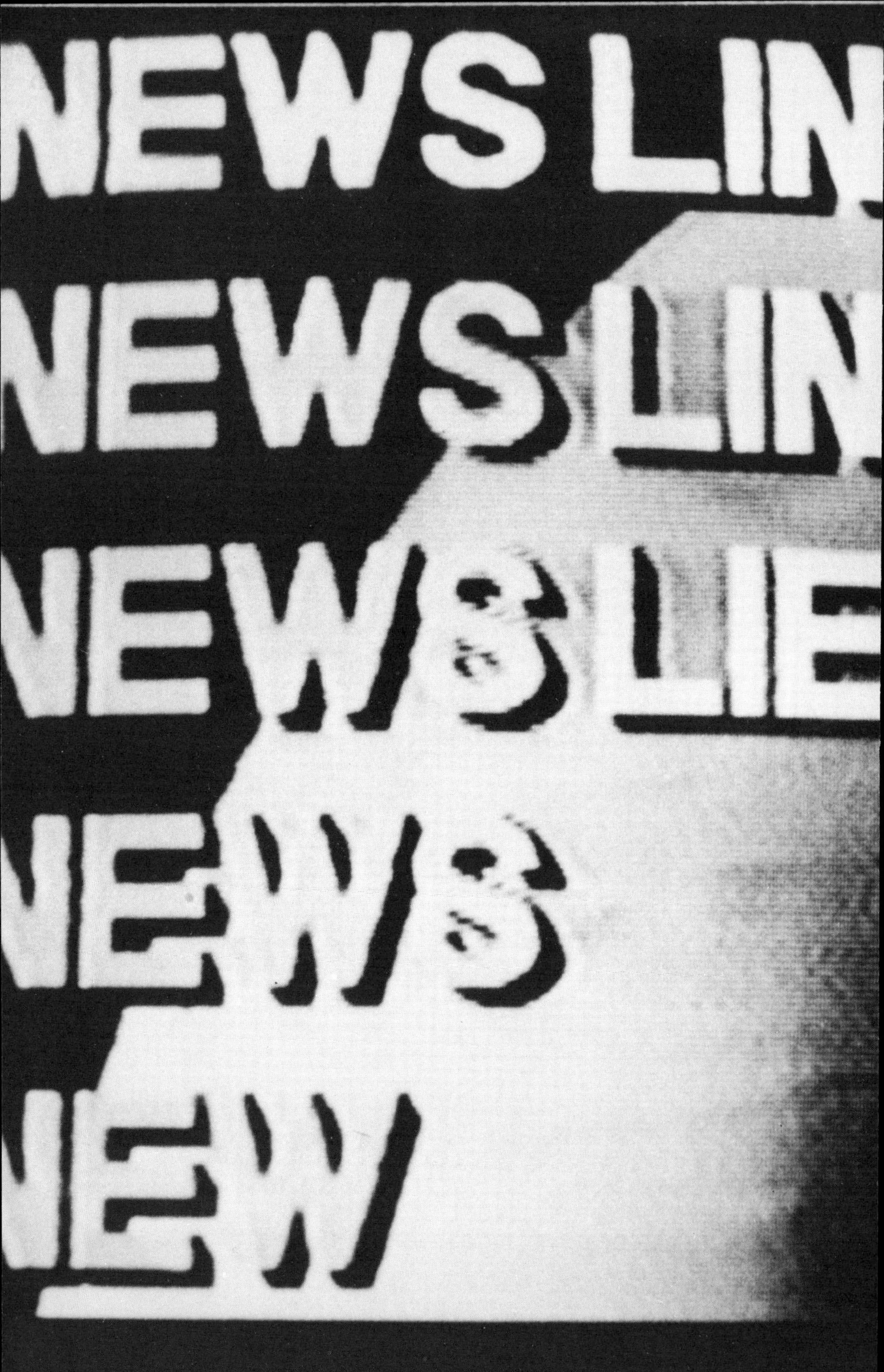

SEDUCTION OR TERRORISM?

Media Health Campaigning: Not Just What You Say, But the Way That You Say It!

Jon Baggaley

A Seventy-year Tradition

In 1921, film was in its infancy. However, it was already apparent that the new medium held great promise for the mass communication of facts about health. Agencies concerned with the prevention of venereal disease were particularly enthusiastic on this score. Yet their plans to distribute sex education films publicly met with strong opposition.

Psychiatric and medical opinion was opposed to the public use of films in sex education, on the grounds that they either give offence, or would unwittingly condone sexual irresponsibility by tending "to break down the sense of reserve, modesty or shame." The need for greater public awareness of sexually transmitted disease was less in question than the explicit manner in which commercial films on the topic attempted to generate this awareness. The controversy, in short, bore a striking resemblance to the arguments raised in the 1980s, concerning the use of mass media for AIDS prevention.

The dilemma of 1921 was tackled in an exhaustive study by noted psychologists Lashley and Watson.[1] Following interview and questionnaire studies of 4,800 people, they concluded that hard facts presented in a serious, straightforward, scientific manner were unlikely to do any harm to anyone. Certain other techniques, however, were liable to have less desirable effects. Gratuitous dramatization and storyline techniques were considered particularly risky, since they "hold attention more through their action than through their relation to (the facts)." The use of popular, colloquial terminologies was also criticized, as tending to diminish a campaign's scientific credibility.

Lashley and Watson also pointed out that young people tend to respond to

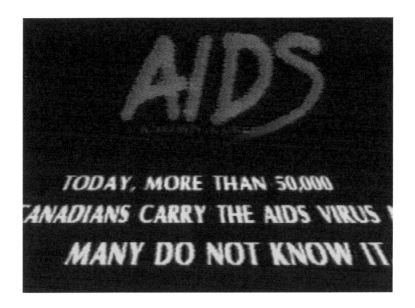

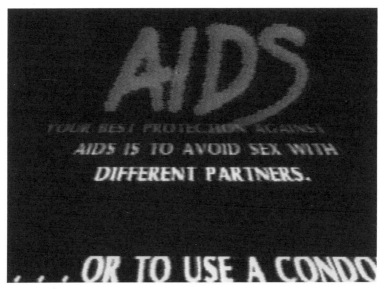

Straight facts and style are popular with viewers, as in this Canadian spot featuring scrolling text. This particular ad was vetoed by Canadian broadcasters on the basis that it described a condom as "your best protection" against AIDS rather than as a means of reducing AIDS risk.

sex education defensively, with "flippancy and innuendo," while with other audiences "the danger of arousing disturbing fears is a serious one." They saw a straightforward expository approach as the only way these contrasting negative reactions could be avoided.

Have we, so far, incorporated these conclusions in our development of public AIDS education? Apparently not. The flurry of international AIDS campaigns since 1986 has run the gamut from hard-sell, dramatic techniques such as those used in Great Britain and Australia to the soft-sell, even lighthearted approach of several Scandinavian campaigns. This range of strategies has been particularly apparent in the contrasting campaigns waged in the electronic medium with the widest of all audiences: that of television.[2]

Has human nature therefore changed since the 1921 study, becoming more amenable to health promotion in all its forms? Numerous studies suggest that this is not the case.

The resistance of prime-target audiences to educational campaigning has been noted with such consistency that, by now, one would have thought something might have been done about it — that, by now, campaign designers would have agreed on the most productive approaches.

The AIDS education literature to date indicates no such action, no such agreement. The consensus of educational research has remained consistent since the Lashley and Watson study in encouraging the straightforward, expository approach to media campaigning, as opposed to more eye-catching, dramatic approaches. However, as Hyman and Sheatsley have pointed out,[3] such evidence seems often to "be overlooked in the general eagerness simply to distribute more information." As Mendelsohn suggests,[4] much of what we see in so-called mass education in public health today is more often designed to please the whims of some well meaning board members than it is to accomplish meaningful effects." In Hinden's words, most media campaigns are "little more than short term propaganda exercises . . . having little impact on the world's major health problems."[5]

Obstacles to Effective Media Campaigning

A major obstacle to media campaigning appears to be the failure of public health agencies and educators to collaborate in the campaign design process. As Job indicates, "the final say in mass media campaigns is often given to bureaucrats who do not have a working knowledge of the principles of behaviour change." Lacking any media skills whatsoever, health agencies typically delegate the sensitive task of campaign design to media advertising agencies; though, as Job discusses in detail, "there is good reason not to expect strong parallels between health promotion and commercial advertising [techniques]."[6]

Advertising agencies, though highly skilled in attracting public attention to a new product or social issue, are conspicuously less successful at creating new psychological needs or altering old ones. Moreover, their traditional research methods — despite an assiduously cultivated myth — are surprisingly inadequate to the task of identifying effective propagandist techniques. Their media production techniques, favouring eye-catching dramatization and popular forms of language, are precisely those which Lashley and Watson described in 1921 as likely to trivialize a health campaign, and to diminish its credibility; and, in the AIDS education context, the predictions which Lashley and Watson made about the potentially undesirable effects of ill-designed public sex education may already be coming true.

By 1988, many of the world's initial AIDS awareness public health campaigns have been evaluated. The general outcome has been a raising of public AIDS awareness, though failure to affect AIDS-related lifestyles, other than in certain high-risk communities where campaigning has been intensive and carefully concerted. The particular resistance of young people to information about AIDS has become painfully apparent;[7] while increases in unwarranted public fears about AIDS, and levels of intolerance towards those who suffer from it, are now matters of common report.[8]

This checkered experience with the mass media — or at least their failure to apply validated media strategies — has led health promoters to a somewhat reactionary view of the value of the media as a campaign tool. This view holds that mass media approaches have little effect on health-related behaviour, and must be combined with other ingredients for a public health campaign to be successful. If media approaches did not continually contradict and conflict with one another, however, there is every likelihood that their effects would be more substantial.

Comparisons of Media Campaign Styles

A rare opportunity to study this hypothesis arose in 1981, courtesy of the Canadian Cancer Society (CCS). Public education about cancer risks and prevention is central to the CCS mandate; it has spent many millions of dollars on the production and delivery of educational campaigns via the local and national media. Subsequently, however, the CCS began to fear that conventional media techniques were failing to communicate with a major sector of the Canadian public — namely, the functionally illiterate members of society for whom cancer risks are maximal.

To investigate this possibility, the CCS commissioned an evaluation of a selection of its most widely used smoking prevention materials. The study was conducted between 1981 and 1985 at Memorial University (St. John's, Newfoundland) and the Université de Montréal under my direction.[9] It emerged that typical smoking prevention materials are indeed ineffective. Readability tests indicated that public print materials were often unintelligible to those readers with less than a college education. Billboard campaigns were either disregarded or ignored outright. Campaign materials in general — even the most expensive film and TV productions — were as likely to increase viewer resistance to smoking-prevention principles as they were to diminish it.

The CCS wished to overcome these problems by identifying the most effective campaign techniques for different types of audience. The major obstacle to media campaigning proved to be less that of public illiteracy, than that of the psychological resistance demonstrated by high-risk audiences. At this point the focus of the study turned to the ways such resistance might be anticipated and overcome.

A wide range of survey techniques were employed, ranging from the questionnaire and interview methods of conventional program evaluation, to a series of innovative research methods associated with the media advertising industry. The latter included analyses of audience responses to media techniques on a moment-by-moment basis, using state-of-the-art electronic methods (continual response measurement, or CRM). They also employed multivariate statistics in the effort to identify the effects of media techniques on specific audiences.

The research indicated that highly defensive high-risk audiences (e.g. smokers) can reject media presentation on the slightest pretext. A momentary turn of phrase or lapse in interest value could generate negative attitudes which persisted for the remainder of the presentation. Such audiences were particularly critical of attempts at dramatic characterization in media productions, and of the realism/relevance of dramatic situations. They suspected all but the plainest of statistical evidence, and where apt to infer a preachy or patronizing approach where none could conceivably have been suspected. In one situation, an actress portraying a doctor was judged to be unbelievable because her performance was too polished!

On a purely negative level, the studies indicated the need for extreme sensitivity in the selection of words, visual situations and even vocal inflections in the effort to penetrate audience defences. On a more positive level, they indicated constructive ways audience defences could be overcome. Even high-risk viewers were positive towards preventive advice which acknowledged the difficulties of modifying high-risk behaviour, and they invariably welcomed practical tips that might be useful in this respect. They proved amenable to symbols of scientific authority, and to subtle suggestions that their behaviour might be harmful to family or friends. On this basis, cancer campaign designers were provided with practical hints on how to overcome the types of resistance their productions might encounter.

Putting Research Into Practice

In one study, for instance, a film on skin cancer was evaluated. A sample of rural male fisherman — particularly the older men accustomed to stripping to the waist in the sun's full glare — indicated intense resistance to the idea of using preventive filter creams. They readily accepted that filter creams were effective, and that their sons should be encouraged to use them; but they seemed embarrassed to apply such measures themselves. These observations were immediately applied by the director of a new CCS film on skin cancer, in inserting a sequence in which a young fisherman was shown using a filter cream while his father watched. On the film's soundtrack, the father cautiously approved the son's behaviour. When the film was post-tested, the older men's resistance to filter creams was found to have been completely overcome.

The film director whose "lady doctor" character had been criticized for being too polished, immediately responded to the finding by recalling the actress and retraining her to deliver the material in an apparently boring monotone. The actress, though surprised, obeyed this directive, and was subsequently judged by a sample of the target audience to be totally believable, an obviously authentic doctor! This particular strategy would not have been apparent without the moment-by-moment precision of the computer-based CRM methods employed in the study. It should be noted that advertising researchers are currently using these methods with increasing fervour in the pilot-testing of beer and hamburger commercials.

Major advantages of the modern computer-based approaches to advertising research are their precision and speed. In the past, campaign designers have been justifiably suspicious of research and evaluation methods, for they have tended to yield results either too blunt, or too late, to be applied. Traditional media research has proved more of a threat than a help to campaign designers for this reason. However, the current methods allow designers to test practical recommendations made during the production process itself, and to insure against unforseen failure. The greatest potential for media research methods appears to be in the "formative evaluation" of campaign strategies.

We are unaware of any use of highly promising CRM research methods in AIDS campaigning to date (though I would be pleased to be proved wrong in this!). It is worth noting that the uses of this technique in the above cancer prevention studies have consistently supported Lashley and Watson's conclusions regarding the merits of straightforward campaign styles, and the frequent pitfalls of the more elaborate dramatization techniques and the particular defensiveness of young people to AIDS education. Via careful formative evaluation, however, it appears that even the most entrenched audience resistance can be overcome.

114

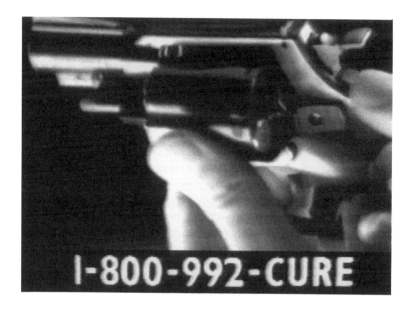

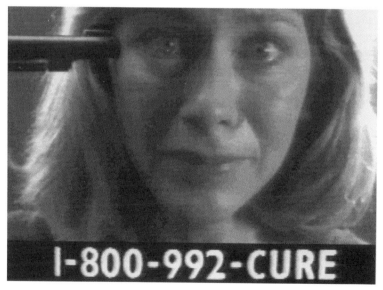

This Russian roulette spot uses fear tactics which the target audience does not regard as an effective approach to AIDS education.

115

It is nonetheless abundantly clear from the smoking and skin cancer studies that, if cancer prevention is a tricky and sensitive matter, the prevention of AIDS is even more so. In the final section of this article, we will review the evidence which we have gained in applying evaluation techniques to the study of AIDS education.

Side-effects of Media AIDS Education

The research team involved in the above studies turned its attention to the need for public AIDS campaigns in 1985. Until then, our grant proposals for funding research into AIDS-campaign methods were predominantly unsuccessful: the topic was officially judged to be of obvious importance, though with a low priority for funding. In 1988, it has become officially recognized as having an extremely high priority for funding; the predictable failure of many official AIDS campaigns may have something to do with this.

However, with the assistance of various international agencies, we were able to conduct several studies on the impact of early AIDS education approaches. A comparison of international public service announcements (PSAs) about AIDS revealed a complete range of TV production approaches, and a correspondingly wide range of audience responses. Audience reactions to PSAs from Britain, Canada, Denmark, Norway, Sweden and the United States were examined. (The study was conducted just weeks before the release of Australia's remarkable "Grim Reaper" campaign, which would have been a fascinating subject for inclusion).

As in the previous studies, the campaign materials that were perceived by viewers as the most effective from an educational standpoint were those which presented hard facts in a simple and straightforward manner. Complex and emotional campaign techniques drew negative responses. The use of light humour was received positively by high-risk viewers, though it was concluded that such techniques should be used judiciously. An unfortunate observation in this study was the announcements judged to be the most successful by our sample (high and low-risk viewers alike) had never been sanctioned for general broadcast use in their countries, owing usually to their relative explicitness. The PSAs which had gained the widest public exposure were the ones our viewers judged to have the least educational potential because they were cautious and vague.

In order to assess whether such perceptions of educational effectiveness have any predictive validity, multivariate analyses were conducted in which AIDS prevention techniques were related to audience knowledge gains and attitude shifts. The effects of three independent attitude factors (knowledge, urgency, and tolerance) were observed in this connection, supporting conclusions by other writers.[10]

For example, it was found that (in 1986 at least) Canadian viewers with a high risk of contracting HIV infection were more tolerant than low-risk viewers on matters concerning civil rights. Not surprisingly, they were also more knowledgeable on AIDS issues generally. Although the film material used in this study received widespread international approval for its effectiveness in increasing public AIDS awareness, high-risk viewers in our study exhibited obviously defensive reactions to it. Following exposure to the PSAs, secondary attitudes exhibited by high-and low-risk viewers on AIDS-related issues were found to have diverged dramatically.

The material had evidently increased (on questionnaire measures) the sensitivity of high-risk viewers to civil rights matters concerning persons with AIDS, while failing to alter the relatively intolerant attitudes of low-risk viewers in this respect. High-and low-risk viewers' attitudes towards the urgency of AIDS as a social issue also appeared to have been polarized. Following the educational intervention, high-risk viewers exhibited a relatively low sense of urgency about AIDS-related matters, while low-risk viewers showed an increased one.

In general, an otherwise useful film intervention was thus concluded to have unwittingly polarized viewers' responses on psychological measures of fundamental social relevance. The polarization of tolerance was assumed to be due to the common instinct of viewers to seek protection for their own individual rights based on personal assessments of their AIDS risk.[11] The reduction of perceived urgency on the part of high-risk viewers was attributed to a denial reaction.

These studies indicated that, in seeking to increase knowledge of AIDS without adequately catering to the related side-effects on public fear and tolerance, educational strategies may well be directly responsible for psychological "boomerang effects" opposite to those intended. Even the best educational materials so far available may conceivably generalize such effects, in view of the extreme defensiveness of their high-risk recipients.

The Need for Sensitivity to AIDS Campaigning Style

In our most recent analyses, direct connections have been established between the unintended boomerang effects, and specific momentary reactions to the educational material, as measured by CRM methods. These results render the need for sensitivity to AIDS campaigning styles even more essential. As with the corresponding samples in our previous studies, high-risk viewers appear liable to judge an educational presentation negatively on the basis of the merest of shortcomings (e.g., a brief digression to explain information they already knew; the use of an unnecessary visual illustration; or the momentary use of a graphic which can be dismissed as ambiguous). Their responses at such moments are found to be significantly related to their overall loss of a sense of urgency about AIDS, and to their increasing self-protectiveness on tolerance measures.

Such effects support Job's recent conclusions regarding the nature of adverse public reactions to smoking and road safety campaigns. Even tenuous evidence, Job indicates, can lead "to quasi-logical support for the denial type of response (by high risk audiences) which alleviates any existing fear." This response leads to assumptions that "the health-promotion campaign is wrong or I am special and immune in some way (e.g., a very good driver)." Obviously, such criticisms are quite unjustified on any reasonable grounds, but on the basis that "the customer is always right," they should nonetheless be avoided.

Our current studies are demonstrating that unintended effects of this sort may easily be avoided by simple alterations to educational films at the post-production editing level, but that such improvements may rapidly be overtaken as old facts, methods and terminologies come into question. The recent fall-from-grace of the term "high-risk group," for example, has been observed in our studies to be sufficient to condemn as useless and insensitive, in the eyes of high-risk individuals, any presentation which uses the term.

For the present, however, we remain optimistic that careful testing of educational strategies by up-to-date program evaluation methods will lead to the development of more efficient AIDS prevention methods. We believe that a more efficient role will be found for the mass media in AIDS education on this basis; and that the growing awareness of psychological responses to public campaign techniques will lead educators, policy-makers, and concerned community members to a united view of the most acceptable educational approaches.

NOTES

1. K. Lashley, and J. Watson, "A Psychological Study of Motion Pictures in Relation to Venereal Disease," *Social Hygiene* 7 (1921).

2. J.P. Baggaley, "Perceived Effectiveness of International AIDS Campaigns," *Health Education Research* 3, 1988.

3. C.F. Hyman, and P. Sheatsley, "Some Reasons Why Information Campaigns Fail," *Public Opinion Quarterly* 11 (1947).

4. H. Mendelsohn, "Mass Communication and Cancer Control," *Cancer: The Behavioral Dimensions*, J. Cullen, B. Fox and R. Isom, eds. (New York: Raven Press, 1976).

5. P. Hinden, "I.U.H.E. President's Message to the World Health Education Conference, *Irish Medical Times* 19 (September 1985).

6. R.F.S. Job, "Effective and Ineffective Use of Fear in Health Promotion Campaigns," *American Journal of Public Health* 78 (1988).

7. A. King, *Report on National Survey on Canadian Youth and AIDS* (Ottawa: Health and Welfare Canada, 1988).

8. Fineberg, "Education to Prevent AIDS: Prospects and Obstacles," *Science* 239, February 1988; and "The Social Dimensions of AIDS," *Scientific American* 259 (October 1988).

9. J.P. Baggaley, "Electronic Analysis of Communication," *Media in Education and Development* 15 (1981); "Developing a Televised Health Campaign: I. Smoking Prevention; II. Skin Cancer Prevention," ibid. 19, 1986; "Formative Evaluation of Educational Television," *Canadian Journal of Educational Communication* 16, 1986; and "Continual Response Measurement: Design and Validation," ibid. 17 (1987).

10. M. Wober, "Informing the British Public About AIDS," *Health Education Research* 3 (1988).

11. J.P. Baggaley, "Campaigning Against AIDS: A Perspective For Southern Africa" (1988), *Media In Education and Development* (in press); "AIDS Education: The Boomerang Effect" (1989), *Studies in Educational Evaluation* (in press).

Flesh Histories

Tom Kalin

I have looked at *Life* magazine's "A Decade in Pictures" for as long as I can remember — the very few photographs "which had been selected, evaluated, approved, collected . . . and which had thereby passed through the filter of culture."[1] I now see an editorial strategy that poses as transparent, framing these photographs, a familiar cultural device made natural by use and repetition. Time — a concept I often experience as a chaotic and disjointed flow of moments — is given an inexorable, narrative order, tied neatly into ten-year bundles. Events and people — things I experience through a myopic and contradictory identity — are endowed with closure and factuality, saturated in History's reservoir of poses.[2]

But this past decade is considerably different from others; for me at least (and certainly for countless others), because of the AIDS crisis. My relationship to my own body — as both physical self and political battlefield — has been profoundly and, perhaps, irreversibly affected by the epidemic of HIV infection. More than just its physical aspects — earlier days of searching for swollen glands and white tongues, coping with and losing a first friend — it is the tissue of texts and images that have constituted the epidemic. Recognizing the inter-textuality of cultural imagery (from words and pictures in newspapers and magazines, to comic books, broadcast news and popular movies), it is important to read across various texts and images to disrupt the dominant media's complex and pernicious mythologies of AIDS and HIV. Within the spectrum of these representations, the pendulum continues to swing between images of dehumanized monsters and blameless saints. To combat these conventions, activists have developed a strategy of resistance to the media's distortions and omissions, as those most intimately affected by the epidemic have begun to take control of their own representations.

The seemingly univocal "mainstream" or "dominant" media so frequently targeted in critiques of representations of the AIDS pandemic is actually a many-headed beast which nimbly evades reductive generalizations about its consistency, voice or audience.[3] Just as activism can range from street protests to peer education, what we might call "oppositional" media means different things

120

across different communities and eras. Senator Jesse Helm's amendments make it clearer than it already was that merely representing my own sexuality is a form of oppositional media, a reminder of the urgent need for a diverse, vital, and strategic media of resistance.

I offer these texts and pictures — stories perhaps — as a testament of how deeply branded we are by the world of images and the signs of social coercion. I offer them as an attempt to interrupt the unending flow of "news" which speaks to a non-existent "general population" in *The New York Times*. I offer them in order to recognize our bodies as the ultimate site of control, where the construction of identity meets the surveillance of the physical. Perhaps most of all, I offer them to freely admit ambivalence, and in an attempt to "not be lost or pushed into the sea of what others believe to be our collective history."[4]

There is an aesthetic to demonstrations making the six o'clock news; there is a politic to representing our own bodies.

1980

As a reminder of just how long ago 1980 seems, one need only recall that at the 1980 Democratic Convention an openly gay African American delegate named Mel Boozer took the podium as a nominee for vice president, focusing the party's attention on lesbian and gay issues.[5] Also in place was an increasingly empowered lesbian and gay nation, one that had perhaps become, post-Stonewall, less "militant" in its tactics while gaining far greater "mainstream" visibility and acceptance. Yet, William Friedkin's film, *Cruising*, remains a pungent reminder that the discourses which construct homosexuality and the subsequent "epidemic of signification"[6] which mythologizes AIDS — as a physical sign of deviance, as a contagion of lifestyle — were fully intact at the decade's start.

Hollywood, indeed, continued as a landscape unchanged: a seemingly endless parade of suicidal 'nellies and nannies' remained the rule, with lesbian and gay independent video and film the under-represented exception. In 1979, during the production of *Cruising* in Manhattan, protesters passed out leaflets declaring, "People will die because of this film," angry that the screenplay (based on a novel by Gerald Walker, a *New York Times* editor) so closely resembled the actual murders of gay men in the West Village during the late 1970s.[7] When a minister's son killed two gay men with an Israeli submachine gun in front of the Ramrod Bar (one of the film's locales), the protesters were chillingly vindicated. Although the national protests, both during the making of the film and after its release, were so highly publicized, no significant changes were effected in Hollywood's representational tactics or unofficial policy.[8]

My own recent re-viewing of the film recalled my furtive viewing of it at the

AIR STEWARD GAETAN DUGAS WAS
IDENTIFIED AS AIDS "PATIENT ZERO,"
BUT THEN A 1969 CASE SURFACED.

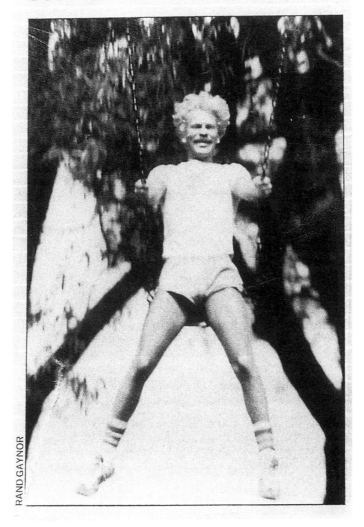

RAND GAYNOR

"Boy on a swing: Gaétan Dugas." Photo: Rand Gaynor.

time of its release, as an eighteen year old — absorbing its homophobia, while seeking some cinematic affirmation of my recently acknowledged sexual identity on the screen. Both the gay and straight press have written extensively about *Cruising*'s pathological and paranoid assertion that homosexuality is contagious. In the context of continuing myths which posit gay men as willful and infectious, I see the leather cap which undercover police agent (Al Pacino) finds while searching the killer's closet (!) as an amulet, an agent of infection.[9] The hat — passing as it does from the head of the killer, to Pacino's head,[10] and finally to the innocent head of his neglected girlfriend — represents the threat that an allegedly corrupt and promiscuous homosexuality poses to the stability of heterosexuality. The body becomes the ultimate costume, socially framed and transformed by the paraphernalia of leather drag.

1981

Although useful in some regards as a narrative document of issues in the early 1980s, Randy Shilts's book *And the Band Played On* is nonetheless a heavily fictionalized account of the earliest years of the AIDS pandemic. Acting as an omniscient narrator, Shilts grants himself unlimited access to a vast array of his characters' private thoughts and emotions, regularly assigning motivations to people he could not possibly have known. This omniscience is especially pernicious in Shilts's treatment of the by-now infamous Canadian airline steward, Gaétan Dugas. Shilts attempts to locate Dugas as the "source" of HIV in this country, and pictures him as the AIDS crisis's "Typhoid Mary." Dugas is dubbed "Patient Zero," an alias of dubious honour fitting for our era of military super-powers and covert operations.[11] Shilts repeatedly exercises his prerogative as *auteur*, fabricating Dugas' internal monologues and conversations to buttress his own theories about willful irresponsibility in the early days of the epidemic.

Quoting from *And the Band Played On*, Judith Williamson tellingly discusses Shilts's use of narrative mythology, linking his account to a traditional fairy tale:

> Gaétan examined himself in the mirror . . . a few more spots had the temerity to appear on his face . . . he smiled at the thought, 'I'm still the prettiest one.' No one within Western culture can contemplate this scenario without understanding precisely in terms of the absent Snow White (for hers is the step-mother who behaves this way), the innocent victim of the Vain and the Bad.[12]

Here, Shilts, the under-appreciated hero of his own novel, becomes Snow White; his heavily touted refusal of "promiscuous" gay sex at the first moments of the epidemic lends him not only moral superiority but the powers of clairvoyance as well.

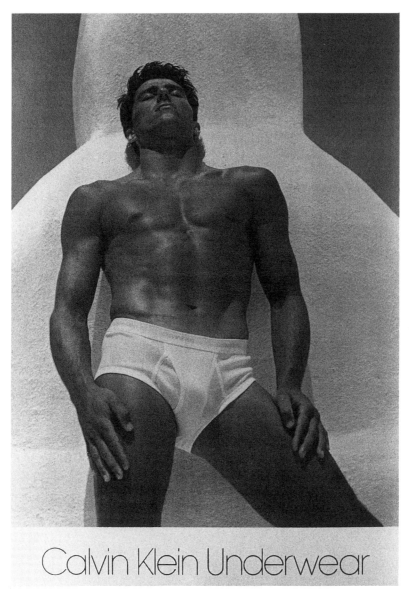

Calvin Klein advertisement, "Brief Commodity Fetish."

A recent *Life* magazine "A Decade in Photographs" spread includes what appears to be a snapshot of Gaétan (taken by a friend? a sister? a lover?) on a swing. Suspended, hair flying, smiling, legs spread, Dugas appears the eroticized jubilant child. His suntanned, extended legs ("Lovers were like suntans to him")[13] propel him towards us, their shape echoed by the fork of tree branches behind him. His image suggests velocity and a sense of threat by the impression of rising forward, the out-of-focus foliage. Infantilizing this "AIDS carrier" (sic) helps to see him as a Bad Seed — a willful, irrational, destructive force. An early related popular convention of picturing bed-ridden people with AIDS as infantile, often wrapped in diaper-like clothing, renders them helpless and pathetic rather than willful. The deliberate editorial selection of this photograph serves to transform personal history into public record. Imagine the snapshots of your youth reprinted in millions of magazines, the *a priori* evidence of a narrative which had yet to be set in motion. (I wonder: who sold this photograph? And for how much?).

1982

The public marriage (on billboards and in magazines) of designer Calvin Klein's marketing genius and photographer Bruce Weber's aesthetic revisionism — one part Herbert List, Leni Riefenstahl, and Edward Weston — introduced an influential marketing obsession with body culture which characterized the 1980s. The model body was a nude body, but not naked; uncovered, but certainly not exposed, clothed in a firm sheath of muscle. The model body could drop the pose of clothes and yet remain styled, a symbol of desire designed by long hours on Nautilus machines.

It was in Andy Warhol's *Interview* (long-time flesh marketplace) and other similar magazines that Bruce Weber's vision of the unattainable, eroticized male first appeared, "fine art" advertising sponsored by the conglomerate Calvin Klein. Ironically, at a time when homophobia was on the rise, Weber, Warhol, and Klein were able to cunningly sell homoerotic imagery to a mass audience. Yet this was a most complicated homoeroticism, it was — contradiction of contradictions — a deeply conservative, homophobic homoeroticism. Klein and Weber exploit their male models' presumed heterosexuality and "natural" masculine beauty. Usually athletes and working class men partially unclothed, their public semi-nudity is excused via accepted cultural modes of male bonding. Free to titillate on the forbidden edge between football's ass-patting and lovers' caresses, these invincible, unattainable members of the master race (always white, often blonde) act as perfect mannequins, able, even in underwear, to remain both fully eroticized and socially clothed.[14]

These three gay men — Klein, Weber, Warhol — were considerably invested in the world of public appearances (consider particularly Klein's marriage during the period when he was rumoured to be sick with AIDS).[15] Their commodity-driven, fetishized vision of the model body as an eroticized, invincible machine collided headlong with AIDS and its signifiers, continuing to yield paradoxes in the marketplace of desire.

1983

1983 introduced the blood scare, a year of national panic calling for a screening of the blood supply. Blood from gay men was widely perceived to posses a "gay taint" (something essentially corrupt or infectious); accordingly, [American] federal authorities requested that gay men with multiple sexual partners should not give blood. Prior to the isolation of the virus that was eventually labelled HIV, mythologies of blood and body fluids were rampant. *Rolling Stone* featured a particularly insidious article which used AIDS as an iconographic dumping ground, liking the "primitive" rituals of voodoo in Haiti (which sometimes involved the use of blood as an element) with the deeply "unnatural" practices of gay male sex. Body fluids became something feared; they represented an unseen arena where a lack of heterosexual, family-centred morality resulted in hidden "time-bombs," tiny corruptions of the blood (flesh) waiting to pour out into the unsuspecting and innocent mass public.

1984

In 1984, American researcher Robert Gallo claimed to have discovered the "probable cause" of AIDS, a virus he labelled HTLV-III. Acting with premature enthusiasm, U.S. Health and Human Services Secretary Margaret Heckler predicted an antibody test in six months and a vaccine within two years. Although widely featured in both print and broadcast journalism, this "discovery" eclipsed the fact that, at the Institute Pasteur in Paris, researcher Luc Montagnier isolated the same virus, virtually simultaneously, labelling it LAV. After a relatively protracted period of scientific debate and dispute over the ownership of this discovery, the two researchers and their respective medical communities agreed to the compromise term "HIV" (for Human Immunodeficiency Virus).

Such nationalism (a system of "bodies," both foreign and otherwise) riddles the global pandemic. The drug AI-721, for instance, a simple food product consisting of egg limpids (a close cousin to mayonnaise), was approved in Israel years ago but had to be subjected to further tests for safety before the Food and

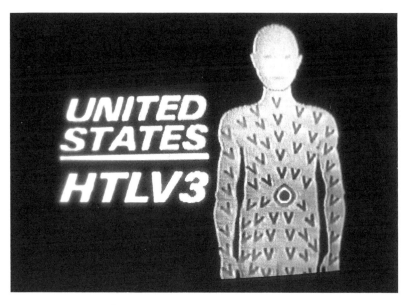

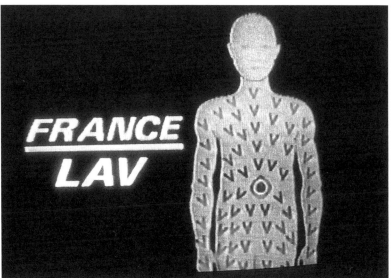

"Viruses and Nationalism," 1984. Stills from television.

Drug Administration would approve its use in the United States.[16] The competitive paranoia of drug manufacturers and U.S. government's devastating inaction have forced many HIV-positive people and PWAs to acquire this drug and others through alternative routes. Inequities in treatment and care between the First World and the Third World continue to proliferate as well: for example, "the cost of treating ten people with AIDS in the U.S. — about $450,000 — is more than the entire budget of one large Zairian hospital."[17] Africa has consistently been blamed in Western accounts for its enormous caseload (primarily heterosexual), blame rationalized either by Africa's lack of a "civilized" health and family planning system or by some vaguely articulated idea of an irresponsible, exotic primitivism. Even as late as 1988, the "discoverer" of HTLV-III, Dr. Robert Gallo, proposed using African men and women to test the safety of potential AIDS vaccines before distribution in the United States.

1985

If you charted a graph of U.S. media coverage on AIDS from 1981 until 1988, you would see a low, flat line stretching between 1981 and 1985, at which point that line would incline steeply. The graph plateaus after Rock Hudson's death in 1985, reflecting the media's temporary infatuation with the crisis of the moment. Hudson's excruciatingly public diagnosis and death produced a new level of collective paranoia that appearances could indeed be deceiving. This resulted in a flood of stories about the star's diagnosis with AIDS and his pursuit of experimental treatment in Paris, and wide speculation about risk to the so-called "general population." However, in late 1987 and into 1988 that anxiety flagged, as the general perception that white middle-class heterosexuals were no longer at risk of infection resulted in a steady decline of media attention. Then, as now, it was perceived that women, people of colour, IV drug users, their sexual partners and gay men were predominantly the ones who would continue to be infected with HIV or living with AIDS.

Images of Hudson were replayed over and over in 1985: the childhood photo of "Roy Schere, Junior," or the perverse surveillance image of Hudson being transferred by stretcher onto an airplane. Nonetheless, Hudson, like Dugas, remained essentially invisible. The images are dominated by predatory glee over a masquerade destroyed — the tabloid celebration of tarnished glamour that comes with the collective sense of ownership and permission that fans grant themselves about stars' private lives. This public unveiling, Hudson's double "coming out of the closet" both as a PWA and as a gay man, continues to characterize public perceptions about AIDS. In the public eye, AIDS has become the physical sign of concealed deviance, the true manifestation of a secret perversion. Thus, Rock Hudson's entire career is now framed by his diagnosis; in the words of *People*, "Perhaps Hudson's success at maintaining a 30 year public front demonstrated that he was a far better actor than he was ever given credit for."[18]

1986

Broadcast journalism deftly compresses image and voice-over into suggestive news bites; the images become miniaturized emblems, the voice-over assumes the intonations of authority (almost always male, frequently Midwestern). Those trusted figures who "bring you the news" were faced with the task of rhetorically representing a familiar litany of so-called risk groups (gay men, Haitians, IV drug users) and their so-called innocent counterparts (hemophiliacs, pediatric AIDS cases, people infected with HIV by blood transfusion), making them identifiable as characters in, and consequences of, the epidemic's narrative.[19] Recognizing this, ABC's "news magazine" program *20/20* repeatedly used a vindictive three-second montage of stock footage to illuminate the "guilty" victim list: Shot from the rear, hands in each other's pockets, two mustached "clone style" white men walk away from the viewer, accompanying the words "Homosexual Males." Shot from above, in a rough, wooden sailboat, approximately twenty Haitian men and women stand packed together; we cannot decipher a single face as we hear the word "Haitians." Shot in extreme close-up, a thumb and forefinger hold a bottle cap of clear liquid (presumably heroin) while another thumb and forefinger hold a match beneath it: we hear "Drug Abusers." The position of these bodies in relationship to the viewer determines our inability to recognize them as people, to assign them identities. ABC quickly establishes a grotesque hierarchy of identification for the viewer, dictated by comparative levels of perceived "exoticism" or otherness and already intact presumptions about class, race, gender, and sexuality.

1987

Newsweek magazine's "The Face of AIDS" issue, pictures 302 people that had died of AIDS-related infections in America between August 1986 and July 1987. At first glance, the distribution of images appears to reflect the epidemiology of AIDS. For instance, the seventeen females (two of them infants) roughly represent the women making up seven percent of people who had died by mid-1987. But the representation of people of colour is far below the percentage of those that had died. When class or racial differences prohibited easy access to photographs or descriptive texts, editors satisfied themselves with only an empty box or a blank area. Women of colour, for example, often have absolutely nothing to gain and much to lose by being identified as PWAs within the fishbowl of the media.[20] *Newsweek* reduplicates this invisibility without commentary, and so these erasures stand unexamined like casualties of war.

In her essay, "Constitutional Symptoms," Jan Zita Grover writes about *Newsweek's* "The Face of AIDS":

> But the peculiar effect of these twelve pages of head-shots and high-school yearbook-like descriptions . . . is to make these people look as if they didn't know what hit them (failed grace) or to make their appearance a consequence of the moral failings often attributed to them (wages of sin).[21]

The moral implications of these collected mug shots are largely dictated by editorial choices of text. Compare for example, *Hustler* magazine co-publisher Althea Flynt's tag line ("a drug addict") with the more neutral and dignified treatment given to an ex-Marine, Walter Leslie ("infected via IV drug use"). And, perhaps most strikingly, fifteen of the seventeen females are tagged with a cause of infection, while the vast majority of men are not (presumed homosexuals). A select few men like Walter Leslie (ex-marine) are saved from gay implication by the naming of IV drug use.

The tabloid voyeurism of these pictures pales beside their great sense of pathos and presence, many faces poised on the verge of recognition. The sense of violating private history in looking at these and other snapshots recalls Roland Barthes' notion of the "flat death" of photography and the collapse of personal history into public record:

> . . . the age of Photography corresponds precisely to the explosion of the private into the public, or rather into the creation of a new social value, which is the publicity of the private: the private is consumed as such, publicly.[22]

1988

In the January issue of *Cosmopolitan*, editor Helen Gurley Brown printed "Good News About AIDS: A Doctor Tells Why You May Not Be At Risk," by psychiatrist Dr. Robert Gould. Gould's devastatingly misinformed article promoted risky health advice (by a psychiatrist with no ob/gyn experience) and inflammatory, racist poison. Gould declared that unprotected vaginal intercourse was a highly unlikely route of HIV transmission, and that Africa's huge caseload of heterosexual men and women with AIDS could be understood because African men "take their women in a brutal way."[23] Outraged, the Women's Committee of ACT UP New York (AIDS Coalition to Unleash Power, an activist group) staged a massive demonstration at *Cosmo*'s headquarters, demanding audience with the publisher and editors, stopping traffic in midtown Manhattan, and showering all present with as many condoms as possible, and the phone and fax lines were jammed for days with practical and specific refutations of the article's deadly lies. The women organizing the protests focused finally on the production of a witty and strategic videotape, *Doctors, Liars and Women*, which documents the organizing process of the demonstration, the women's confrontational "interview" with a flabbergasted Gould, and the appearance of both Gould and the protesters on a New York talk-show.[24]

In the spring of 1988, ACT UP New York joined many activist groups across the country in a coordinated series of protests intended to focus national attention on the AIDS crisis. Gran Fury, a collective which creates public projects in order to "inform a broad audience and provoke direct action to end the AIDS crisis,"[25] produced a series of posters to help bring attention to the events. For the day targeted as "AIDS and Women," the Women's Committee organized a protest at Shea Stadium, determined to bring safer sex information to Mets baseball fans. By renting blocks of seats, the activists were provided free time on the Spectacolor display for messages such as "No Glove, No Love." Those in the rented seats entertained both the crowd and the television cameras with massive banners reading "Men: Use Condoms or Beat It." Their high-spirited appropriation of the five o'clock news served as an effective intervention not only for those at the Mets game that day, but for the millions of viewers tuned in to the evening sports as well.

1989

Carl M. George's super-8 movie, *DHPG Mon Amour*, is a profoundly moving, quirky and difficult film which narrates a day in the life of two men, David Conover and Joe Walsh. Following Walsh as he leaves his job at New York's Community Research Initiative [26] and shops for food, the film opens with Ella Fitzgerald's *Nights in Tunisia* played beneath Walsh describing himself and Conover, his lover of eight years. Joe was diagnosed HIV positive in 1985; David has been living with AIDS for several years and is currently dealing with CMV retinitis, a condition which can lead to severe impairment of vision and possibly blindness. Refusing to accept standard and "official" medical advice on appropriate drug treatments and methodology, David chooses instead to self-administer the medication DHPG Gancylovir, opting for an infusaport applicator (which remains under the skin) rather than a bulky and physically prohibitive Hickman catheter.

Although flushed with nostalgia, its colours richly saturated and grainy, *DHPG Mon Amour* firmly locates the extraordinary conditions of living with AIDS in the late 1980s within the daily life of these two men. We see them washing apples, lighting a barbecue grill, watering houseplants, sterilizing needles, preparing medications, and self-administering DHPG Gancyclovir. The filmmaker refuses to be overcome by either the lush seduction of super-8 (by nature infused with romanticism and a home movie aura), or by the powerful, visceral sight of someone self-injecting medication. *DHPG Mon Amour* successfully appropriates current nostalgia for the 1960s (read here through the super-8 grit of "underground" filmmaking) and, though placing it in a vastly different context, visually recalls the spectacle of injection in films like Andy Warhol's and Paul Morissey's *Trash*. Focusing precisely on the ordinary minutiae of David's and Joe's daily life, *DHPG Mon Amour* shows the struggle for self-determination and control over one's own body, and resonates on both an intimate and more broadly political level.

The soundtrack, a strong and simple mix of David's and Joe's voice-overs with music, was recorded three months after filming; as we see David mixing medication we hear that he has — in these three months — lost most of his vision. The film pierces our indifference again and again; our ability to see is contrasted with David's loss of sight, a loss that he and Joe remind us could have been delayed or halted altogether if DHPG Gancyclovir was used earlier. The very real result of the federal government's unresponsive system of health care and drug approval is made visible in this movie, and is effectively brought home. Later, when David swabs his nipple to sterilize it, applies a bandage to his chest, the rich, grainy image troubles a clinical reading of the footage. The image is tugged in several directions, at once subtly erotic, physically disturbing, emotionally moving. *DHPG Mon Amour* insists on a vision of the body that is not wrenched from either personal or collective histories.

All of us impacted by the epidemic of HIV infection and AIDS demand recognition that our relationships to our bodies are shaped not only by the physical factors of illness, but by a socially and culturally determined history of the body as well. To effectively combat this global pandemic, everyone affected — activists, health care workers, journalists, legislators, the "general public" — must reconsider the interrelationships between access, entitlement and the power to control one's own life. For those already painfully aware of the inequities of class, race, gender or sexuality, this epidemic has demanded coalition-building between communities with often vastly different concerns. Locating this coalition-building within a context of what has come before is critical, recognizing as the following quotations by Angela Carter and Roland Barthes attest, that flesh and histories are inseparable:

But our flesh arrives to us out of history, like everything else does. We may believe we fuck stripped of social artifice; in bed, we even feel we touch the bedrock of human nature itself. But we are deceived. Flesh is not an irreducible human universal.[27]

History is hysterical: it is constituted only if we consider it, only if we look at it — and in order to look at it, we must be excluded from it. As a living soul, I am the very contrary of History, I am what belies it, destroys it for the sake of my own history.[28]

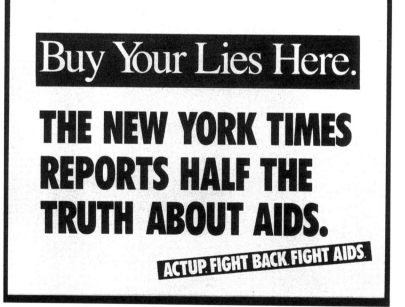

ACT UP Outreach Committee, *Buy Your Lies Here*, 1988. Poster.

NOTES

1. Roland Barthes, *Camera Lucida* (New York: Hill and Wang, 1981): 16.

2. A reworking of a piece by Barbara Kruger.

3. See Paula A. Triechler, "Seduced and Terrorized: AIDS and Network Television," in this anthology, and John Greyson, catalogue essay in *AIDS: The Artists' Response*, exhibition and catalogue organized by Jan Zita Grover.

4. This is a modified version of an unpublished text I have used to describe my videotape, *They are lost to vision altogether* (1989). Some of the images in this piece (years 1983, 1984, and 1986) appear in the tape, which serves as a conceptual basis for this article. This tape is distributed by Video Data Bank as part of its six-hour compilation *Video Against AIDS*.

5. For a particularly insightful reading of the history of biomedical discourse and the signifiers of AIDS and HIV infection, see Paula A. Treichler, "AIDS, Homophobia and Biomedical Discourse: An Epidemic of Signification," *AIDS: Cultural Analysis/Cultural Activism*, Douglas Crimp, ed. (Cambridge: MIT Press, 1988).

6. *The Washington Blade*, 20:52. (December 29, 1989): 3.

7. Vito Russo, *The Celluloid Closet* (New York: Harper and Row, 1987, revised ed.), pp. 236-38. Russo's excellent overview contains a longer account of the protest against *Cruising*: "I'm trying to present a portrait of a group of people who get their sexual kicks in ways society decisions which equated gay male sexuality with pathological contagion.

8. Although films like *Making Love* and *Victor/Victoria* were produced in the early 1980s and appear to espouse a "positive image" approach to representations of gay male sexuality, both are (to my mind) more concerned with domesticating queer sexuality, making it conform to upper-middle-class heterosexual values, rather than articulating the possibilities of difference.

9. For a further discussion of images of the body as closet within the film see Peter Brown, "The Body As Closet," 1990.

10. Pacino flirtatiously dons the cap moments before he has the murderer prepare to have sex (in Pacino's words, "lips or hips?"), then chooses instead stabbing over sexual penetration.

11. Contrary to convenient mythologies, Dugas was not the first person in North America found to be HIV positive. See Douglas Crimp, "How to Have Promiscuity in an Epidemic," Douglas Crimp, ed., op. cit., for an extended discussion of Shilts's book and its conceits.

12. Judith Williamson, "Every Virus Tells a Story: The Meaning of HIV and AIDS," in *Taking Liberties: AIDS and Cultural Politics*, Erika Carter and Simon Watney, eds. (London: Serpents Tail, 1989).

13. Randy Shilts, *And The Band Played On: Politics, People and the AIDS Epidemic* (New York: St. Martin's Press, 1987).

14. I am indebted here to Richard Meyers' unpublished paper, "Artistic Immunity."

15. Consider these entries from the diaries of Andy Warhol:

Saturday, July 17, 1982:
Went to see *Young Doctors in Love* (tickets $10) and it was really good . . . and there was a funny scene where the guy in the Calvin Klein ad is wheeled into the operating room in his jeans in the same position he's in the ads, and so that's funny if you get it.

Saturday, July 31, 1982:
Then we went for pizza, and you could really see in the light who the dogs were (pizza $20). Then we went back to Calvin's but we walked in on Calvin and Steve who were with those two porno stars Knoll and Ford and so we were embarrassed and left and went back to the party down the street.

Saturday, September 18, 1982:
I couldn't work with Jon because he had to go to a gay cancer funeral, at Paramount, it

was a secretary there — a male secretary. And, I mean, I got so nervous, I don't even do anything and I could get it.

And even as late as 1987, weeks before his death, Warhol's paranoid disavowal continued

Monday, February 2, 1987:
Worked and then they picked me up for the black-tie dinner at the Saint that Rado Watches was giving and it was all built around the paintings I did and Sara Vaughn singing. And we were all afraid to eat anything because the Saint has the gay taint from when it used to be a gay disco. It was so dark in there and they were serving the food on black plates.

16. This policy derives from the Kefauver Amendment of 1962, which was prompted by the incident in which American women use Thalidomide (which had been approved in Great Britain to ease pregnancy complications) and which later proved to cause birth defects. AIDS activists have been effective in demanding change on both a corporate and governmental level: for instance, pressuring Burroughs Wellcome to reduce the price of AZT and pressuring the FDA to allow importation of drugs such as Dextran Sulfate. Corporate profit margins and federal bureaucracy have obstructed access to potentially life prolonging/life saving treatments. AIDS and other health crises are forcing reconsideration of conventions such as placebo trials and lack of a national health care system in the United States.

17. From *Let The Record Show . . .*, ACT UP/Gran Fury's piece as it was displayed in Berlin, 1988.

18. *People* (Summer, 1985).

19. Unfortunately, the dominant media continues to do little about specifically informing its audience of the risky behaviours — anal and vaginal sex with a rubber, oral sex without a rubber, needle and works sharing — which can transmit HIV, preferring, still, nine years later, to refer to "risk groups" and a non-existent "general population."

20. I do not mean to imply that any person with AIDS has more or less at stake by making themselves visible within the media than any other PWA, but rather that people occupy varying relationships to access or visibility often due to class, racial, or sexual difference. Many PWAs and HIV positive people publicly identify themselves in a gesture of empowerment and to combat stereotype.

21. Jan Zita Grover, "Constitutional Symptoms," Carter and Watney, eds., op. cit., 155.

22. Roland Barthes, op. cit., 98.

23. Robert E. Gould, "Reassuring News About AIDS: A Doctor Tells Why You May Not Be at Risk," *Cosmopolitan*, January, 1988.

24. The women were literally thrown off the show ("escorted" in the studio's parlance) because they refused to honour the white male authorities on the stage and came up from the audience to join the "experts" while cameras were rolling and a hysterical host struggled to regain order. *Doctors, Liars and Women*, produced and directed by Jean Carlomusto and Maria Maggenti, distributed by Gay Men's Health Crisis (G.M.H.C.), New York.

25. From a statement written by Gran Fury. Gran Fury is an eleven-member collective (named after the Plymouth automobile used by police as an undercover car) of which I am a member. The group was formed in January 1988, shortly after the installation of *Let the Record Show . . .*, an installation by ACT UP New York in the windows of the New Museum of Contemporary Art in 1987, a project many of the members had worked on.

26. The CRI is an alternative to the Food and Drug Administration's sluggish bureaucracy, a community-based group who runs experimental drug trials and acts as a vital source of information and resources to people with AIDS concerned with treatment options.

27. Angela Carter, *The Sadeian Woman and the Ideology of Pornography*. (New York: Pantheon, 1979): 9.

28. Roland Barthes, op. cit,. 65.

Seduced and Terrorized: AIDS and Network Television

Paula A. Treichler

> We had no such thing as printed newspapers in those days to spread rumors and reports of things, and to improve them by the invention of men . . . Such things as these were . . . handed about by word of mouth only; so that things did not spread instantly over the whole nation, as they do now.
>
> — Daniel Defoe, *A Journal of the Plague Year*, 1722

> If it bleeds, it leads.
>
> — Media maxim

There is a particular breed of monkey that, like other monkeys, is curious by nature; it is also, even in captivity, terrified of green snakes, an evolutionary enemy. If you put a green snake in a brown paper bag on the floor of the monkey's cage, the monkey, irrepressibly curious, will slowly approach the bag, open it, and look in: a green snake!!! The monkey will fly to the top of the cage and cling there, terrorized. But as its panic gradually subsides its eyes will be drawn, seductively, back to the paper bag. What could be in it? Slowly the monkey descends, approaches the bag, opens it: a green snake!!! To the top of the cage again, clinging and terrorized.[1]

Like the monkey confronting the green snake, many of us may recoil in terror when we encounter the AIDS epidemic on the major television networks; yet we are also aware of the medium's seductiveness and indeed experience it whenever we return to see what the brown bag contains. But should we care? Why analyze network television, an industry increasingly corporate and uniform? Patterns of AIDS coverage on the networks are at times so identical that one imagines their representatives all at the same AIDS workshop — learning how to give events the same conventional interpretations, select the same AIDS experts, use the same misleading terminology, and track down the same live footage from the people who were *really* there. This is satirized in the independent video *Rockville Is Burning* (Bob Huff and Wave 3, 1989), in which AIDS activists take over a television station and begin broadcasting a radically different version of the epidemic. Yet television, including the three major networks and PBS, is not monolithic. Rather, like every cultural form, it offers openings and opportunities for intervention. Further, television's unique seductiveness and power to shape public opinion mean that in the current crisis we cannot afford to dismiss it as unsalvageably bourgeois. Rather, a brief inventory of problematic approaches to the AIDS epidemic suggests, in turn, how television could more intelligently engage, educate, and galvanize its audience.[2]

What Kind of Story?
The AIDS Narrative as Always Already Written.

Whereas the *Los Angeles Times* and the *San Francisco Chronicle* printed stories about a rare pneumonia among gay men within days of the Centers for Disease Control's first official report in June 1981, television network news did not cover AIDS until June 1982. Television coverage of the epidemic remains largely passive, relying on an inherited as-told-to narrative format that does not encourage careful, complex, and original reporting or analysis. The AIDS epidemic, by contrast, is unprecedentedly complex, and a prototypical challenge to current social systems. Some media organizations have accordingly assigned a "point person" to coordinate AIDS coverage, but this remains the exception rather than the rule. Media specialists say that the AIDS epidemic has generated twenty-two official sub-issues for the mainstream media.[3] These are the "pegs" that reporters require to hang stories on. This narrative division of labour has the advantage of keeping AIDS and HIV in the news because each issue (children, virology, blood, drugs, etc.) has its own narrative trajectory, its crises and dead periods. But if a story does not fit on one of the established pegs, it is typically doctored or dropped. Of course, what is not covered as news may be carried elsewhere: an *L.A. Law* (NBC) episode addressed ethical questions of euthanasia; *The AIDS Connection* was a viewer call-in show; and *Nightline* (ABC) has staged several debates over controversial AIDS issues. But individual components of the epidemic are always part of the larger story and it is this larger story that network television, addicted to simplicity and convention, never gets right. Stories begin portentously: *AIDS is the plague of our times; AIDS continues its deadly spread; the Third World is devastated by AIDS; AIDS: Is a cure at hand?* They end predictably: *Will the plague be stopped? Only time will tell; We may be closer to a cure, but it will not come in time for people like John Smith.* Though often undermined or even

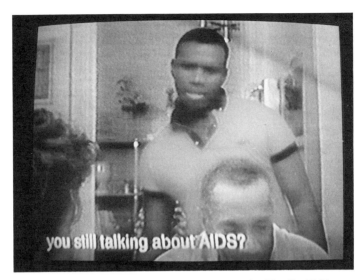

Patricia Benoit, Haitian Woman's Program, *Set Met Ko*, 1988. Still from colour video.

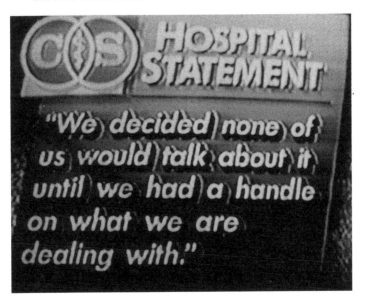

Statement by friends of Jaqueline Corianne Shearer, *Cori: A Struggle for Life*, 1989. Still from colour video.

contradicted by the story they surround, these bookends nevertheless promote an illusion of control. Even stories *about* controversy get packaged in this univocal way.

One could argue that this is not bad. Physician and writer Marshall Goldberg asserts that, though flawed by sensationalism, melodrama, inaccuracy, and a desire to entertain, television nonetheless succeeds in teaching the basics: AIDS is believed to be caused by a virus, the virus is not transmitted by casual contact, and so on.[4] But the problem is that AIDS 101 — AIDS by the book — is always an already written narrative. Although treatment experience now suggests that people with AIDS today may live many years beyond their diagnosis, perhaps indefinitely, the Spring 1989 edition of *The AIDS Quarterly* (PBS) calls AIDS "finally fatal." Apart from the obvious fact that life itself is finally fatal, actual footage within the report challenges this doomsday judgement in several ways: a number of experts characterize AIDS as a chronic, manageable condition; people with AIDS are shown living their lives, taking considerable responsibility for treatment choices; and a group of physicians emphasizes the importance of refusing the orthodox scenario, of "not looking down the end of the film." Yet the program's prior declaration of inevitable doom has already been established by the opening visuals — electronic green images of the human immunodeficiency virus (HIV) invading white cells over a *Jaws*-like soundtrack; a weeping female IV-drug user crying to the camera that "I'm breaking out in sores all over my body — open sores."

By not challenging the dominant account of AIDS, television reduces subsequent contradictions to mere errata slips tucked discreetly into the formula narrative. A 1987 *Nova* (PBS) program on AIDS vaccines says nothing about government inaction in testing drugs, nor challenges the U.S. Food and Drug Administration's (FDA) single-minded focus on AZT. Such programs on the epidemic conform to the formula attributed by Dorothy Nelkin to TV science documentaries in general:

> In an effort to personalize science, the scientist is made a star; the tweed and turtleneck chic of Carl Sagan and Jonathan Miller represents a contrast with the eccentric and dangerous figures on entertainment programs, but these scientists are equally idealized. Many documentaries, such as those produced by NOVA, are thick with awe and reverence; while explaining science carefully, with elegant visual images, they . . . perpetuate the images of science as arcane.[5]

In 1989, Peter Jennings ended an *AIDS Quarterly* piece on treatment options with an upbeat comment: "So, for a change, at least all the news about AIDS is not all bad — in part because we have the financial resources in America, and also because there has been enormous pressure to mobilize those resources." The grammatical structure of Jennings' "there has been" disguises the facts concerning just who has exerted the pressure and how long they have been doing it. Outstanding exceptions such as a *MacNeil/Lehrer News Hour* segment of May 2, 1989, entitled "AIDS: Drug Dilemma," demonstrate that TV coverage can be bolder — and effective. Leading off the *News Hour,* Spencer Michaels of station KQED in San Francisco chronicled the enormous pressure gay activists have placed on the FDA, and some of the successes and failures activism has produced; the segment opened and closed with shots of the familiar SILENCE=DEATH button of the AIDS activist group ACT UP.

Public Broadcasting: The Nonalternative Alternative

The above examples suggest that public broadcasting has the potential to challenge the commercial networks, but rarely does so. "PBS?" asks independent video artist John Greyson,

> Don't get me started. After nearly a decade characterized by benign neglect and not-so-benignly horrendous coverage . . . their big contribution to America's number one health priority is . . . a 2.5 million-dollar quarterly newsmagazine, that will update viewers on the "facts" . . . interview "experts" . . . and feature profiles of AIDS "heroes" . . . In other words, over $12,000 per minute to replicate what the commercial networks do so offensively already as a matter of course . . . This, from the same network that has a Congressional mandate to buy substantial amounts of independent work, but has so far aired only one of the over 100 independent works produced on AIDS to date.[6]

Public television's role could be to provide critical and interpretive commentary on the prevailing stereotypes of the commercial networks; instead it reiterates professional wisdom, merely performing such tasks as translating scientific language into baby talk and generally reproducing the most conventional views about the function and role of "art." Douglas Crimp writes that "AIDS and the Arts," a July 1987 feature aired on *MacNeil/Lehrer,* reinforces the stereotypical equation of AIDS with homosexuality, suggests that gay people have a natural inclination toward the arts, and "implies that some gay people 'redeem' themselves by being artists, and therefore that the deaths of other gay people are less tragic."[7] Yet simultaneously, in omitting mention of the wide range of artistic responses, PBS deprives its viewing audience of some of the most exciting video works being produced today. These include Greyson's 1987 *The ADS Epidemic,* his 1988 *The World is Sick (Sic)* and his 1989 *The Pink Pimpernel,* as well as Mark Huestis' and Wendy Dallas's 1986 *Chuck Solomon: Coming of Age,* Isaac Julien's 1987 *This Is*

Not an AIDS Advertisement, Barbara Hammer's 1987 *Snow Job*, Stashu Kybartas' 1987 *Danny*, and Tom Kalin's 1988 *They Are Lost to Vision Altogether*.[8]

What's Wrong with This Picture? Television and Representation

Network television consistently doles out orthodox blocks of AIDS-related content like a series of bricks:

AIDS is caused by HIV, or "the AIDS virus"
AIDS is spread by those infected with HIV, or AIDS "carriers"
Those infected with HIV will develop AIDS
Those with AIDS (or "AIDS victims") will die
AIDS is a gay disease
AIDS is everybody's problem
Fear of AIDS is worse than AIDS itself
Science is conquering AIDS
Conquering AIDS may be impossible
The face of AIDS is changing
The general population is still safe

From such bricks is network AIDS built; and with bricks so old, no wonder the building is crumbling. Instead of such stereotypes, television could be providing state-of-the-art bricks; better yet, it could provide knowledge and analysis about the construction process. It is nonsense to think such knowledge is too complicated for television audiences or too hard to communicate visually. For example, Colman Jones's 1987-88 radio programs on AIDS for the Canadian Broadcasting Corporation's *Ideas* series explored sophisticated notions such as the social construction of reality, representational icons, and discursive strategies that disguise homophobia. *Will Sex Ever Be the Same Again?*, produced in 1990 by Jane Ryan and Helen Thomas for ABC Radio National in Sydney, Australia, addressed equally difficult questions of representation and reality. Such examinations of the construction of knowledge are not beyond the grasp of the average American listener; nor are such independent video documentaries as Jean Carlomusto's and Maria Maggenti's 1988 *Doctors, Liars, and Women: AIDS Activists Say No to Cosmo* and the several productions since 1987 of the Testing the Limits Collective. In *All of Us and AIDS*, a 1987 educational video produced by Catherine V. Jordan, high school students make a video about AIDS; the film-within-a-film device effectively raises questions about representation. In contrast, the networks appear to believe that the real world, simple and accessible, is out there waiting for prime time; processes and decisions about representation — what

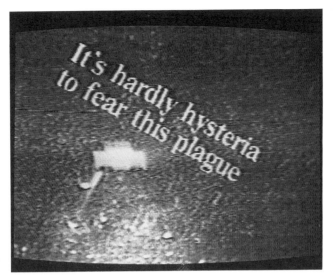

Barbara Hammer, *Snow Job: The Media Hysteria of AIDS*, 1986. Still from video.

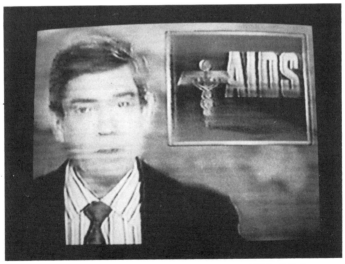

Tom Kalin, *They Are Lost to Vision Altogether*, 1989. Still from colour video.

Brazilian writer Herbert Daniel calls the staging of the epidemic — are ignored.[9]

This is unfortunate, because television's analysis of representation might graphically demonstrate and deconstruct its own recurrent conventions in representing persons with AIDS: the emaciated gay man in a hospital bed, the "innocent" transfusion victim surrounded by loving family, the Third World prostitute, always wearing red. We know that counter-examples to these canonical AIDS victims are systematically excluded from the reports of people with AIDS who are rejected by photographers because they do not look sick enough. Such an analysis could examine how disjunctions between text and image affect AIDS stories: for example, while Mervyn Silverman argued on *Nightline* in the early 1980s that AIDS was not "caused" by gay men, the television audience saw shots, not visible to Silverman, of gay men kissing; more recently, a report, in contradiction to all existing scientific evidence, that mosquitoes transmit AIDS was accompanied by footage of virologist Robert Gallo lecturing on a completely different subject; Timothy E. Cook cites an early NBC report which tells us that "homosexuals say that AIDS victims are being discriminated against, evicted by landlords, and feared by health workers"; but the accompanying visual footage shows gay men in bikinis sporting in the sun on Fire Island.[10]

It is not that network television is incapable of illustrating its own representational processes. The cable network C-Span regularly describes the conditions of media production, and even in such highly charged contexts as the presidential campaigns, television has been willing to devote time to the way candidates are packaged for the mass media. Perhaps this coverage is neither so complex nor as politically incisive as we might wish, but it shows clearly that the networks grasp the concept of representation, have indeed put it to work in representing their own operations, and believe that viewers will get the point.

What's Wrong with This Picture? The Representation of Gay Identity

The human interest of an individual's story can capture viewers and challenge stereotypes about the epidemic. TV often does this well. What is more difficult is linking these individual stories to the collective social crisis, and showing accurately the complexity and contradictions of individual and social identity. *An Early Frost*, the first feature-length drama about AIDS on network television which premiered on NBC in November 1985, features an appealing yuppie attorney with an attractive gay lover; but when the attorney finds out he has AIDS (possibly infected by his lover, who turns out to have had occasional "promiscuous" episodes), he returns to the bosom of his nuclear family to die, with limited signs of the gay community or its support. *An Early Frost* demonstrates television's tendency to dissolve the gayness of the gay person with AIDS into a homogenized and universalized person facing death. Without denying that this universalizing process may sometimes be valuable, I would suggest that it enables television both to dramatize death and to escape a fate worse than death: showing gay people being gay. *TV Guide*'s story on lead actor, Aidan Quinn, was entitled "Why This Young Hunk Risked Playing an AIDS Victim." The story spells out what the "risk" is: "Back in Chicago, Quinn's home town, acquaintances couldn't understand why their gruff friend wanted to play someone so . . . unmanly, an outcast with such a vile disease. 'You gotta be courageous to play a fag, Aidan,' one told him."[11]

In retrospect, despite its unsatisfactory emphasis and resolution, *An Early Frost* seems downright benign compared to the March 1986, *Frontline* (PBS) program *AIDS: A Public Inquiry*, which includes within its two-hour framework the crashingly homophobic film *Fabian's Story*, or to the infamous December 1988, episode of *Midnight Caller* on NBC. Both programs present gay men as dangerous "AIDS carriers," pathological and sadistic "Patient Zero" figures who continue to have unsafe sex even after they are diagnosed and warned. Both the documentary and the drama kill off their villains before the end. And neither clearly distinguishes HIV infection from the multiple clinical conditions that warrant a diagnosis of AIDS.[12]

Television could provide a great service by finding ways to convey the relationship between self-identified identity, perceived identity, fantasy and desire, and actual behaviour — as well as between one's identity in acquiring HIV infection, transmitting it, and experiencing its consequences. Interestingly, television soap operas, which thrive on the paradoxes and complications of identity, have easily incorporated the AIDS epidemic into ongoing narratives. The 1987 video *Ojos Que No Ven* (Eyes That Fail to See), produced primarily for Spanish-speaking communities, though now also available in English, uses the popular *telenovella* format to weave together several different themes about AIDS and to embed them in the story of an extended Latino family. Such a clarification of identity would be especially useful for women, for at present, despite thousands of cases of AIDS and HIV infection, they remain largely invisible in terms of the epidemic. Even given educational efforts, many women continue to believe they are not at risk; nor are most AIDS agencies set up to provide treatment or social services for women. Further, many women, "at risk" or not, are still unaware that the epidemic indirectly threatens all women's rights (routine testing of all pregnant women already occurs at some sites) — a threat spelled out clearly in Pratibha Parmar's 1987 *Reframing AIDS* and Amber Hollibaugh's *The Second Epidemic*. Finally, a different kind of media coverage could show people speaking for themselves, thus acknowledging political, sexual, cultural, social, ethnic, gender, and class identities as something more than "special interests."

Safe Sex, Safe Texts, and the Market

Although many individual TV stations readily accepted ads and public-service announcements on both birth control and AIDS, the commercial networks initially refused to do so on the grounds that accepting them would violate their First Amendment rights of free speech. Their refusal exemplified what Greyson calls "the ADS epidemic": acquired dread of sex, which you can get from worrying about AIDS or watching too much television. The ADS epidemic encompasses a formidable array of phobias, including homophobia, erotophobia, fear of the exotic and unknown, fear of death, and fear of conservative retribution. The networks' uncharacteristic prudery reflects their stance that a political position is a bad thing and that something called "neutrality" can actually be achieved. One irony in this moralistic prudishness is that the networks spend vast sums developing ways to commodify people, products, events, and phenomena for the viewing public. To an industry equipped for the market, condoms should not have presented a major challenge.

In part, individual television journalists created their own reporting problems. The first network story on AIDS, by NBC in June 1982, took the line that "homosexual lifestyles" had triggered an epidemic. This angle on AIDS lasted, presenting reporters with the ongoing problems of covering a group — the gay community — not usually covered on the nightly news. They also had to find suitable language to communicate the facts of transmission and prevention, and to educate viewers about their own potential risk without causing panic. Accordingly, television coverage evolved a kind of visual and verbal shorthand that allow "the facts" to be telegraphed: two men together in an urban setting, in shops or among crowds; phrases like "the exchange of bodily fluids," "homosexual acts," "safe sex." The dreaded phrase "anal intercourse" was finally uttered (on PBS) only after the way had been paved by detailed broadcasts about Ronald Reagan's colon surgery.[13] The problem of conveying information without causing panic handled through messages that mixed fear with reassurance. Thus, ever popular "spread-of-AIDS" stories quick to reassure viewers that the epidemic's spread remained confined to isolated groups and locales: newly identified people with AIDS, in other words, were efficiently relegated to the (still) growing category of contaminated Other while the presumed category of the viewer, the "general population," though (still) shrinking, remained pristine and pure.

By the time network television finally broke down and told viewers to "use a condom," this once explicit piece of advice had become a euphemism, a symbolic stand-in for the difficulty of talking frankly about AIDS and sex, a piece of technical information to be moved from group to group, culture to culture, as though isolated from the social, political, economic, cultural, and moral understandings and commitments of those to whom the advice was given.[14]

Spectacles of AIDS, Regimes of Truth

Michel Foucault uses the term *regime of truth* to describe the circular relation between truth, the systems of power that produce and sustain it, and the effects of power it induces, and which it in turn reconfigures. Truth, in this sense, is already power: we can forget the fight for or against a particular truth, and instead interrogate the rules at work in a society that distinguish "true" representations from "false" ones. Media accounts of AIDS conform to such regimes; they come to seem familiar, true, because they simultaneously reinforce prior representations and prepare us for similar representations to come. Media research often contributes to these regimes, for example by studying media coverage of the epidemic without examining gay or alternative media. These studies often plot the quantity of media coverage in relationship to some "real world" variable like the number of AIDS cases or scientific findings. That Rock Hudson's illness and death provoked the most dramatic increase in coverage is then deplored, as though it revealed a deep moral weakness in the American psyche. But the Hudson case is more than simply the first major case of Celebrity AIDS: it provides significant evidence that the media and "the masses" alike will pay attention if something interests them.

The networks excuse their haphazard, reactive response to the AIDS epidemic with direct appeals to the market. "The public is sick of AIDS," says the director of research at one of the major networks. "It has lost its market value." If we think we can overcome that reality, "we exaggerate our own importance." This new-found humility camouflages a fair degree of cultural and institutional imperialism. Moreover, the statement "the public is sick of AIDS" depends upon the us/them dichotomy by now virtually universal in the social construction of the AIDS epidemic; "the public," of course, is our old friend "the general population," here constructed as a media market assumed to be heterosexual and to be (or to want to be) white and middle-class. The networks could aggressively examine how to present televisually the complex aspects of this epidemic, seeking advice from more creative and knowledgeable videomakers than themselves. Instead, caught in the production and reproduction of over-determined images, journalists reflexively phone predictable requests to the nearest AIDS service organization: "Can you get me a black prostitute with two kids who shoots drugs and is still on the street spreading AIDS?"[15]

Conclusion and Afterward

In the interval since this essay was first published, television coverage of the epidemic has not dramatically changed. As Cook, Rogers, Kinsella, Thompson, and others report, the quantity of U.S. media coverage of the AIDS epidemic appears to have peaked with the widespread concern over heterosexual transmission among the "general population" in 1987.[16]

In terms of quality and selection, however, some specific improvements can be identified. Most noticeable, perhaps, is the introduction of alternative viewpoints into regular news coverage — for example, AIDS activists, scientists and clinicians who disagree with federal policies. This was especially evident at the Sixth International Conference on AIDS in San Francisco in June 1990, when many media outlets assigned reporters to cover the activists as well as scheduled conference activities. A model of AIDS programming during the conference was provided by San Francisco network affiliates, encompassing live interviews and commentaries on the conference, regular "town meetings," and independent documentaries and feature videos on a range of topics. Though such efforts may not alter the format or authoritative stance of network coverage, they do allow diverse voices to be heard. Similarly, several recent segments of The AIDS Quarterly have moved toward a more critical and investigative stance, for example demonstrating how federal AIDS funds are actually spent and in some cases wasted at the state and local level.

International reporting and programming have improved. Another segment of The AIDS Quarterly examined the epidemic in Poland and Eastern Europe, a story that requires resources unavailable to many videomakers. The AIDS Quarterly also offered Born in Africa, which followed what happened when Ugandan rock star Philly Lutaya announced that he had AIDS. Even more imperative is international coverage that moves beyond familiar American perspectives. To its credit, Born in Africa included information about the conditions of and constraints on its own production, brought about in part by prior sensationalistic coverage of AIDS in Africa by the Western press. In the United Kingdom, the BBC produced an excellent program on AIDS and art, moving far beyond the humanist perspective familiar in U.S. reporting. Programs from the U.K. series Out on Tuesday, independently produced by Mandy Merck for Channel Four, are rarely accessible in the U.S. outside lesbian and gay film festivals.

In January 1991, shortly after the United States declared war on Iraq, AIDS activists from ACT UP disrupted the start of the CBS Evening News with Dan Rather and the MacNeil-Lehrer News Hour on PBS. "Fight AIDS, not Arabs!" shouted the protestors at CBS as the network cut hastily to a commercial; at PBS, the group carried a sign reading "Act up, Fight back! Fight AIDS, not Iraq!"[17] The takeover, however brief, enacted Rockville is Burning in real life, reminding us that the mass media are capable of experimental and electrifying coverage. This was demonstrated by CNN's live coverage of the events in Tienamen Square in China, C-Span's live coverage of various AIDS events, and the popularity of alternative and resistant films and videos at the Fifth and Sixth International AIDS Conferences.[18] Television's coverage of war in the Persian Gulf, particularly by CNN and

C-Span, suggests its power not only to provide the resources for near-saturation coverage but also to educate the viewer about the conditions of televisual production. We also glimpse the potential, via satellite access, for global perspectives that are, at this point, virtually unavailable to the average viewer. Rather than accept hopeless judgements from research and marketing departments that "AIDS is a dead issue" or "we can't say 'condom' on television," network executives and individual reporters can look at what interests people, what they watch, what they find compelling. They can repeatedly communicate the simple and undisputed messages about AIDS that are still widely misunderstood. They can make clear that you can't get HIV infection or AIDS from giving blood. They can aggressively seek international and alternative perspectives. They can be courageous enough to do what network television has failed so dismally to do thus far — provide programming and public service announcements directed at the general population in its *true* diversity, including gay men and women, poor people, middle-class and working-class people of colour, drug users, sexually active adolescents, and so on. Any of these possibilities would be far more welcome than the green snake.

NOTES

1. The green snake phenomenon was described to me by Leland C. Clark, Jr., Ph.D., professor of pediatrics and director of neurophysiology, University of Cincinatti College of Medicine.

2. Selected readings on television (and media) coverage of the AIDS epidemic include Keith Alcorn, "AIDS in the Public Sphere: How a Broadcasting System in Crisis Dealt with an Epidemic," in *Taking Liberties: AIDS and Cultural Politics*, Erica Carter and Simon Watney, eds., (London: Serpent's Tail, 1989): 193-212; Dennis Altman, *AIDS in the Mind of America* (Garden City, NY: Anchor/Doubleday, 1986); Douglas Crimp, "AIDS: Cultural Analysis/Cultural Activism," *AIDS: Cultural Analysis/Cultural Activism*, D. Crimp, ed., (Cambridge: MIT Press, 1988); Crimp, "Portraits of People with AIDS," *Cultural Studies*, Lawrence Grossberg, Cary Nelson, and Paula A. Treichler, eds., (New York: Routledge, forthcoming); Jan Zita Grover, "Visible Lesions," *Afterimage* (Summer 1989), 10-16; Claudine Herzlich and Janine Pierret, "The Construction of a Social Phenomenon: AIDS in the French Press," *Social Science & Medicine* 29:11 (1989), 1235-42; James Kinsella, *Covering the Plague: AIDS and the American Media* (New Brunswick, NJ: Rutgers University Press, 1989); Timothy Landers, "Bodies and Anti-Bodies: A Crisis in Representation," *The Independent* (January-February 1988), 18-24; Robert Norton and Jim Hughey, eds. "Communication and the AIDS Crisis," special issue of *Communication Research*, 17:6 (December 1990), especially "Language Discrimination of General Physicians: AIDS Metaphors Used in the AIDS Crisis," by Fobert Norton, Judith Schwartzbaum, and John Whear, 809-26; Cathy Packer and Susan Kauffman, "Reregulation of Commercial Television: Implications for Coverage of AIDS," *AIDS & Public Policy Journal*, 5:2 (Spring, 1990), 82-8; Randy Shilts, *And The Band Played On: People, Politics, and the AIDS Epidemic* (New York: St. Martin's Press, 1987); John Tagg, *The Burden of Representation* (Amherst: University of Massachusetts Press, 1988); Paula A. Treichler, "AIDS, Gender, and Biomedical Discourse: Current Contests for Meaning," in *AIDS: The Burdens of History*, Elizabeth Fee and Daniel M. Fox, eds. (Berkeley: University of California Press, 1988); Treichler, "AIDS, Homophobia, and Biomedical Discourse: An Epidemic of Signification" in *AIDS: Cultural Analysis/Cultural Activism*, Crimp, ed.; and Simon Watney, *Policing Desire: Pornography: AIDS and the Media*, (Minneapolis: University of Minnesota Press, 1987). See also Todd Gitlin, ed., *Watching Television* (New York: Pantheon, 1986), and Sharon M. Friedman, Sharon Dunwoody, and Carol L. Rogers, *Scientists and Journalists: Reporting Science as News* (Washington: American Association for the Advancement of Science, 1986). Several papers on television were presented at "AIDS: Communication Challenges," a day-long conference held in conjunction with the annual meeting of the International Communication Association, San Francisco, 27 May 1989, including David C. Colby, "Mass Mediated Epidemic: AIDS and Television News 1981-87"; Pat Christen, "The Impact of Television on the Development of AIDS Public Policy and Funding"; David Perlman, "The Print Media's Response to AIDS"; Everett M. Rogers, "Diffusion of AIDS Information through the Electronic Media"; Mervyn Silverman, "The Impact of National Television on AIDS Funding"; and Jorst Stipp, "An Analysis of Trends in NBC's Coverage of AIDS."

3. Dearing, James W. and Everett M. Rogers, "The Agenda Setting Process for the Issue of AIDS," presented at the annual meeting of the International Communication Association, New Orleans, 28 May-2 June, 1988.

4. Goldberg, Marshall, "TV Has Done More to Contain AIDS than Any Other Single Factor," *TV Guide* 35:48, 28 November 1987, 4-7. The value of such control becomes especially clear when it is absent — as it was, for example, on a November, 1986, segment of *Wall Street Week* where a guest expert was asked by a visiting panelist to recommend stocks that might go up as a result of the AIDS epidemic or on an April 1989 segment of the conservative Washington talk show *Tony Brown's Journal* where several AIDS conspiracy theorists presented their views to a largely black audience with virtually no challenge or contradiction. Eva Lee Snead, for

example, listed as "Dr." and author of *Win! Against Herpes and AIDS*, argued that "AIDS is a figment of the media," that the "HTLV virus" was deliberately used to contaminate Zairean gamma globulin, and that the World Health Organization (WHO) is behind it. She was supported by a young black man in the audience who feverishly documented places in the *Congressional Record* where this could all be verified. He also supplied the motive, about which Dr. Snead was murky: to obtain the natural resources of Central Africa by killing off the black population there and in the United States. At this point the largely black audience burst into applause. In the entire half hour, reservations were expressed only twice: a representative from WHO forcefully but briefly took issue with Dr. Snead's theory, and a young black woman in the audience said, "I do AIDS education and what you're saying in this room would set me back ten years; I'd like to know what credentials, what business you have saying what you're saying?" Both were ignored. The program ended with a Lyndon LaRouche follower (white) rising from the audience to commend the entire event and attempt to fill in a few missing links (e.g., the role of the Trilateral Commission). Important theoretical questions asked why conspiracy theories are so appealing and in precisely what ways (and on what grounds) they are to be distinguished from scientific theories.

5. Dorothy Nelkin, *Selling Science: How the Press Covers Science and Technology* (New York: W.H. Freeman, 1986): 74-5.

6. John Greyson, "Proofing," in Jan Zita Grover, ed., *AIDS: The Artists' Response* (Columbus: Ohio State University Press, 1989): 22-5. The *AIDS Quarterly*, to which Greyson refers, has greatly improved in recent installments. At the time of Greyson's comments, the single independent feature aired by PBS was *The A.I.D.S. Show*, Peter Adair and Robert Epstein, 1986. Since then, additional independent videos have been aired.

7. Crimp, *AIDS: Cultural Analysis/Cultural Activism*, op. cit. 4.

8. Many of the alternative films and videos I refer to in this essay are now compiled on *Video Against AIDS*, a set of three tapes curated by John Greyson and Bill Horrigan, produced by Kate Horsfield, and available from Video Data Bank in Chicago and New York and from V/Tape in Toronto. Likewise, many are described more fully in Jean Carlomusto, "Focusing on Women: Video as Activism," and Catherine Saalfield, "AIDS Videos By, For, and About Women," both in *Women, AIDS, and Activism* by the ACT UP/NY Women and AIDS Book Group (Boston: South End Press, 1990:), 215-18 and 281-8; Jan Zita Grover, ed., *AIDS: The Artists' Response*; "In conversation: Isaac Suken and Pratibha Parmar," and Roberta McGrath, "Dangerous Liaisons: Health, Disease, and Representations," both in *Ecstatic Antibodies: Resisting the AIDS Mythology*, Tessa Boffin and Sunil Gupta, eds. (London: Rivers Oram Press, 1990): 96-102 and 142-55.

9. Herbert Daniel, *Life Before Death* (Rio de Janeiro: Tipografía Jabot, 1989).

10. See Silverman, "Impact of National Television"; Shilts, *And the Band Played On*; and Cook, "Construction of Homosexuality."

11. Michael Leagy, "Why This Young Hunk Risked Playing an AIDS Victim," *TV Guide* 34:17, 26 April 1986, 34-38. As actor Tom Hulce said in his presentation at SIDART (June 1989), what shocked audiences at Larry Kramer's play *The Normal Heart* was not "the medical details about AIDS — the seizures, the lesions, etc. — they're used to medical stuff. What shocked them was seeing two men kissing." Concern about job discrimination in Hollywood was addressed on *Saturday Night Live* in 1986; linking AIDS panic to McCarthy-era blacklisting, a skit showed a gay male actor worried about being "pinklisted" and trying to establish his heterosexual credentials by swaggering into a bar, flirting with the waitress, and talking about the Dallas Cowboys. Ironically, Aidan Quinn told *TV Guide* that since his performance in *An Early Frost* he has gotten more scripts calling for him to play "more normal, human guys" instead of the narrowly typecast rebel hunks he played before.

12. *Fabian's Story*, widely criticized as unethical, nonrepresentative, and exploitive, shows a

black male prostitute who continues to have unsafe sex even after his diagnosis: Martha Gever, in "Pictures of Sickness: Stuart Marshall's *Bright Eyes*" (Crimp, ed., *AIDS: Cultural Analysis/Cultural Activism*), notes in contrast that a positive film about a man with AIDS, *Chuck Solomon: Coming of Age*, 1986, by Mark Huestis and Wendy Dallas, was turned down by PBS (though shown by Channel Four in Britain). The figure of "Patient Zero," a Canadian flight attendant represented as a kind of Typhoid Mary character by Randy Shilts in *And the Band Played On*, is discussed by Crimp in *AIDS: Cultural Analysis/Cultural Activism*.

13. The evolution of explicit usage is discussed by Cook (1989), Kinsella (1989), and Packer and Kauffman (1990). Generally, "penis" and "anal intercourse" are considered to be the most sensitive words and some stations, even now, have not permitted them. Interestingly, the only phrase prohibited by the relatively liberal National Public Radio was "full-blown AIDS," which they considered to be sexually suggestive. Michael Callen, "Media Watch (And It's Still Ticking)," in Crimp, ed. (1988) writes that "One distressing presumption that runs through this asshole coverage is that anal intercourse and male homosexuality are synonymous. When will someone point out that heterosexuals can *and do* engage in anal intercourse?" (p.150)

14. As Brooke Grundfest Schoepf and her colleagues in Project CONAISSIDA point out, discussing their experiences working with women in Zaire, condoms present cultural difficulties for women in the context of their countries' deepening poverty: for many women, only the provision of new income-generating activities would provide real alternatives to multiple-part-ner sex. See Schoepf, Fukarangira wa Nkara, Claude Schoepf, Walu Engundu, and Payanzo Ntsomo, "AIDS and Society in Central Africa: A View from Zaire," in Norman Miller and Richard C. Rockwell, eds., *AIDS in Africa: The Social and Policy Impact*, (Lewiston, NY: Edwin Mellen, 1988): 218.

15. Pat Christen, "The Impact of Television," reported that the San Francisco AIDS Foundation regularly receives such requests from the media.

16. See Cook, "Construction of Homosexuality"; Rogers, "Diffusion of AIDS Information"; Kinsella, *Covering the Plague, and Larry Thompson*, "Commentary: With No Magic Cure in Sight, Dramatic Epidemic Loses Luster as News Story," *Washington Post*, 13 June 1989, health section, 7.

17. Associated Press, "AIDS activists disrupt start of television news shows," *Daily Illini*, 23 January 1991:4

18. Screenings of activists' and artists' videos at the Montréal conference consistently played to overflow crowds; after the conference, with little additional publicity, many orders for *Video Against AIDS* (see note 8) came in to Video Data Bank and V/Tape from community health organizations and health educators — precisely the viewers conventionally believed to require "straight" materials.

Short-Term Companions:
AIDS as Popular Entertainment

Simon Watney

This new world may be safer, being told
The dangers and diseases of the old . . .
  — John Donne

My purpose is to tell of bodies which have been transformed into shapes
of a different kind.
  — Ovid

Introduction

In an important article about the cultural construction of the social meanings of AIDS, Judith Williamson has observed how:

> . . . [W]hile it is relatively easy to counter hysterical conservatism, it is less easy to pin down the wider sense in which AIDS takes its place within the narrative systems along whose track events seem to glide quite naturally, whether in news reports, movie plots or everyday explanations.[1]

Such narrative systems provide the basic structures through which we communicate and make our various senses of the world. They range from the plot-lines of TV soap operas to the conventions of historical fiction, the logic of jokes, and the ordering of events of the main TV evening news. From the beginning of the epidemic, a particular set of mass-media narratives was engaged to "handle" a topic which was almost universally regarded as scandalous, drawing attention to the lives of social groups which are generally marginalized — gay men, prostitutes, and injecting drug-users.[2]

The "scandal" of AIDS, however, was never publicly recognized in terms of the terrible tragedy of the epidemic *within* those groups. Rather, it was regarded from the frightened perspective of the rest of the population whom these groups were erroneously held to threaten. All those narratives deal with fantasy, such as the story of the imagined "AIDS carrier," setting out deliberately to infect other uninfected people; the story of the family whose young child received an infected blood sample; the faithful wife infected by her bisexual husband; the deserted African village; the HIV positive female prostitute who says she is not having safer sex with her clients; the courageous scientific quest for the virus, and subsequently for a vaccine; and so on.

These stories all make sense in the broader context of the expectations audiences have in relation to different types of publications, different types of TV programs, different types of films, etc. Thus the "AIDS carrier" story belongs to a cluster of similar stories, well known from popular fiction and film, about vampires, mysterious killer-diseases, dangerous strangers, illicit sex, etc. Similarly, the story of the stricken young family belongs to the wider order of narratives about terrible, undeserved medical tragedies, as does the story of the faithful wife. In relation to AIDS however, such narratives carry a heavy cargo of assumptions that do not need to be spelled out literally, but that are strongly implicit: the unseen, but nonetheless signified, image of the HIV positive blood donor, and the equally invisible-but-signified "unfaithful" husband, whose "dark" sexual secret is held up as the cause of his wife's tragedy. The deserted African village serves its purpose as an image of mysterious catastrophe, the exotic, non-Western suggestion of the possible source of the epidemic, while the image of the prostitute functions as the narrative site for a vast array of sexual anxieties on the part of many heterosexuals about the whole subject of non-marital sex, and its imagined dangers.[3] Finally, the documentary format provides a familiar narrative of scientific discovery and technological achievement just around the corner in the form of a "breakthrough." The message is also reassuring: we know the boffins are out there in their labs, so there's nothing really to worry about. As long, that is, as one doesn't perceive oneself or one's peers as being at any real risk of contracting HIV.

This rather arbitrary list suggests something of the range of forms of narrative that have dominated the shaping of most Western perceptions of HIV and AIDS. Such agenda-setting may of course be analyzed in much greater detail, and doubtless a full taxonomy of AIDS narratives could be established. The most immediate point, however, is that for the better part of a decade, AIDS coverage across the mass media has consistently positioned readers and viewers alike in contradictory ways, implying that they both *are*, and *are not* at risk. This is the context in which gay men appear as threatening rather than threatened, and in need of punitive control rather than support. However, this agenda has not been established without some resistance, and several attempts have been made over the years to "de-sensationalize" coverage of the epidemic, both in the press and on network TV. Nonetheless, most coverage continues to regard gay men as if they were members of a uniform culture, with a shared "gay lifestyle," and identical sexual needs. We appear simultaneously as villains and as victims, but never as a social constituency facing the worst natural disaster in the history of any minority group within many Western societies. Anti-gay prejudice has been widely mobilized by divergent institutions, ranging from churches to political parties of both the Left and Right.

De-sensationalizing strategies tend to take the form of "human interest" programs, such as talk shows, and biographical features, although these only very rarely confront the actual circumstances which make them necessary. Only a handful of investigative programs such a Britain's *Hard News*, and *The Media Show* (both on Channel Four) have attempted serious, in-depth analyses of the wider biopolitics of mass media representations of HIV/AIDS issues. The great majority of print features and TV programs about AIDS may, however, be regarded as a form of macabre entertainment, which provide a limited series of heavily moralized *tableaux* that tell us much about the complex moral management of modern sexuality but little or nothing about the complex, shifting realities of the epidemic as it is lived all around the world. In such circumstances AIDS becomes a cipher, rather than a syndrome. The epidemic is staged as if it were a form of public morality play about guilt, judgement and damnation, rather than a terrible ongoing catastrophe to which governments and international institutions around the world, from the United Nations to the European Community, have signally failed to respond adequately or sufficiently.

One strategy intended to correct the relentless homophobia of dominant AIDS commentary has been concentrated in the more independent domain of feature films, initiated by the late Arthur J. Bressan's *Buddies* (1985), and Bill Sherwood's *Parting Glances* (1986). Both films were set in New York City and dramatize aspects of the epidemic as lived by gay men, who continue to make up the great majority of AIDS cases, cumulatively. *Buddies* tells the story of a young, successful yuppy, who "buddies" an older gay man dying from AIDS. The man with AIDS is an ex-hippie, whose outlook and identity had been forged in the early 1970s period of Gay Liberation. The film movingly describes his buddy's gradual recognition of the extent of anti-gay prejudice in the U.S.A. and its baleful influence on the course of the epidemic, and his new friend's life-expectancy. It is an extremely ambitious allegory of the difficult social relations between different generations of gay men, and the divisions of class within the gay communities in the U.S.

Parting Glances is less overtly political, and has the rather different, if equally ambitious aim of locating AIDS (and gay men in general) within contemporary

Manhattan society. Yet the aim of *Parting Glances* is not simply "normalization," but a demonstration of the actual diversity of urban New York life, and the centrality of gay men in the social life of the city. Thus the tragedy of AIDS comes to be seen as a tragedy for the entire city.

Since 1986, the epidemic has of course deepened and widened in New York, as in most other major Western cities. For example, by the summer of 1987 there had been 1,000 diagnosed cases of AIDS in the United Kingdom as a whole, whereas there had been more than 10,000 cases in New York alone.[4] At the time of writing this article there have been approximately 100,000 deaths from AIDS in the U.S.A. but only around 2,000 deaths in the U.K., which nonetheless has a quarter of the overall population of the U.S.A. The gradual changes in the demography of the epidemic in the course of the 1980s make it increasingly important to challenge the authority of the mass media's response, which still seems largely frozen in the postures and narratives established in the early years of the decade. By reducing AIDS to a kind of ghoulish spectacle, media coverage has been responsible for many of the misunderstandings that continue to frame beliefs and attitudes. Thus the recent acknowledgement of the impact of HIV amongst injecting drug users and their sexual partners has frequently been presented in such a way as to imply that the epidemic has somehow "moved on" from gay men, though nothing could be further from the truth. The same media industry which for many years refused to accept even the possibility of hetero-sexual transmission, now tends to ignore all other modes of transmission, even though the prevalence of HIV among gay men means that we are still far more vulnerable than any other social constituency in most first world countries. This is the immediate, pressing context in which the most recent major feature film about AIDS appears.

Like its predecessors, *Longtime Companion* sets out to realign perceptions of AIDS, and to narrate the history of the epidemic from a gay male perspective. Yet the worsening of the AIDS crisis around the world forces us to consider whether the conventions of Hollywood melodrama, now crossed with the conventions of TV soap-opera, are sufficiently resilient to effectively undermine the by-now solidly accreted cultural agenda of AIDS which has been established for almost ten years by the press and TV alike, with an unusual and significant degree of unanimity. How does one narrate an epidemic in process? How might one deploy one narrative in order to discredit another? Can a film contest one set of inadequate explanations of an immensely complex social phenomenon, and at the same time establish its own superior explanatory authority? How, in other words, might it be possible to use the narrative forms of the entertainment industry to call into question its own stubborn fears and prejudices?

Longtime Companion

By the summer of 1988, AIDS had struck the fictional worlds of three major American network soap-operas — CBS's *The Young and The Restless*, ABC's *All My Children*, and NBC's *Another World*. Yet as *New York Times* critic Deborah Rogers has pointed out, "all three AIDS plots on these television serials feature patients who are women — and women with no history of drug abuse."[5]

A year earlier, Britain's Central TV produced Alma Cullen's four-part mini-series, *Intimate Contact*, which, four years later, is still slated for a possible movie remake. *Intimate Contact* tells the story of a philandering businessman who contracts HIV from a prostitute in New York, and is more concerned with the snobbery and hypocrisy of his family's responses than with his illness. It is thus rather like a Victorian "improving" fiction, intended to edify its audience, and to dispel prejudice. Perhaps the most fascinating aspect of *Intimate Contact* lies in its depiction of the sick man's wife, Ruth, played by Claire Bloom. Ruth is totally shut off in her house-proud middle-class world, and the extent of her inability to deal with her husband's diagnosis is shown as a direct result of her smug, complacent Thatcherite world-view and class position. However, as a result of meeting a gay couple and an HIV positive haemophiliac boy and his father, she learns the lesson of "compassion." In other words, *Intimate Contact* finds in AIDS only an example, albeit extreme, of the supposedly universal problems of ignorance and prejudice. The husband with AIDS dies conveniently early on in the series, which finds its closure in the moral "improvement" (and new likability) of the heroine. Indeed, one almost comes to regard AIDS as a blessing in disguise, at least from Ruth's point of view. AIDS is not seen to possess any real specificity of its own here, and this, to a great extent, reflects British liberal opinion to the present day.

In narrative and ideological terms this duplicates the problems raised by NBC's made-for-TV movie, *An Early Frost* (1986). As Vito Russo pointed out:

> In *An Early Frost*, we see how AIDS affects a young man's mother, father, sister, brother-in-law and grandmother. There is no consideration given to the fact that this is happening to him — not them.[6]

An Early Frost narrates the simultaneous coming-out of a young gay man to his family alongside his dilemma of living with AIDS. Yet the extraordinary level of violent prejudice this brings out in his family is understood by the film to be quite natural and inevitable, if ultimately susceptible to reason and "love." Prejudice is seen as a kind of free-floating universal, able to be attracted to almost any object in an arbitrary fashion. Thus both *An Early Frost* and *Intimate Contact* were entirely unable to confront the specific, concrete issues raised by homophobia, and by AIDS. The "problem" of the epidemic is thus posed for heterosexuals as a question of rationality, familial stability and how "well" they can behave, rather than the real issue facing millions of gay men about how long we or our closest friends will manage to stay alive.

This is the immediate *representational* context in which *Longtime Companion* was made and is viewed. In recent months, I have seen the film in New York, London, and Melbourne and various audience responses provided an especially keen sense of the enormity of the differing experience of the epidemic in these three cities alone. The American TV critic in *People* magazine found *Intimate Contact* genuinely shocking in terms of its "frankness," and "amazing" because "the victims are at first unlikable." Such issues are not raised by *Longtime Companion*, for the simple reason that its narrative structure is not organized around exemplary victims and *individual change*. Rather, it sets out to narrate a *collective experience*, and this is its greatest strength.

In New York, the great majority of gay men have already lost many friends to AIDS, and will know many more who are ill. The lowest estimates suggest that at least 36 percent of all gay men in New York are HIV positive. In London however, far fewer gay men have had any direct experience of AIDS, though very many know somebody with HIV. Throughout the 1980s, the American urban experience of AIDS has increasingly involved a grim routine of visits to people in acute hospital care, deaths and mourning, whereas in Britain the overwhelming experience has been of people with HIV who seem, for all intents and purposes (it is widely perceived), perfectly well. Melbourne, like its sister city Sydney, has a worse epidemic than London, but the situation is nowhere near as bad as in New York. Yet the internal cohesion of the Australian gay communities means that the epidemic is felt in a far more immediate way than it is in London. This is largely a result of different political histories.[7]

For example, the Australian government's response to AIDS has been far more practical and pragmatic than government responses in either Britain or the U.S. More than 80 percent of Australian AIDS cases have been among gay men. Acknowledging the risk of HIV infection to gay men, the government set up community-based AIDS Councils in all Australia's States and Territories. As a result, AIDS education has been based on the demonstrably effective principles of community development rather than the familiar types of anti-sex scare-mongering that have been so typical elsewhere. Thus, Australia probably has the best-educated and serviced gay communities on earth. Moreover, the political struggles for the decriminalization of homosexuality which were fought there throughout the 1970s and 1980s on a State-by-State basis have resulted in a clear, well organized gay infrastructure which the government now recognizes as legitimately representative of a social constituency with its own specific needs and entitlements. The Australian ideology of multiculturalism thus traverses racial, ethnic, and sexual boundaries, unlike in the U.S., where lesbians and gay men are

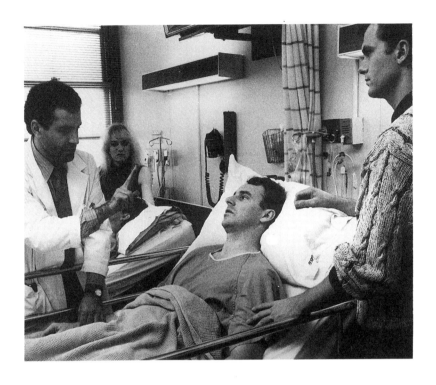

Norman René, *Longtime Companion*, 1991. Film still, American
Playhouse Theatre. Photo: Gabor Szitanyi.

by no means accepted by local or national governments on a par with other social/racial groups.

In Britain it goes without saying that multiculturalism has never existed as an "official" legitimating national ideology, either for the Asian and Afro-Caribbean population, or for lesbians and gay men. On the contrary, multiculturalism remains distinctly unfashionable, except in limited Leftist versions. This, in turn, is reflected in the timidity of British non-governmental AIDS service organizations with regard to gay men's health education — a timidity that is rationalized in terms of the supposed threat of funding losses, or prosecution. There is no equivalent whatsoever in Britain to the vast array of HIV/AIDS education materials and projects which abound in Australia, and one would be extremely fortunate to find so much as a poster or leaflets in a London or Liverpool gay bar in 1991. Nor are British gay men accepted as a valid social constituency in the U.K., with the result that HIV/AIDS education is still surrounded with anxiety about possible consequences for service organizations that provide it. Such fears largely outweigh anxieties about the epidemic itself and its future impact on the lives of gay men.[8]

The sheer scale of AIDS in the U.S. has resulted in a growing awareness of the terrible shortcomings of the American private medical system, which in turn has given rise to the AIDS activist movement, ACT UP, in recent years. Furthermore, increasing numbers of American lesbians and gay men have come to question the dismal track record of the U.S. government in all areas of HIV/AIDS work, from the planning of clinical trials for potential new drug treatments to housing and social security benefits. In other words, gay communities in different countries perceive AIDS not simply in terms of local statistics, but also in relation to the position gay men held in those societies before the epidemic began, and in relation to the respective degrees of confidence in gay identity and political organization which historically characterizes each place/community. These same factors have also largely determined the ways in which heterosexuals think about the epidemic, according to national variations in the acceptability or otherwise of frank, public homophobia. All of this in turn shapes both the production and reception of "information" about HIV/AIDS, whether in the form of explicit, targeted health education campaigns, newspaper reports and features, or feature films.

Such objectives, if shifting in their conditions, constitute the backdrop over which cultural producers struggle to narrate AIDS, either against the grain or on the terms of "popular" consensus, beliefs and attitudes. In such circumstances it is hardly surprising that all along, death has played the most significant role in AIDS narratives. However, one must at once distinguish between approaches to AIDS which proceed from entirely fatalistic assumptions concerning the rate of progression from HIV to AIDS and the life expectancy of people living with AIDS, and other approaches which attempt to question and problematize precisely such fatalism. Indeed, among all the uneven and conflicting public responses to AIDS, it is the widespread Anglo-American indifference to the deaths of tens of thousands of young gay men that is perhaps most unacceptable and also frightening to AIDS activists.

Longtime Companion is in many important respects a film about the deaths of gay men. It is also a film which attempts to explain how gay men live, or at least how middle-class white gay men in New York live. It positions itself somewhere between the dominant media's gloating fatalism and the opposite extreme — often found, understandably, among gay men in the tendencies to heroize, sentimentalize or even deny death altogether. Furthermore, we should note that the death of gay men is not an entirely new topic. On the contrary, the picture of the supposedly lonely, miserable old age and expiration of gay men has long been a central warning trope held up to young gay men throughout the modern period. This projective fantasy evidently overlooks the types of social solidarity and organization that exist among older gay men, who are in fact far less likely to experience the systematic neglect and isolation that are the increasingly common fate of their heterosexual peers.

Nonetheless, homophobic ideology seems to require the motif of the pathetic, isolated, aging gay man as a form of sadistic wish-fulfilment. In this respect it appears that there is a close social and psychological relationship between the cultural image of the sordid, older gay man, and the parallel one of the gay "AIDS victim." Both are expressions of vengeful emotions, and the policing of the boundaries of individual and collective sexual identities. In effect, they result in a not-imprecise inversion of existing social realities in relation to aging and death in most Western societies, as experienced by gay men and by heterosexuals. However, when we talk of homophobia we should not theorize it solely in relation to the explicit, conscious projects developed by those relatively few people who deliberately and maliciously target the lives and happiness of lesbians and gay men. On the contrary, we need to think about the broad mass of perfectly decent people who thoughtlessly, and more or less automatically reproduce the values of a culture which identifies homosexuality in an extraordinarily narrow range of ways. Most people are not ogres of homophobic hatred, and there is thus an urgent need to develop cultural interventions which challenge the logic and rhetoric of homophobia, whether it comes from governments, or in gossip. In other words, the cultural legitimacy of homophobia must be a central target in effective cultural work concerned with the meaning of AIDS, among gay men and heterosexuals alike.

It is entirely understandable that much has been made of the difficulties in getting *Longtime Companion* to the screen in the U.S.A. and elsewhere, but this should not lead one to suspend all one's ordinary critical faculties. It is not, as we have seen, the first commercial feature film about AIDS, as falsely claimed in much of the publicity surrounding the film's launch. Nor will it be the last. However, for this very reason it is important to try to think about the film's real achievements, as well as its problems and occasional failures.

Longtime Companion sets out to chronicle how a group of relatively affluent white gay men in Manhattan were effected by AIDS in the course the 1980s. By the end of the film, most of the central characters have died, while the survivors have come to realize the full extent of the failings of the U.S. health care system, which is shown to have put even white middle-class men in much the same grim position as the poorest black injecting drug users from Brooklyn and Harlem. In New York the film was criticized by some gay critics on the grounds that it neglects the experience of AIDS in the city's black and Hispanic populations, while one heterosexual critic objected to the absence of heterosexual families. Both complaints strike me as beside the point, for surely there can be no good reason why a film should not be made specifically about the experience of the social group which all along has been worst affected in the U.S.A. Besides, there is a bitter irony in gay criticism that only serves to reinforce the fundamentally homophobic notion that it is wrong to make a film which takes gay lives and feelings seriously for once. The second objection was even stranger, since it so obviously stemmed from a complete inability to understand why such large numbers of gay men choose to live in cities such as New York and San Francisco, rather than in the small towns and suburbs that refuse to accept them.

Certainly *Longtime Companion* is very good indeed at the level of everyday life during an epidemic, and one could hardly come away without an awareness of the relentlessly accumulating centrality of biomedical issues in the lives of most urban American gay men. For by now, most gay New Yorkers are only too familiar with the full range of ghastly, life-threatening illnesses to which HIV may make one vulnerable. Toxoplasmosis ("toxo"); *cytomogalovirus* ("C.M.V."); *mycrobacter-ium avium intracellulare* ("M.A.I."); *pneumocystis carinii* pneumonia ("P.C.P."); *cryptospiridiosis* ("crypto") . . . the names trip off our tongues like those of old friends, old friends from another planet as far as most other people are concerned. We also see and hear about the vast array of treatments with which so many are also increasingly familiar: acyclovir (against herpes); AZT and DDI and DDC (against HIV); foscarnet and DHPG (against CMV retinitis); nebulized pentamidine (against PCP), and on and on and on. Indeed, the routine nature of care, and the casual way in which these men face, discuss, and share appalling illnesses is one of the most striking aspects of the film, together with its depiction of the gradual pauperization to which AIDS so frequently leads, even for those who are adequately insured. These are not issues that have surfaced elsewhere in the mass media. Way back in 1984, Richard Goldstein in the *Village Voice* in New York in which he compared AIDS to the Blitz in London, noting however that

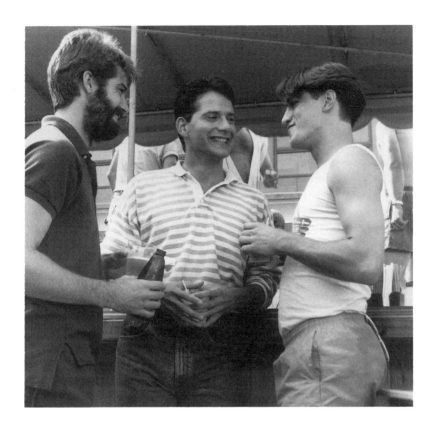

Norman René, *Longtime Companion*, 1991. Film still, American
Playhouse Theatre. Photo: Gabor Szitanyi.

AIDS is more like a Blitz taking place in a city where most people are walking around like tourists, as if nothing were happening, utterly unaware of the disaster all around them. This is the sense that *Longtime Companion* never quite manages to achieve, for the simple reason that it doesn't look beyond the world of gay men, save in the person of Lisa, a heterosexual woman played by Mary-Louise Parker, in what is much the best performance in the film.

Critics also seem to have entirely missed the significance of the film's depiction of gay relationships, love, friendship, and sex, and the full extent to which these are *taken for granted* as facts of life rather than matters of "controversy." *Longtime Companion* ends with a dream sequence, as Lisa and her two closest surviving gay friends walk slowly along the beach on Fire Island in 1989, where the beginning had been set eight years earlier. They are discussing a forthcoming ACT UP demonstration which they are going to attend, which is simultaneously a measure of their politicization and their friendship as men and women, gay and straight. In the dream, all their dead friends come pouring down the tow-path onto the beach, where they embrace and are reunited. At the New York screening I attended, most people seemed unmoved, and if anything, angered at what they saw as a gratuitous determination to give the film some kind of upbeat "happy ending" at whatever cost. In London and Melbourne, however, people all around me were in tears, evidently deeply moved.

This in itself tells us something about the extent to which New Yorkers have been hardened by AIDS, something about the extent of suffering and the numbing that so frequently goes with loss on this scale. Obviously AIDS has no "happy ending." The dead do not come back to life. But I don't think the filmmakers were trying to pretend this. On the contrary, the sequence works precisely on the level of its cathartic release of long-pent-up emotions, themselves frequently conflictual. For example, in one of the film's more powerful yet understated sequences, we see how one of the central characters, Willy, is simply terrified of possible contagion in the early stages of the epidemic, and consequently neglects his responsibilities to a dying friend. This is not a judgment. It is an observation of how things were, and how sometimes they still are. For gay men have no automatic or magical access to superior information than that generally available on TV and in the same newspapers other people read. The dream-sequence at the end of *Longtime Companion* seems to me to speak of the rarely stated scale of horror all around us, and the certainty of worse to come. It also speaks of the most simple and passionate wish that none of this had ever happened, that our dearest friends might indeed come back to life again, that we miss them horribly. This is surely not to be dismissed as "denial" or "delusion," but should be understood as a necessary catharsis, and moreover a catharsis that binds our communities ever closer in the fight to save lives.

This is not to say the film has no problems. For example, it is inexplicable to me how a film about AIDS released in 1990 cannot even bring itself to so much as mention safer sex. Yet criticisms that it fails to deal adequately with the rise of AIDS service organizations or AIDS activism again seem beside the point. This is a film about mainstream, non-political, ambitious young gay New Yorkers, and it seems to me to represent that large population with more than a little insight. In other words, it deals with precisely those people least able to understand what was going on around them in the early stages of the epidemic. If such bright, successful, young white gay men had little opportunity to understand the epidemic, what hope was there for the rest of the population? This seems to me a vitally important, underlying theme in *Longtime Companion*, and one which we neglect at our peril. It is also that same population which has been systematically denied effective health education, whether gay or straight, that is the film's proper intended audience. An old friend of mine in New York reacted furiously to the sight of an ACT UP sticker in the film in a sequence set a year before it actually appeared. At the time, Vito Russo whispered in my ear that the heart of someone who could only care about dates must have shrunk to the size of a pea. Yet at the same time we in other countries have to try to remember what gay New Yorkers have been living through during the past decade. With so little apparent concern, and so little material support, it is hardly surprising if many American lesbians and gay men have developed thick protective carapaces around their feelings as a straightforward matter of emotional survival. Undoubtedly many will come away from *Longtime Companion* with mixed feelings similar to those of Jewish audiences watching postwar films about the rise of the Nazis.

In the course of the 1980s gay men in America have moved from shock, to grief, to fury at the enormity of the failures of government and mass media responses to AIDS. This guarantees a heavily over-determined response to *any* feature film dealing with the epidemic. However, our entirely justified anger at the previous failures of the film industry and TV to deal fairly or truthfully with AIDS should not blind us to the achievements of a film which at the very least begins to redress serious sins of omission. In 1989, I attended a public discussion in Montréal at the SIDART section of the Fifth International AIDS Conference on the vexing subject of AIDS and the film industry. The panel included actor Tom Hulce, *Longtime Companion*'s producer Lindsay Law, and other professional representatives from the North American TV and film industries, as well as Vito Russo.

It was deeply depressing for me to witness the sheer scale of anger in the audience against the TV and film executives. In retrospect, it became clear to me that the furious barrage of American criticism had less to do with individual panel speakers than with the feeling of total exclusion from the mainstream mass media on the part of gay men, feelings for the most part accumulated over lifetimes. It seemed obvious to me that no individual was going to make the public recantation, as it were, which was effectively being demanded. Unfortunately, the intensity of anger prevented what might have proved to be productive dialogue. This is not to say that such anger is intrinsically wrong, only that it should be appropriately targeted at culpable institutions, especially when the opportunities for such dialogue are evidently so very rare for Americans. It was particularly tragic that the Canadians in the audience were infuriated by the Americans' refusal to permit any genuine discussion to take place, and were thus prevented from coming to any real understanding of why the Americans felt so deeply aggrieved in the first place. There are certain parallels here with the reception of *Longtime Companion*.

However bad the epidemic is in Canada or Britain or Australia, we in these countries at least have advantages that remain all but unthinkable in the U.S.A., whether in terms of socialized medicine, good government-funded AIDS service organizations or regular access to network TV audiences on our own terms. While it is far from clear to me what American audiences might possibly learn from an out-of-date British TV mini-series such as *Intimate Contact*, it seems clear that *Longtime Companion* does succeed in communicating a specific American experience in international terms. It helps non-Americans to begin, at least, to understand the nightmare of the American epidemic, and for the first time, allows straight Americans to think about gay men as people in many respects like themselves. This is no mean achievement. Sadly, the publicity materials for the film in both Britain and Australia managed to erase quite literally the film's wider political significance with posters that cynically removed that ACT UP READ MY LIPS slogan from the T-shirt of one of the leading men as seen in the film and on the original American advertisements. Nevertheless the film itself seems to me to offer a genuinely effective bypass around anti-gay prejudice, and within its own conventions to remain both accessible and truthful to the complex and terrible issues raised by AIDS. We should not, of course, expect too little of a major feature film, but by the same token, nor should we expect too much.

165

NOTES

1. Judith Williamson, "Every Virus Tells A Story," *Taking Liberties: AIDS And Cultural Politics*, E. Carter and S. Watney, eds. (London: Serpent's Tail Press, 1989): 69-70.

2. Simon Watney, *Media*, (Minneapolis: University of Minnesota Press, 1987).

3. Simon Watney, "Missionary Positions," *Critical Quarterly*, 31:3 (1989); also Cindy Patton, *Inventing AIDS* (New York: Routledge, 1990): ch. 4; also Paula A. Treichler, "AIDS and HIV Infection In the Third World: A First World Chronicle," *Remaking History*, B. Kruger and P. Mariani, eds. (Seattle: Bay Press, 1989).

4. "AIDS chief killer of NY women," *The Guardian*, London, 9 July, 1987; Andrew Veitch, "AIDS cases exceed 1,000," *The Guardian*, London, 8 September, 1987.

5. Deborah Rogers, "AIDS Spreads to the Soaps, Sort Of," *The New York Times*, 28 August, 1988. I would like to thank Charles A. Barber for drawing this article to my attention.

6. Vito Russo, *The Celluloid Closet: Homosexuality in the Movies* (New York: Harper and Row, 1987), rev. ed.: 277.

7. Simon Watney, "The AIDS Community: An Interview With Dennis Altman," *Gay Times*, London, February 1990, 47-8.

8. Simon Watney, "Introduction," E. Carter & S. Watney, eds., op. cit.

On ReFraming AIDS

Pratibha Parmar

I would like to preface this article with a few comments about *ReFraming AIDS*, a documentary video which I made in 1987. As the title suggests, one of my concerns was to wrest the discussion of the AIDS crisis away from the conservatives and the Right who had been unashamedly using it to further repress and terrorize what they saw as marginal and disposable communities. Women, gays, drug users, and racial minorities were coming under increased state repression and oppression in a multitude of ways which were specific to each one of these communities. For me, the political moment in the summer of 1987 in Britain was characterized by the escalation of a virulent backlash against the lesbian and gay communities. Newspaper headlines were screaming for compulsory testing, for quarantine, for isolation, and in one instance a conservative MP went on television and suggested in all seriousness that people who were HIV positive should be shipped off to camps on deserted islands.

There were no forums as yet where lesbians and gay men could be heard or seen, where our voices were coherently arguing and articulating our concerns regarding the disease. There was some very interesting work that was being done in this area by writers, activists, and media workers, and I wanted to bring these voices and images together in one space. Stuart Marshall, Simon Watney, and Isaac Julien were some of the people whose work was exemplary in setting the agenda and the parameters for a discussion on our own terms and using our criteria.

My other concern in the video was to show the diversity of discourses around sexuality, racism, representation, and AIDS. For instance, *ReFraming AIDS* shows, specifically, how lesbians and gays of colour in England have been affected by the government's responses to the AIDS crisis, through increased state surveillance, police harassment, and ultimately as an immigration control mechanism. Britain is an extremely racist, nationalist and homophobic society and the media has played a crucial part historically in perpetuating these retrograde attitudes and practices. The AIDS crisis is no exception. The government mounted a media campaign supposedly to educate people about the virus, but in effect the campaign further perpetuated fear and ignorance. In the video, I was concerned with deconstructing the messages of the media campaign mounted for television.

The video shows the work of filmmakers, writers, and photographers who were creating their own representations as a direct challenge to the retrogressive messages of State-controlled media. Isaac Julien's short video, *This is not an AIDS advertisement*, an important intervention at the time, showed desirable representations of gay men at a time when they were equated with notions of illness and disease. The media campaign's message about safe sex was anti-sex, and about control over people's sexuality, desires. and sexual behaviour. Isaac's video was a challenge to that in its celebration of gay male desire.

Sunil Gupta's photographs of gay men in India showed how the notion of AIDS as a white gay man's disease had spread internationally to the detriment of local populations. Both these artist's work was included in the video as a way of attempting to recontextualize the debates around race and sexuality. There are many historical links between ideas about racial difference, social difference and sexuality. In British colonial history, just as homosexuality was seen as a disease, so was colour — racial "types" other than white were considered outside the norm. If AIDS has created the current backlash, it is within existing historical contexts using prejudice, notions of racial type, sexual type, and sexuality.

Feminists have a long history of critiquing State responses and methods of control over women's bodies, whether through abortion laws or reproductive technologies. Lesbians and feminists have been at the forefront of AIDS activism because many of us have already experienced the ways the media and the State attempt to control women's bodies and minds. The experience of political activism and articulating challenges to the dominant political moral agenda has been extremely useful for recent AIDS activism.

The AIDS crisis has dramatically effected many Third World countries, and while it has been thrilling and strengthening to see the extent of AIDS activism both in North America and in Europe, it has been of some concern to me that such activism has lacked an internationalist perspective. It is crucial to have a global perspective, to move away from parochialism and inwardness. In Africa, AIDS is pervasive: whole populations are dying, and have been dying for a number of years, yet there is very little coverage of it. When there is, it constructs Africa and Africans as the "Other," removed from the rest of humanity. Poverty and economic devastation in many African and other third world countries, caused by First World economic policies, are also partly responsible for the lack of resources and funding for health care facilities.

Furthermore, some of the divisions and fragmentations that exist around issues of race and culture within the lesbian and gay communities are sometimes duplicated within AIDS activism. There is not enough acknowledgement of lesbians and gays in black communities and communities of colour who are not only struggling against the racism of their white lesbian and gay peers, but also against the homophobia within our own communities. As AIDS continues to effect all sectors of all communities, it is imperative to work on several fronts.

Recently, I read a U.S. government report which said that twenty-five percent of all reported AIDS cases in North America had been diagnosed in black people, although black people comprise only twelve percent of the total population. According to the same report, fifty-two percent of all women infected with the AIDS virus are black, sixty-one percent of all babies born with AIDS are black, and the statistics get worse . . . Every two hours a black person dies of AIDS. These are statistics which should give us real cause for concern yet I haven't seen much evidence of what things being done, not only by the government, but also by various communities who are organizing around AIDS in order to stop the decimation of all people, regardless of sexuality, race or gender.

I made *ReFraming AIDS* several years ago, yet I feel that the points it raised are entirely relevant today, particularly within the context of the Fifth International Conference on Aids.

Postscript : March 1991

Since June 1989, and since making the video *ReFraming AIDS*, I have continued to be active in issues around the AIDS crisis. In these intervening years I have met activists from ACT UP in New York, from whom I have learned a lot about anger, loss, and grief. It has also been positive to see a maturity in political organizing where coalitions are being developed at between different communities.

In August 1988, black youth Yusuf Hawkins was murdered by white youths in the Benson Hurst area of New York. There were public rallies and demonstrations, one of which I went to, and marched with the ACT UP banner. It was a bizarre situation: we were being "protected" by lines of policemen on foot and on motorcycle. During the two hours we marched, a group of men followed us shouting the most continuous stream of virulent homophobic invectives I have ever heard. Yet the resolve of ACT UP members to be out and visible at an anti-racism rally organized by the black community did not falter. This solidarity helps "keep the faith" in knowing that the AIDS crisis has given birth to a generation of activists for whom there is no time to waste.

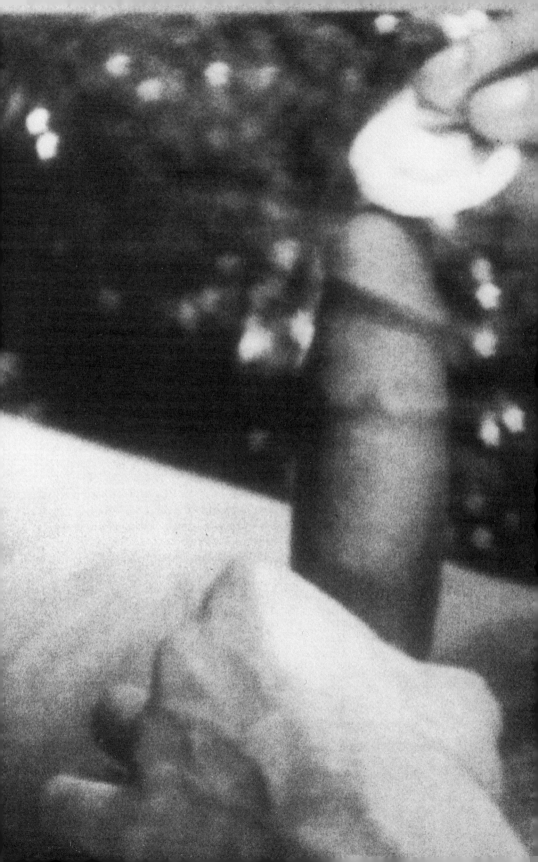

PORNOGRAPHY AND BEHAVIOUR CHANGE

Erotica and Behaviour Change:
The Anthropologist as Voyeur

Bernard Arcand

We are often reminded that we inhabit a world that enjoys, and even promotes, quick judgements and short-term analysis. New ways of understanding social phenomena, and indeed new theories of society, appear to emerge from public opinion polls, from the latest topics of discussion in the street cafés of Paris, or the most recent trendy exhibitions in New York.[1] An anthropologist, however, should not be concerned with such fashionable modes of ready interpretation, and I intend to comment here on the long-term historical context within which AIDS must be located when considering sexual behaviour.

By now, we have all heard the suggestion that AIDS has modified people's sexual behaviour. According to some analysts, *because* of AIDS, the sexual revolution is truly over and the time for relatively careless experimentation has passed. This suggests, of course, that we have been thrust into a new era: a time for restraint and for careful conservatism — a time when the ideal model of the safest possible sex would advise making love to oneself (someone we *really* love, as Woody Allen once said). In this context, then, pornography could easily be seen and understood as somewhat of an alternative and a useful stimulant for masturbation: a means of escaping from a more active sexuality that has become too uncertain, if not blatantly dangerous.

Such analyses are in fact as narrow as the opinions we usually expect from fashion magazines, public opinion polls or letters to the Editor. The causal relationship between AIDS, pornography and sexual isolation is largely an illusion or, more precisely, a coincidence. Indeed, I would go further and claim, with care, that AIDS probably could not have fallen on a more appropriate society. By this I mean that its impact would have been far worse in societies other than our modern post-industrial world (it indeed is much worse today in other societies). Furthermore, I propose that a society that generates pornography is also best suited to face such an epidemic, and that the relationship between the two phenomena is only a coincidence.

In other words, we should be more careful before crediting AIDS with having modified sexual behaviour. It seems more likely that these changes, which we have been able to predict for a long time, have now come about, and continue to occur, quite regardless of any epidemic. What we are noticing now appears to be the result of the conjuncture of a number of cultural elements that have developed progressively over the last few centuries. What follows is a summary of four of these long term trends.

First, and with all due respect to Susan Sontag, long before AIDS could be turned into a metaphor, we in the West convinced ourselves that pollution and danger come to us from others. As Claude Lévi-Strauss learned from his grandfather, the Rabbi of Versailles at the time, the outside world is a permanent menace and source of disease: an idea which is typical of our culture, and contrasts sharply with the beliefs of many South American Indians, namely that the danger to the world resides within us. In other words, at the same time that our notion facilitated, and even advanced, the destruction of the environment (the destruction of nature as well as the elimination of other societies), our culture prepared us to close in upon ourselves in the face of external danger. We are thus easily convinced that avoidance is safer and, when facing urban violence for example, it becomes quite appropriate to warn children that foreigners are dangerous.

Secondly, we should not be very surprised by the link between sex and illness. Human sexuality has been essentially a medical matter in Western culture since at least the eighteenth century. Taking over many of the traditional roles of the religious moralists, medical officers have generally become the accepted guides for appropriate behaviour.[2] Some opinion polls have even shown that most people's *first* concern about sex is health. Sex, which used to be fun, or scary, useful for survival, sinful and evil, has now turned into a bodily concern. And thus, most people seem very well prepared to listen to the sexual advice of medical science, whether this comes from psychiatrists or epidemiologists.

Thirdly, we have recently become the first society (known to anthropology) which actually promotes masturbation. All other societies consider this activity a rather marginal, secondary and minimal form of sex. Masturbation may be tolerated with mild contempt or declared an offence punishable by death, but in all cases it is seen as something done in the absence of a better solution. Yet, modern sexology recently changed all that by offering the radical proposition that sex is fundamentally an individual and egotistical act, one in which the partner is first and foremost a *means* to achieving self-expression and fulfilment. In other words, the sexual partner should serve as an aid, comparable to tools, or gadgets, or pornography.[3] We have become convinced, along with the vast readership of the Hite reports and Nancy Friday's books, that masturbation represents the ultimate and best possible sexual experience. Either that or, as recent trends would have us believe, the notion that no sex at all is cool.

174

The great success of pornography between 1950 and 1980 was not simply the result of years of accumulated frustration from the repression of sex. It was (it had to be) also supported by a parallel transformation of sexual behaviour, indeed of social behaviour in general, which reflected a shift in emphasis from the reproductive and communal interests of society to the fullest expression of individual concerns. These were the days when the notion of essential human rights took on new meaning, and deviated from collective and shared rights to focus on the protection and defense of the individual person. In this respect, the authorities who censored the pornography that was rampant in London towards the end of the eighteenth century[4] out of their fear of seeing the working class reproduce too fast and increase in a way that was perceived as a threat, were probably misguided: not so much because one doesn't usually read while making love, but because pornography is associated with declining birthrates.

Finally, and possibly most importantly, all these modern trends offer the radical view of sexuality as something that can be considered, in and by itself, an activity which is divorced from the rest of human experience. This is another example of the unique fragmentation that industrial society invented, and which was necessary to allow the reduction of human beings to a labour force; once muscles and brains became commodities that could be bought or sold with little regard for the rest of the person, sooner or later, sex was bound to follow. Without this segregation, pornography would be impossible. And the fragmentation is maintained: masturbation is not something one does at the workplace.

The struggle against AIDS is easier in a culture that is prepared to deal with sexual experience on its own and in relative isolation, thus not requiring, or even claiming (as most other societies would), that in order to modify sexual behaviour one must at the same time transform every other facet of life, from inheritance rules to the cosmological ordering of seasonal variations. When I stated that AIDS could perhaps not have found a more appropriate target, I was referring to a culture that is prepared to have medical officers formulate the official advice and rules of sexual conduct — a society where one third of the population lives alone and where masturbation is recognized as a valid and often sufficient form of sexual expression — in other words, a society that seems remarkably well suited to instruct the individual to stay home, close the doors, and wait until the doctors declare it safe to come out again. But we must also be aware that this society began to emerge some two or three hundred years ago and that it had been following the course I have described long before there was a social or health problem demanding an urgent reaction. Modern man has been made ready for AIDS.

NOTES

1. Gilles Lipovetsky, *L'empire de l'éphémère* (Paris: Gallimard, 1987).

2. The social management of human sexuality has long been a focus of scientific enquiry. References here are easy to find and I wish to mention only Michel Foucault's rather massive history of sexuality *Histoire de la sexualité* (Paris: Gallimard, 1976, 1984 and 1984).

3. André Béjin, "Crépuscule des psychanalystes, matin des sexologues," *Sexualités occidentales*, P. Ariès and A. Béjin, eds., *Communication* 35 (1982): 198-224.

4. Paul-Gabriel Boucé, ed., *Sexuality in Eighteenth-century Britain* (Manchester: Manchester University Press, 1982).

Do It! Safer Sex Porn for Girls and Boys Comes of Age

Jean Carlomusto & Gregg Bordowitz

There's a scene in a kitchen. In the middle of the night a guy gets up to get a snack. He is joined by his lover who gives him a rim job through a dental dam. Then one of them licks whip cream off the other's balls. Finally, one puts a condom on the other, squirts honey all over the condom-covered cock and sucks the hard candied dick.

In another scene, a woman is lying on the couch watching television and masturbating with a vibrator. She looks up to see another woman standing over her holding a towel. She unfolds the towel to reveal dental dams, gloves, sex lube and a dildo. One goes down on the other using a dental dam. The other dons a glove to finger-fuck her partner. The two spend the rest of the night exploring possibilities.

This is our job. As the Audio/Visual department of Gay Men's Health Crisis (GMHC) in New York we're charged with the task of producing safer sex video educational materials for the purpose of getting the message out that you can have hot sex without placing yourself at risk of AIDS. These videos are to be instructional. They have to demonstrate how specific acts, such as anal, vaginal, and oral sex can be made safer. The material has to be culturally relevant — rendered in ways that are meaningful to specific audiences. Lastly, the material has to exist in a form that makes it easy to distribute as widely as possible. And, with all this to consider we still have to make the girls wet and the guys hard. To start, we had to come to a clear "safer sex" definition.

Safer sex, of course, is a means of disease prevention. Too often discussions of safer sex are reduced to debates about various modes of HIV transmission — debates that overlook the fact that there are many sexually transmitted diseases and viruses that may compromise one's immune system. Safer sex is a set of individual decisions one makes about one's sexual life in view of one's health

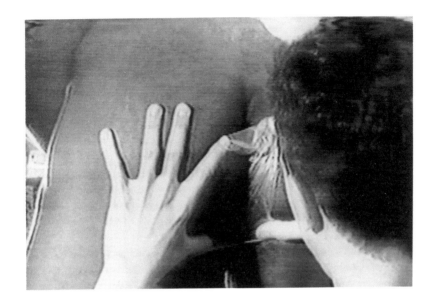

GMHC, *Midnight Snack*, 1990. Safer Sex Short, still from colour video.

concerns. And since pleasure — the ultimate goal — also contributes to one's wellbeing, the message has to make clear that any sexual act can be made safer; that we can get laid safely, get it on, get off and do it!

The safer sex videos we produce are a series of "shorts," approximately five minutes each. The "shorts" are like music-videos — extremely slick images rapidly edited in a variety of ways, on different formats, to resemble some of the most current trends in video production. The "shorts" are non-narrative in structure and dialogue is kept to a minimum, as every explicit scene is guaranteed hot and explosive.

Each video is designed by a task group which chooses the scene, the situation, and the acts to be performed. Each group produces a short with a specific community or audience in mind. There is a black men's task group, a latino task group, and a lesbian task group. In addition, there are scenarios developed to represent the many ways we all get turned on: anonymous sexual encounters (two boys meet and fuck safely in a public bathroom); bisexuality (two guys and two girls get in on safely sharing sex toys as they work on an infinite number of possibilities); sadomasochism (heavy bondage and discipline, between two BIG MEN); and drag (a drag queen fucks her hairdresser before the big show. Safely, of course).

> A construction worker uses leather straps to put a cop in bondage. The worker puts a condom on his erect cock and ass fucks the cop. After, he puts on a glove and fists fucks the cop. End.

Although we will all admit to having fantasies, few of us ever disclose what is actually running through our heads as we make love or masturbate. We are very protective of these fantasies for obvious reasons: our partner may feel threatened if the fantasy doesn't involve him or her, or we fear that bringing these dark fantasies out into the open will somehow lessen their clandestine allure. We internalize our own brand of homophobia that shies away from images of sex because they seem inappropriate. Instead these images stay in our minds where they can remain suppressed except during moments when we want to fan the coals. As safer sex educational video makers, we must employ fantasy to teach about safer sex.

The recognition of lesbian sexuality and the Centers for Disease Control's persistent refusal to include data on woman-to-woman transmission of HIV were the primary motivations in creating the lesbian safer sex video, *Current Flow*. Lesbian-defined sex positive imagery is scarce. While there are hundreds of porn tapes for gay men, there are few created for lesbians. Videotapes depicting lesbian sex created for straight men are available on the shelves of even the most mundane video rental stores. These tapes cater specifically to straight male fantasies about lesbians. Only a few tapes trickle in slowly from the West Coast made for, by and about women, and even fewer of these deal with safer sex for lesbians.

This is both oppressive and dangerous because in order to educate lesbians about safer sex we have to establish what it is. Saying "use a dental dam" is not the same as saying "use a condom," since many women don't know what a dental dam is. And how could they possibly know? It is a latex square manufactured for dentists performing oral surgery! (People like Denise Ribble and the women from ACT UP's Women's Caucus are getting the word out that this little square of latex can prevent transmission of HIV and other sexually transmitted diseases and viruses in vaginal/cervical fluids, or in menstrual blood. This task is enormous.) Our goal was to show some ways lesbians could have safer sex.

In a short for black men who have sex with other men, directed by Charles Brack, a businessman gets into a cab. The driver flirts with him. He reciprocates. When they arrive at the destination, the man in the suit can't find his wallet. Searching his pockets for money he finds some condoms. The driver accepts this currency and fucks his fare on the back seat. Taxi!

Undoubtedly, the AIDS crises necessitated revolutionary action by the lesbian and gay community. Countering the repressive forces behind State-sponsored "just say no" campaigns, the community produced its own discourse about sexuality. Now, with this experience in mind, safer sex education must be developed to address ever widening circles of people among the communities hardest hit by AIDS. Resources must be made available for communities to develop their own forms of education.

Safer sex educational video is a form of direct action. We recognize that sexuality cuts across socially constructed boundaries between races, classes and genders. We make representations that legitimate specific acts — anal, vaginal, oral sex — and we can create an atmosphere conducive to sexual experimentation. In the face of increasing censorship amidst a morally conservative climate, we militantly advocate sex — in beds, kitchens, bars, restrooms, taxis, anywhere you want. If it's safer sex, do it! That's the message.

Reflections on Safer Sex Porn

If the safer sex videotape has become a bona fide genre it has become one in an atmosphere of reactionary censorship and punitive morality. Consider the history behind this criminal lack of [American] governmental responsibility and leadership ten years into the AIDS crisis.

On October 9, 1987, 800,000 people marched on Washington for gay and lesbian rights. Three days later Senator Jesse Helms passed an amendment through the Senate, as part of a Health and Human Services bill, that would eliminate any federal funding for AIDS educational material that promotes or encourages homosexual behaviour.

The materials that Helms found particularly offensive were the *Safe Sex Comix* books published by Gay Men's Health Crisis. The *Safer Sex Comix* are a series of small, eight-page comic books that depict safer sex. The creator of the comic books, Joey Leonte, summed them up in this way: "The idea was that guys would pick them up in the bar and bathhouses, get turned on and realize that all they were seeing was safer sex."

What Helms was attacking was educational material that related specifically to homosexuality and explicit safer sex information. He couldn't make a direct health argument against funding the comic books because there wasn't one. Instead he used a smokescreen of public morality: is homosexuality right or wrong? Is this something you want your federal tax dollars going towards? The irony of the situation was that no federal money had been used on the comic books. Yet the backlash of the Helms initiative was so strong that within days GMHC underwent a stringent and disruptive audit to confirm that no federal money was being spent on sexually explicit materials. Consequently, a study funded by the Centers for Disease Control, one designed to gauge the effectiveness of sexually explicit educational materials, was not renewed.

Currently there are over 90,000 people diagnosed with AIDS in the United States. In the face of this staggering figure the federal government is pushing prudish morality instead of prudent government health policy. We believe that the federal government should be funding a wide variety of community efforts to create culturally relevant AIDS educational materials, regardless of value judgments about sexual explicitness.

The lack of resources to produce educational material, coupled with a repressive atmosphere, has necessitated a guerilla-type production of safer sex "propaganda" that renders options and pictures possibilities. In their form, these low-budget videos are short, fast-paced, visually arresting, militantly graphic pieces that can be distributed in as many ways as possible. The producers steal conventions and add to it a queer sensibility. This work is informed by a rich history of queer avant-garde counter-culture. Thus, there is a keen sense of the ridiculous, self-mockery and appreciation for masquerade in all the tapes.

Safer sex video is a body of work forged through queer resistance to violent heterosexist repression. Any discussion of safer sex materials must start by recognizing that the producers of this material have been seriously limited by two factors: the use of AIDS by right-wing conservative forces in an attempt to repress gay and lesbian sexualities, and the perception by conservative forces within the lesbian and gay liberation movement that the AIDS epidemic is an opportune moment to revise radical thinking on sexuality.

The convergence of these forces has shaped the work being considered here.

The limits placed on the production of safer sex materials explains the form of safer sex video.

There are three principles that are fundamental to the production of safer sex material:

- No representation can instrumentally institute behaviour change. Representational practices can only render options and picture possibilities. The objective of the safer sex shorts is to present a set of options for sexual behaviour that are not pictured within the dominant field of representation.
- We are not the origins of our fantasies. We are constantly mediating, or negotiating, between our desires and images provided to us in culture.
- There is a distinct difference between fantasy and actuality. One may dream of fucking someone else without using a condom. Yet, when one actually fucks, one uses a condom.

Issues of ethnicity and race relations are engendered by the *Safer Sex Shorts*. Everyone involved with the project is committed to producing tapes that legitimate relations between blacks, between latins, between asians and between whites. We are also interested in producing tapes that depict sex between people of different colours.

The inter-racially cast videos reaffirm a number of stereotypical views of race relations. In the beginning of the project, members of a black men's group requested that none of the videos depict a black man getting fucked by a white man. Their reason was that this was a reoccurring theme in industry produced porn that merely recapitulated racism. This view presents interesting contradictions. It assumes that there is something wrong with getting fucked, or being on the bottom. It assumes that an image of a black man fucking a white man does not reaffirm notions of race relations.

In *Current Flow*, the lesbian short, a black woman plays the aggressor with a white woman initially taking a passive position. To some, this scene reaffirmed stereotypes of black lesbians as butch. For those who are aware of this stereotype, this scene can reaffirm this notion. Some may find that stereotype sexually exciting, others may feel trapped by it.

A burden of responsibility is placed on the few safer sex tapes that managed to get produced in the current repressive atmosphere. Ultimately, the answer to many of the questions raised by these tapes is the production of more tapes. Many of the questions raised by the *Safer Sex Shorts* point to important issues about the depiction of sex between people of different colours and the lack of representations of people of colour and women. These questions warrant a continued commitment to the provision of resources to groups of people of colour and women to produce safer sex videotapes for themselves.

We have learned that it is the controlling interests of the producers that determines the politics of any piece of pornography. In the dominant pornography industry the controlling interests are largely those of white straight men, thus most pornographic materials represent the desires and fantasies of white straight men.

Imagine if there were equal access to the resources needed to produce films and videos about sex. Women could make porn for and about women. Black gay men could experiment with many different ways of picturing their sexualities. Marginal groups could develop many different ways to picture sexuality. The limited category of pornography would be exploded and whole new genres and categories would be developed representing the diverse interests and desires comprising sexuality.

Use a dental dam for eating her out.

Cut a condom lengthwise to make a latex sheet.

GMHC, *Current Flow*, 1990. Safer Sex Short, still from colour video.

Working with the Film Language of Porn:
A German View of Safer Sex

Wieland Speck

The first feature film about AIDS — *Buddies*, by New York filmmaker Arthur Bressan — was shown at the Berlin Film Festival in 1984, and I had the opportunity to speak with Bressan. He explained to me that many of his friends were ill. This was something that in Berlin, and in Europe in general, was virtually impossible to imagine at the time. Bressan's film shows gay men struggling to combat the effects of a still very puzzling disease with what few resources were then available. Tests were still unreliable, and people could only guess at how the disease was transmitted. Nonetheless, it was becoming clear that gay men would have to change their sexual behaviour. What was not clear was to what extent.

Buddies was shown in West German cinemas in 1985, but few people seized the opportunity to find out how AIDS was going to affect the everyday lives of gay men. That same year I made my first feature film for television: *WESTLER — East of the Wall*. I had written the story in 1983-84, setting it in 1982-83. I found it hard to deal with AIDS in the framework of an East-West Berlin love story, because in the East the disease simply did not exist. I wrote one scene of a TV talk-show in which reactionary moralistic politicians and a gay rights activist engage in a heated debate about the impact of AIDS on the gay community, but in the end I realized this would just not fit into the film. Instead, I did a sex scene in which an actor ejaculated onto the screen rather than into his lover. Though less than pleased with the stunt, the television station grudgingly accepted it.

As a "substitute" for the scene about AIDS which I had to leave out of the film, after shooting I began working on the problem of how to induce gay men to change their sexual behaviour. I wanted to get as close as possible to the notions of sex as a sensual and emotional experience, rather than an intellectual one. The gay porn industry had not reacted to AIDS at all; the actors in porn videos were still merrily screwing away as if nothing had changed. I also wanted to reach beyond "my" audience, to the home video and commercial nightlife markets. I thought up ideas for six short films in which sexy men have fun with condoms. The watchword from AIDS researchers by then was, "No more exchange of bodily fluids!" Even deep kissing or the slightest scratch was considered very risky.

In 1986, I began to look around for funding. I realized that the videos would have to be technically very good for the industry to take them on, since the idea was to run them as shorts before regular porn films. I regarded this as an interim solution until the industry finally started producing feature-length videos in which the actors put the new safer sex rules into practice. My immediate goal was simply to raise the profile of condoms in gay porn. I wanted viewers to see porn actors using them; I wanted them to realize that safes and sex go together.

While plenty of "straight" skin flicks were being made in West Germany, virtually no gay porn was being produced. I spoke to a Hamburg producer and to West German condom manufacturers, but no one was interested. From 1987 on, fundraising agents of mine tried to persuade producers and distributors in Paris, San Francisco and Los Angeles to put up funding ("Do something so your clientele doesn't die out!") but to no avail. A few porn distributors did tell me they might be able to use the shorts once they were available.

Around this time the AIDS support groups in West Germany were working flat out to ensure that the steady flow of new information about the transmission of HIV was disseminated to the general public. Posters, pamphlets, etc., were produced: all media directed at our understanding rather than at our emotions. Using gay porn as a medium was still out of the question. Then the first safer sex video came out of New York: *Chance of a Lifetime*, by the Gay Men's Health Crisis (GMHC). I discussed the film with gay men and asked them about their attitude towards safer sex. The video, they said, did not solve the main problems, and it was simply not erotic enough to work as gay porn (which it should have been). Like the posters and pamphlets, it was directed primarily at our understanding. I decided I had to get some notion of the imagery of pornographic films.

Pornographic films are a depiction of the sex that is suppressed in the movies we see at the cinema or on television. It is the stringing together of the sequences missing from regular films. But with their own compulsory happy end, skin flicks are as far from the "truth" as the mainstream movies which deceive us with their false representations of our sex life. If our culture were capable of exploring sexuality on film the way it explores the other human instincts, pornography would probably never have developed as a genre. What we get in regular movies is a substitute: after some initial stimulation, the scene fades out and viewers are left to fill in the gaps with conventional ideas of what sex is. This amazingly simple artifice prevents the audience from reflecting on sexuality; the development of sexuality is thus uncoupled from the living organism of culture. The law which all media obey is: "Sex belongs in the bedroom and shall remain as it has always been!" No limits, however, are set on the power games played in the resulting sexual vacuum. Advertising succeeds very well by deceitfully alluding to sex through initial stimulation but finally substituting consumer products for it. We can see killing on TV everyday, but no lovemaking.

This means that pornography cannot depict sex as we experience it in our everyday lives, but only endless variations of the sex act, taken totally out of context, with a rudimentary story-line that follows an inevitable course. Society's desire for perfection is usually well served in porn films. The actors are always young, beautiful and in a state of erection. Since, by definition, pornography consists of the missing sequences from regular films, there is no room for context or character development. Male logic amounts to: if you rub it, it spurts. How could consciousness of vital changes in behaviour be blended into this pro-grammed dream world?

In interviews, the arguments I most frequently heard against the use of condoms were:

- "The safer sex rules are just too complicated, so I don't bother."
- "A rubber can rip, so why use one?"
- "Whenever I try to put one on, I lose my erection."
- "Less sensation when having sex."
- "Putting one on in front of someone is too embarrassing."
- "Buying them is too embarrassing."

All the men I interviewed in 1988 knew more or less what safer sex was. Whether or not they practised safer sex was another matter. In the beginning, safer sex rules were repeatedly revised to reflect new findings about HIV transmission, but they have remained fairly constant since 1988. From a very involved set of purely rational instructions that were difficult to incorporate into everyday life, safer sex was reduced to a few basic principles that were considerably easier to live with. I wanted to make videos that dispelled the old prejudices and showed the safer sex principles being put into practice.

Several Safes are Better than One — Don't Forget Your Lubricant

In the video, *Don't Forget Your Lubricant*, I wanted to show the worst-case scenario of a condom breaking in the middle of anal intercourse. My strategy was to expose the greatest danger right from the start, and not try to gloss over it. A second topic addressed in this video was that of buying condoms. A third topic intended to show that a guy who has only one rubber with him is not properly

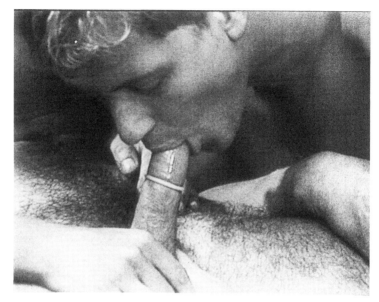

Wieland Speck, *Make Friends with Rubber II*, 1988. Still from colour video.

equipped for safer sex. And the purpose of the fourth topic was to show that a lubricant increases safety.

In this video we see a man trying to buy condoms from a vending machine but he doesn't have the right change. Another man finds a lone remaining rubber in his apartment, puts it in his pocket, and goes out. Next we see the empty condom package, then the two men having anal sex. A picture of a spinning car tire signals "Danger: hot rubber!!" The condom breaks, but the men don't have a second one. Their only option is to seek satisfaction some other way. We see them masturbating each other to orgasm. Another sequence shows a man putting coins into a condom vending machine and shoving several safes into his pocket. In the final shot, the passive partner from the earlier scene advises, "Play safe, take two with you." The film ends with the number two starting a countdown which fades out at nine.

Practice Makes Perfect — Discover Your Rubber

The aim of *Discover Your Rubber* is to prompt viewers to learn about condoms by playing with them on their own. Young men should do their own private "rubber

187

test" before they get into a situation where they have to use one. The embarrassment men, especially young men, might feel when buying condoms is addressed. Other topics are how to put on a condom properly, what it tastes like, how resistant it is, and how to take it off after use.

This video takes place in a typical large city. A young man chooses a pack of condoms from the display in the supermarket. He goes to the checkout counter and puts the pack on the conveyor belt. The cashier rings up the sale without blinking an eye. When he gets back home — we're assuming he still lives with his parents — he immediately tries one on. He wants it to look like the one he sees on a model in a gay men's magazine he has. Then he puts on a second, black safe on top of the first one, plays with it, tests the strength, and pulls it until it rips. He sees that the sperm goes into the reservoir tip. Then he takes the rubber off, ties a knot in it, and disposes of it. He knows the score.

Make Friends with Rubber

Here the rubber itself is the focus of the film, since it brings the two actors together. The first version is shorter than the second and is designed to be shown when a succinct, hard-hitting message is wanted. The second, longer version shows actual intercourse so that a more complex picture of safer sex can be conveyed. The extra time it takes to put the rubber on and take it off, the use of a lubricant, and minor handling problems are not obstacles to pleasure.

As in the previous videos, the characters are introduced in typical porn-film style: a man is on his way home from grocery shopping, and the bag he is carrying rips. A second man helps him pick the things up, including a pack of condoms. The men end up having sex together. One of them inadvertently puts a condom on the wrong way — a "problem" easily solved. We see how a condom should be removed after intercourse. Finally we see the two men relaxing, and the title of the video appears.

Porno 90

This video, just under twenty-five minutes in length is not a short to be shown before regular porn movies, but rather an independent film. It is shown at safer sex workshops for gay counselling and in porn cinemas, and can be borrowed free of charge from sex video shops. Although there are now videos available in which safer sex is practised, whether customers can get hold of them is more or less left to chance. The film therefore seeks to show, not didactically put purely pornographically, that practising safer sex is possible and that it does not limit

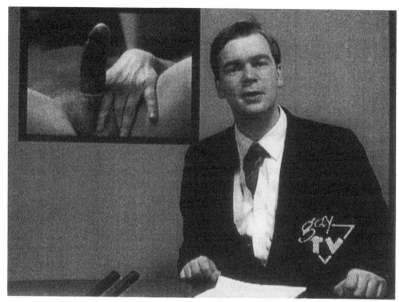

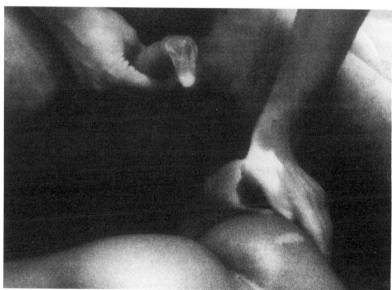

Wieland Speck, *GAY TV*, 1988. Stills from colour video.

sex in any way. Everything that was possible before — oral sex, sex in public places, group sex — is still possible. It doesn't matter with whom you have sex or with how many people; following the rules of safer sex is the only way to help prevent the transmission of HIV.

GAY TV

This film differs from the other videos in that it is intended primarily for the general public. It is a TV special feature, presented as a statement by four Berlin artists (poet Max Goldt, writer Detlev Meyer, composer Eschi Rehm and myself) in which both audio and video components are used to convey basic information about condom use. An overview of products from around the world is provided, and the advantages and disadvantages of each are discussed. Models present the main types of condoms.

GAY TV can be shown where porn films cannot. For instance, it was shown on a giant wall screen in the lobby at the official opening of the German-speaking Young Filmmakers Festival, the Max Ophuls Preis in Saarbrucken. Significantly, the only complaint came from a delegation from Georgia, USSR, who objected to the public presentation of what they regarded as the unpresentable lower half of the male body. Perhaps they were envious of the vast array of condoms, which are notoriously hard to come by in the USSR. Or perhaps it was the culture shock of seeing what they know only as a liberating white spot between a man's legs suddenly come to life in full colour on a Western movie screen. In any event, the question of saving lives by increasing condom use and changing sexual behaviour went completely over their heads.

Since all the other videos were intended as porn films, this one had to be made so that it could be used for discussions at public events. Discussing pornography proved to be impossible. Porn either works or it doesn't. And whether it works depends essentially on the individual, who reacts instinctively rather than rationally. Opinions, although they can be influenced in discussions, do not have any demonstrable, lasting impact on sexual behaviour.

Whenever the whole series of videos was shown at public screenings, running GAY TV first had a positive effect on the audience, helping them to relax and be more receptive. Because of the taboos about depicting sex, these screenings always attract a large audience, from all social classes and sexual orientations. Yet viewers are under a lot of stress because they are afraid their own sexual desires will be exposed.

This was evident when the series was presented in the symposium Erotica, Safer Sex, and Behaviour Change, at the Fifth International Conference on AIDS in Montréal, 1989. The medical corps came in such droves that we had to switch rooms, and video monitors in the hall and on the rooftop terrace had to be turned on. Many of the physicians present were seeing for the first time explicitly what their international reputations had been founded on: men having sex together.

After my presentation, I received stacks of business cards from doctors and social workers who wanted to use the videos for AIDS prevention programs in their own countries. Representatives from Latin America, in particular, but also from Southeast Asia, said that it was very important to show the videos, but that similar material could not be produced in their own countries. This has resulted in the cooperation between international agencies and the German AIDS support group, *Deutsche AIDS-Hilfe*, which are doing everything within their power to help distribute the videos. It is definitely to the credit of the organizers of the Montréal conference and its parallel cultural event called SIDART to have included aspects of AIDS other than the purely medical. These efforts have enabled some crucial steps to be taken in transferring knowledge about prevention from the informed, affluent West to the Third World. That these are only initial steps goes without saying.

Even in Western countries, prevention efforts are constantly facing new challenges: the "success" of safer sex education campaigns among white, adult, gay men is being offset by the increase in the incidence of HIV infection in ethnic groups, drug users, prostitutes, and gay adolescents socialized as heterosexuals by their families. The drive to educate people must be continually renewed, since the media quickly lose interest and show little sense of responsibility in informing the public. In Germany it is now more difficult than at any other time in the last five years to get coverage of AIDS in the press or on television.

Translated from the German by Jim Cookson

Designing Safer Sex: Pornography as Vernacular

Cindy Patton

Going Too Far

In the spring of 1989, I was asked to intercede in a controversy over a sexually explicit advertisement which had been placed in the gay and lesbian community newspaper of Ottawa, the capital of Canada. The ad — which was, in my view, tasteful in the extreme — featured a frontal nude male sporting a condom on his not-very-hard cock. The ad had been produced by a local gay photographer in conjunction with the local AIDS community organization. The photographer's work is widely known in the Ottawa community — portraiture, erotica, news photography, and recently, safer sex posters. His work and his style were so eminently recognizable in the local gay and lesbian community that a Phillip Hannan photograph would seem "natural," would feel as vernacular as a Keith Haring drawing might in New York City.

But this particular photograph created controversy from two fronts: radical feminists were outraged by the appearance of a documentary dick in the pages of their local rag and the safer sex pedagogues were concerned that the dick wasn't hard enough. They feared that condom novices might try to apply a condom before a proper erection. Poor Phillip was caught in the middle: in order to make the ad more acceptable in the pages of a serious newspaper — in order to make the ad visually distinguishable from, say, pornography or bar ads — he had agreed to photograph a model who was at half mast.

The regionally distributed newspaper, *GO*, is published by the Gays of Ottawa, the local gay and lesbian council, but is governed by a somewhat autonomous editorial board. *GO* is somewhere between a house publication and an independent periodical — the latter being the tradition in gay community newspapers.[1] The ad in question was approved by the lesbians and gay men of the editorial board, folks savvy about local political trends.

After publication of the ad, a group of lesbian feminists levied strong accusations: the ad was deemed pornographic, and thus available to the wealth of controversial analysis about the role of such representations in the oppression of women. The women argued that the ad, as a depiction of male sexuality, was assaultive to women, especially to female victims of male sexual violence. Although the hardline anti-pornographers were a minority in the community and among the membership of Gays of Ottawa, other women felt torn by a more inarticulable discomfort with the ad and wanted to maintain their allegiance to their sisters. These women weren't particularly interested in having naked men in their newspaper but had, at least initially, believed that the ad constituted valid risk-reduction education.

The crux of the controversy, at least in terms of the politics of representation, became clear in my conversation with one of the hardline anti-porn women. The woman made clear that she did not oppose risk-reduction education. (I was officially there to lecture on AIDS and during the question period we had a heated discussion about whether monogamy and working toward "deeper" relationships, her favoured solutions, were effective. Her views on the ad were framed by two beliefs — that monogamy is equivalent to safer sex and that pornography leads to uncaring, promiscuous relationships.)

> "What did you feel was wrong about the ad?" I asked.
> "It exposed male genitals," she said.
> "Oh," I said, with an air of conclusion. "I thought you said he was wearing a condom."

"The only weapon we have. . ."

When AIDS emerged as an epidemic in which "prevention is the only weapon we have," new demands were placed on both the imagination and on the languages of sex. The apparent need to define unequivocal methods of conveying and reinforcing safer sex information[2] collided with arguments about the limits of good taste, the nature and offense of pornography, the meaning of sexual representation and the role of fantasy. "Your brain is the biggest sex organ," became a cry of the 1980s.

The different styles of safer sex information-giving parallel closely the forms of sexual representation and representation of the body which emerged in the 1970s and 1980s. At first, categorical information (in the cool, we've-heard-it all rhetoric of sexology) declared that promiscuity, anal-penile penetration, and oral-genital contact were suspect practices. Very soon, a Methodist how-to rhetoric took over as men pursued workshops and exercises designed to "eroticize safer sex." But cultural and subcultural variations in "gay" sexual and

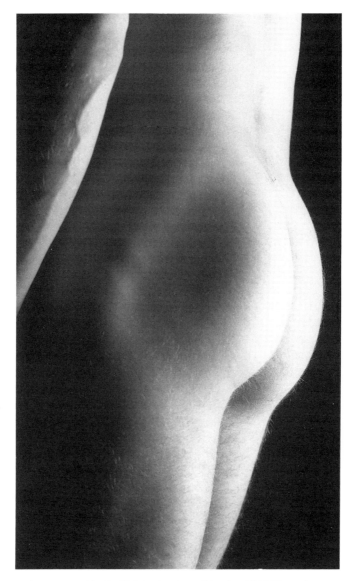

Images used in the Risk Reduction ad for the AIDS Committee
of Ottawa campaign, published in *GO Info*, November 1988.
Photo: Philip Hannan.

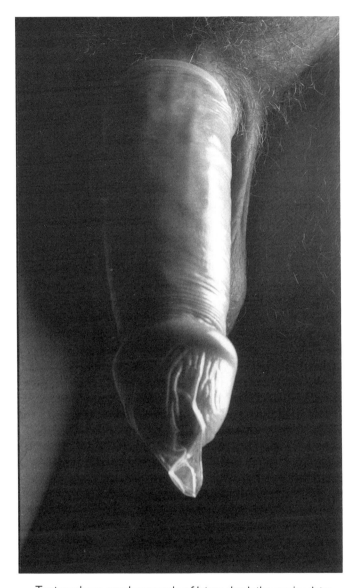

Text read: use condoms made of latex; check the expiry date; practice while jerking off; use water-based lubricant — a drop in the tip; place at the end of the cock; pinch out the air at the tip; roll it onto the base of the cock; use lots of water-based lube before inserting; pull out soon after coming — hold the rubber at the base of the cock; never re-use a condom.

learning styles threw up obstacles to the largely middle-class, psychobabble-oriented "Hot, Horny, and Healthy" and "Meeting Men" style of workshops (however successful these were/are at introducing a new set of relational styles, values, and terminologies to a core group in the most visible gay male communities). There was a recognition that "outreach" had to occur, and the programs needed to be changed and expanded; the terms "culturally sensitive" and "sexually explicit" were bandied about as if the former were a category of narrative preference and the latter were a marker of realist representation.

Both terms, however, were already overdetermined; they cut both ways. On one hand, "culturally sensitive" suggested a hands-off, community self-determination ethos. Sexuality is not largely considered a culture in itself, but rather an artifact *of* cultures. By the time "cultural differences" were a common concern in gay community-based AIDS groups (around 1985 or 1986 in the hardest hit dozen cities), the hegemonized "clone"[3] cores of the gay community were well into a new sexual austerity. It had complex roots attributable most obviously to the multiple problems of the AIDS epidemic (care for friends and lovers, fear, and despair) but also related to the aging of and the career demands on an upwardly mobile baby-boom cohort. This "austerity" was visible in many ways: in the closing of many bars, declining attendance in other gay clubs and entertainment-oriented businesses, an apparent increase in monogamous relationships (or at least reversal of stated values about monogamy and "leisure sex"), and in the increase in concern about "sexual compulsion" and "substance abuse."[4]

Cultural sensitivity came to mean the way those people who couldn't understand straightforward medical terms talked about sex. Outside the gay communities grappling (however badly) with their own diversity, "cultural sensitivity" became a new form of voyeurism for public health officials and clinicians who mastered the quaint vernaculars of their charges. Both within the discourse of the gay community and in public health practices, those who "need" cultural sensitivity are measured against a middle-class, white norm; they are more than simply "different," they are lacking in both the decoding skills and the behavioural and social values of the mainstream society. They are deficient at best (gauged by whether they "change" once they receive a "culturally sensitive message") and potentially recalcitrant.

The practices that were deployed under the rhetoric of "cultural sensitivity" therein worked in two directions and provided part of the basis for the bifurcation into categories: those who had a right to (and could be counted on to respond to) education, and those who could be held legally (through arrest) and medically (through denial of full possibilities of health care) liable for the lack of knowledge which their "risk" behaviour was presumed to represent (regardless of whether they received education, sensitive or otherwise).[5]

In some areas this meant softening medical terms that might seem offensive for some groups, notably those not perceived to be "truly at risk." Thus, when speaking to mainstream heterosexuals, we were to talk of "making love" rather than penile-vaginal intercourse. In other groups, like gay men, it meant not blinking an eye when speaking of rimming or fisting as opposed to anal-oral contact or manual-anal insertion. In all cases, cultural sensitivity entailed scientists begrudgingly giving up their stuffy clinical terms in order to water down the "real" and "specific" language *for* sex into derivative popular terms considered less accurate, and thus at the opposite pole from "documentary," on a realist representational continuum.

Despite the nod toward pluralism, the culturally sensitivist framework, which I want to criticize on specific points here, posits the reality of acts as existing prior to the meanings created around them, and constructs a double-entry system that equates acts with correspondent, technically-correct words. Science-language for acts are more correct than folk terms, which are slightly confused translations. The task of the culturally sensitive educator is to match up existing folk terms with their corresponding science term in order to insure that message conveyed is true to its ideal form. The process involves treating folk concepts as "found" and static artifacts of a pre-or proto-scientific thought system: the educator is "sensitive" when s/he leaves such language as is and covertly determines its match to the ideal terms.

Ignored are the ways the polysomy of folk terms enrich, alter, or are reinvested once they are linked to the dominant discourse through an enforced equivalency that is determined and policed by the culturally sensitive educator. Like the subtle imperialism of late twentieth century anthropology, uncritical cultural-sensitivist educators and clinicians unconsciously accept their own science-language as the standard for reality effects. This acceptance takes place even as they celebrate the "richness" of the speech of the *indigene*, in pseudo-aesthetic appreciation that masks their inability to understand the meaning-potentials of folk terms that indeed constitute a surplus in their own system of equivalencies. Although the talk occurs in the folk language, cultural violence occurs in terms of ripping loose the sexual folk languages (vernaculars) from the objects of scientific/educational intervention.

Using folk terms in the charts and graphs of scientific conferences and educational materials that circulate outside the space of the original vernacular may serve as an authenticating mark for the outsiders because it suggests a qualitative intersubjective validity that shores up mistakes in quantitative measurements of sex. However, this serves to flatten out the folk terms, which lose both their linguistic polysomy and their temporal specificity, and seem like a foreign language when they are pronounced back into the folk culture, no matter how proficient the accent.

An interesting study in England showed,[6] for example, that people preferred being addressed by interviewers in medical sounding language, even though they often did not fully understand these terms. Likewise, injecting drug users and street teens feel offended when outsiders use their vernacular, and sense that even the most sensitive professional is using the "street terms" inside quotes. Vernaculars cloak group identification; *indigene* defences are diminished when vernacular is colonized.

The idea of sexual explicitness, too, bore this scientific/realist mark; it was as though there were a bare, mirror representation or language of sex. But instead of filtering "correct terms" through a posited "culture," the sexual-explicitist framework views the downest, dirtiest words as most accurate to the user: anything less than unvarnished prose is marred by repression. Bawdy terms place sex in a bodily context rather than a clinical context; they were used within clinical discourse in rather the same way as foreign terms, which are always used but remain italicized to indicate their otherness and their magic power to convey meaning, all the while remaining untranslatable. But because bawdy terms are perceived by explicitist translators to have a privileged relationship to a bodily or sexual reality, there is no mechanism for deciding which bawdy terms to use, no assessment of the context of mode of address in which the terms are conveyed, no appreciation for the ways in which sexual rhetorics reinscribe systems of power.

In this framework, linguistic transgression is equated with realism: rather than evaluating specific, local bawdy terms as they operate doubly and performatively in their contexts, the most naive sexual explicitist uses his/her own discomfort or amusement with "dirty words" as the criterion for closeness to sexual reality. This constitutes an inverted, romantic imperialism. Dominant culture's rejection of the validity of "talking sex" in bawdy terms is taken as a validation of these terms. When a subaltern population, unconsciously idealized as "naturally" less "uptight" about sexuality, rejects those very same terms, however, the *culture* of the group is viewed as lacking in the verbal tools to express their unhegemonized sexuality. That the "dirty words" of one culture function to police, constitute, resist, and protect sexual identities and subgroups is lost when these words are stripped of context and inserted into another culture's system of linguistic/sexual constructions.

From 1981 and well into the present, community educators worked from these two frameworks (or practically speaking, from both) in the shadows of U.S. government silence about AIDS. The downside of no government response was no government funding. On the other hand, no government response meant no government interference — education by and for gay men and injecting drug-users could stay within the borders of these fragile communities. The first federal funding to community groups in the United States for risk-reduction education became available in late 1985 under the "Innovative Programs" section of that year's AIDS-related allocations. This came more than four years after the identification of the first cases of what came to be called AIDS. The $400,000 that was eventually granted came with restrictions, including potential censorship by a "community standards" review board modeled on local obscenity-law enforcement, and a requirement that the then-new anti-body testing had to be an integral part of the package.[7]

With the badly needed funding came the inevitable clash over how to do safer sex education. In 1987, Senator Jesse Helms of North Carolina displayed on the floor of the Senate some sexually explicit, culturally sensitive brochures from Gay Men's Health Crisis in New York City. The particular pamphlet that drew the most ire was a cartoon book by a recognizable gay artist, about s/m sexuality. It embodied fringe sexual culture; it was explicit in visuals and language; and, Helms argued, the American taxpayers had paid for it. (In fact, no federal funding had been used on the project, as Gay Men's Health Crisis demonstrated with their scrupulously kept books. This led to an attempt to withhold funds from organizations as a whole, rather than only denying funding to particular programs within an agency.)

Pornography of Life

Most educators from within the hard-hit gay community were convinced that explicit, sensitive material was essential, and that bondage was not the solution to HIV.[8] Helms' outrage had a chilling effect on gay male health education. The gay community, however, had already suffered through long periods alternating between silence and blackmail threats of closet-blasting. In sorting out how far to go in producing material "direct" enough to be useful without bringing down wrath on the gay community, two questions emerged. Were realist portrayals of gay male sexuality inevitably pornographic by definition to a mainstream who wanted to hear nothing about it? Was conventional pornography (as a one-hand sex) "safe" regardless of whether it had transferable didactic value?

Porn producers, educators, and community activists became divided over these questions. The questions themselves ran through a range of discussions — Is sex a drive, a compulsion in some people? Could wo/men make choices about safer sex? Did certain environments lessen one's ability to stick to safer sex? Could someone consent to unsafe sex? Whose responsibility was an individual incident of safer sex? Who was responsible for establishing new norms?

These questions prompted controversy, anger, and accusations of, on one hand, denying the reality of an epidemic, but on the other, denying the demands of desire. Did they promote unsafe sex or promote paranoia about sex? These arguments were intransigent both within the gay community and among anti-pornography feminists. In both arenas, debate was thwarted by a failure to clarify assumptions about sexuality and about representation. Surely groups ("audiences," "target populations," "subcultures," "hegemonic culture") bring a range of readings to a particular representation of sex, and safer sex educators must work within the logics of interpretation that are established and/or evolving within communities. The theories that inform approaches to safer sex (both personal approaches and organizing strategies) must begin to accommodate the lessons of gay social constructionist theory and decades of folk knowledge gained by gay/lesbian community activists.

Community Organizing for Safer Sex

Popular and formal analysis of safer sex organizing begins with the premise that sexuality is learned through immediate communication and observation in both "public" and "private" social venues, and through mediated observation and communication, including medical texts, popular press, how-to books, and pornography. For each person, the particular matrix (of public/private, communication/observation, texts, identification with social categories, and subsequent punishments and pleasures experienced "from" a range of subject positions in a range of social fields) creates a set of registers, or decoding strategies, or a hermeneutic, which in turn positions him/her in a network of policing, advice, sexual possibilities, styles, erotic preferences, and closets.

Every culture, and sub-groups within every culture, has public and private sexual languages with strong rules concerning the appropriateness of speaking such languages "out of bounds." Dirty jokes, double-entendres, and sexual leers are probably the classic and nearly universal modes of public sexual discourse, but medicalized discourses about the sexual (like the charts of Ronald Reagan's colon in an era obsessed with anality), as well as graffiti, euphemism, and pointed polite silence, are also forms of public sexual signification.

Sexual languages vary dramatically and are important in some cultures — gay culture, for example — and unimportant in others. Sexual languages vary by class, gender, ethnic group, age, by location and even time of day. Sexual language employed in the marketplace is not the same as that used late in the evening in the bar, even between the same interlocutors. Thus, determining what is "appropriate" use of sexual language, or how a set of sexual ideas will be interpreted, requires an understanding of the register of usage and the people likely to recognize that register.

Furthermore, gendered and class-based differences in terms of access to "the public" intersect with public/private languages so that, for example, men engage in a public language (for example, porn film viewing in XXX cinemas) in the absence of women. It is precisely this absence of women that constructs as "public" those particular words/texts/performances on that particular occasion. Likewise, men of different classes use public language to signal their status and to domesticate other men, for example, obtaining labour from a repairman during a board meeting. Here "public" becomes a social construction doubly defined by the absence of a certain class of people and by pre-existing social power differentials that enable the dominant class to display and enforce exclusion. Indeed, in the first case, exclusion is enforced by the very "public" language used (i.e., by producing a social logic in which a woman harmed in the vicinity of the XXX theatre is liable for her transgression of the "space" corresponding to the "language") unless a man appeals to a countervalent language, for example, "She's my wife."

Now, some would argue, "If you don't like it, don't look at it." Unfortunately, public and private collide in contended areas of social power: the live and let live, "peek-a-boo" politic of pluralism is impossible in a society penetrated by circulating symbolic capital (taxes, money) and by mobile media that threaten previous linguistic cordons (*Playboy* at the 7-Eleven; gay newspapers surveilled and rendered as "evidence" in right-wing publications). The curious ideology of taxes, which constructs the public will within the collectivity of purchasers, made the Gay Men's Health Crisis pamphlet fair game for public debate. Direct-mail letters informed right-wing supporters of the details of the pamphlets which the *New York Times* did not find "fit to print." While the language in the GMHC pamphlet was "targeted" and considered "private" by participants in s/m culture, the right wing considers it not a language to be left within its intended venue, but a language to be scrutinized in order to reveal the hidden truth about homosexuality and AIDS.

Sexual vernaculars are learned contextually. Members of such language communities experience cultural recognition not through visual, ethnic-like identification, but when *what you say* is meaningfully decoded by another person. Sexual vernaculars are the identifying characteristic of liminal or threshold sexualities — being "in the life" historically precedes more visual markers of subcultural affinity. Only when a vernacular reaches hegemony does it seem to be a "natural language," a coherent language with a legitimate parentage. Thus the dominant language of heterosexuality, by its claim to naturalness, intimidates those who operate within the liminal space of minority sexual vernacular.[9]

People from certain subgroups become afraid to speak their native tongue when their "texts" — a red hanky, a turn of phrase or cut of suit, a pamphlet, a book, an ideology — though private, suddenly come under scrutiny and become public, rendering the inner language and symbols of the micro-culture vulnerable to unanticipated readings by an Other with greater discursive power. On the other side, members of hegemonic language communities feel their territory has

201

been invaded with languages they do not wish to acquire (perhaps because these languages highlight, sometimes for the first time, their experience of the space and irregularity of the borders of their arbitrary and unjustifiable coalition of power).

New Right moralists sound every bit as pained as feminists when they speak of being forced to confront pornography. Neither their differing definitions of pornography, nor any quality of rhetoric or empirical analysis of the quantity of their pained, personal testimonials, can be used to adjudicate demands for censorship. It is also nearly impossible to demarcate acceptable and "obscene" language through literal zoning because dominant society, in fact, already "contains" the micro-cultures dispersed in its landscape of sexualities. To zone is to excise, demand speech from and then quarantine the sexualities that reverberate in the register of suppressed bodily pleasures. But we need not construct an ethic that valorizes any/all policed sexualities just because we do not yet have a basis for deciding between conflicts over sexual rhetorics and the harms/privileges they claim. It will seem relatively clear to sympathetic readers of this volume that Jesse Helms is trying to suppress legitimate sexual vernaculars; but how to adjudicate access to and control over the narrow space of a counter-culture, as in the pages of the *Gays of Ottawa* newspaper, is another question. Can the common outrage at Helms and the diverse and conflicting outrage at the *GO* episode be differentiated within an ethic that takes seriously the responsibilities and rights of autonomous groups? We can imagine many ways of keeping Helms' hands out of our business, but can we construct an ethic that enables us to critique and learn across our own divisions and vernaculars?

In this context then, "sexually explicit materials" — deemed "pornographic" or obscene by outsiders — are but vernaculars formed within the hermeneutics of communities or micro-networks. There is no spectrum with repressed sexuality on one end and liberated sexuality on the other, each with its own "natural" language. That pornography has been useful as a mode of communicating concepts and values about safer sex among some sectors of the gay male community does not mean that "pornography" should be used with everyone (or even that other groups should identify their own "pornographies" and reproduce them in a safer sex form). Rather, it suggests that pornography is a vernacular form for some networks of men. Pornography works not because it is "explicit" and leaves no room for doubt, but rather, because it is a richly ambiguous mediation within a complex vernacular.

Every group has sexual vernacular that is internally "explicit" in the sense that terms have some correspondence to meaningful gestures, acts, or concepts within the sexual imaginary and practices of the group. Embarrassment or discomfort occurs when the traditional limits of a group's vernacular are transgressed, when the "line is crossed" — but the line is specific to the group in its relationship to the mainstream culture. What is important is to identify how values and concepts about sexuality and sexual practice have been effected within a community or micro-network. The mediated and situated aspects of that symbolic process — whether rap songs, dirty jokes, girl-talk, how-to books — are the material templates for safer sex organizing.

Imitating or reproducing such vernacular does not represent a move away from "euphemism." Rather, it represents a dangerous step into the most intimate cultural process. In order for such vernacular productions to be rich and useful to sexual cultures, in transition as a result of the new needs of the HIV epidemic, they must be consistent in *form* (oral, written, pictorial, gestural), in *aesthetic*, and in *mode* of cultural circulation. The last is probably the least examined area, and the one most often violated in the quest for "cultural sensitivity." Outsiders can often catch on to form and aesthetic (acquire a "second language" of sex), but rarely, or only after considerable time and error, can they master the choreography and pathways of group symbolic interaction. By the same token, however, the ways of being within sexual cultures are difficult to articulate for members of the culture, precisely because the processes of acculturation are performative and unformalized (indeed, forming acculturation processes that are invisible in a critical line of defense for marginal sexualities).

"Safer sex" is a cultural intervention which may work entirely within existing cultural economies, or may stretch the edges of the economy, but cannot be imposed from outside. Mediated forms are not more "real" or "accurate" material thrust upon a repressed or ignorant group: that amounts to sexual imperialism. Mediated forms work within the conceptual logics of a group and must circulate within the borders of the micro-culture to renew and inform the symbolic processes of groups as they struggle to make changes and make sense of the new demands on sexuality of HIV and related political backlash. The task of safer sex organizers requires committing members of another sexual culture. It requires participants in cultures to risk articulating some other way of life in order to work together to reform sexual cultures that resist both disease and social oppression.

NOTES

1. Newspapers for the lesbian/gay community have emerged worldwide since the early 1970s. There was a handful of news- and feature- (as distinguished from literary or avant-garde) publications devoted to gay/lesbian issues from the mid-century homophile movements in the U.S. and Scandinavia — luscious, underground or coded "skin" magazines (largely physique magazines which only ambivalently acknowledged that their aesthetic was desired to be easily appropriated by working-class, subcultural homosexuals), and the longstanding *Advocate* from California which slightly predates gay liberation. The increase in new periodicals stems from the inspiration of gay liberation and from the importance of the radical and underground presses of the new social movements of the 1950s and 1960s. Newspapers linked geographically dispersed homosexual groups — some highly organized and longstanding, some little more than transient social networks — with little in common beyond the as-yet unspoken scars of a shared history of oppression, and a vague idea of a homosexual desire or essence. There emerged an "imagined community" (to extend Benedict Anderson's notion) which debated political strategy, the meaning of "being gay," producing a set of core values and social mores that gave rise to a sense of "lifestyle," social (if not geographic) place, and accompanying identities. The importance and role of the gay media in generating the gay/lesbian subject in postmodernity has yet to be theorized. On media, see John D'Emilio, *Sexual Politics/Sexual Community* (Chicago, 1983), and Michael Bronsky, *Culture Clash* (Boston: South End Press, 1984). For a possible conceptual source on the relation between media, language, "nationalism" and community see Benedict Anderson, *Imagined Community* (London: Verso Press, 1983). A fruitful materialist account of the relationship between lifestyle/community and cultural artifacts is Pierre Bourdieu's *Distinction* (Cambridge, MA: Harvard University Press, 1984).

2. Unequivocal, but not univocal: the "education" for gay men was initially offered as a mode of breaking the silence about AIDS promoted by the mainstream culture. It was recognized that the information could and should be offered in a variety of forms. As control over this enterprise of "spreading the word" shifted away from a small number of well informed and politically engaged groups to mainstream news media, and as divisions in strategy arose between AIDS groups, educators began seeking something like "teacher/learner-proof" ways of communicating about safer sex. The media and government — and many gay groups — were initially criticized for their silence. After about 1985, "safer sex information" materials were criticized for undercutting "neutral information" with encoded moral judgements. Use of the term "promiscuity," for example, with its longstanding cultural meanings, was said to misdirect risk-reduction efforts toward reducing partners and producing an inefficacious "trust," instead of toward condom use, or not practising penetrative activities. The problematic of safer sex information has shifted over time in relation to the investments of the producers of the information. But nearly all the arguments were based on a belief in the potential neutrality of information, and on the belief that anti-body testing produced a relatively uniform experience which could form the common basis for the later integration of the information that, together, would produce behaviour change.

3. Clone culture is, roughly speaking, the "new" image of gay masculinity, circa 1980, made common by mainstream media representations of these "ordinary men." The style can be characterized by 501 Levi jeans, the work shirt, the bushy mustache and short, neat hair. In addition, clones characteristically dated clones, creating a kind of homo-gender role homosexuality in contradiction to the contemporaneous popular that gay male culture comprised butches and queens. There was more than a little anti-queen sentiment in clone culture, which generally also tended to be middle-class and white. While clone culture ushered in a more positive mainstream image of gay men, this came at the cost of disdain for homosexual men

who veered outside the masculine gender role which clone culture only slightly stretched. The clone image has been widely, diffusely associated with a lifestyle that "causes AIDS" since this was the first group of men represented as "having AIDS."

4. Whatever the numerical realities of the latter, the rise in concern about excesses of pleasure marched lockstep with the mainstream, Reaganite views on drugs and sex. Some effort was made to articulate drug and alcohol abuse as an effect of homophobic oppression rather than individual pathology ("addiction is a disease"), but this view was difficult to assert relative to sex (no doubt because of its centrality to gay identity) without appearing to claim that gay men are, in some essential way, self-destructive. Within the gay community, sex was perceived to be more importantly linked with HIV/AIDS, as both the pre-condition for the epidemic, and the mechanism — in the form of "safer sex" — for stemming the epidemic. Thus, "sexual compulsiveness" had a different valence, and was less accepted as an "issue" than gay substance abuse, although the latter appeared as a separate issue. Indeed, an advertisement for a major gay-operated detox. and therapy unit claims that more gay people die each year from chemical dependency than from AIDS, an obviously problematic set of rhetorical equivalences. This stands in marked contrast to rhetoric of the Black Power movement in the 1960s and, to a lesser extent, the African-American political infrastructure, which asserts that drug-control patterns have resulted in a disproportionate, negative effect on drug use and trade within urban African-American neighbourhoods.

5. I take up this complex issue of the cultural/political economy of safer sex education in my book, *Inventing AIDS: Discourse/Resistance* (New York: Routledge, 1990).

6. Kay Welling, "Preliminary Report on a Pilot Study," presented at The Social Aspects of AIDS, conference, South Bank Polytechnic Institute, London, February 1989.

7. It is important to the history of the political economy of AIDS education and the access to clinical trials and prophylaxis to recognize the ideological significance, in 1985 and through the present, of linking anti-body testing with "risk behaviour change." It was assumed, with this first funding requirement, that anti-body status knowledge would change and reinforce behaviour: no data supported this view and health education wisdom was divided on this type of "confrontation with reality"-style of education. The original testing mandates were an experiment in social engineering, and one which most current data suggest failed. Studies by the Centers for Disease Control, and recently by the National Cancer Institute, find no correlation between knowledge of anti-body status and behaviour change. Certainly such knowledge affects individuals in a wide variety of ways related to health beliefs, social and psychological support, community attitudes, to suggest only a few. With new calls for early testing in order to take advantage of early advances in PCP prophylaxis and with the hope that low-dose AZT can hold off immune system depletion in asymptomatic people until a better drug can be developed, it is critical to understand how behaviourist ideas are embedded both within the testing system and in public attitudes toward HIV policy development. It will be a difficult task politically (and educationally) to transform the testing system, designed as a sexual behaviour change experiment, into a system for early diagnosis of HIV. The relationship between the testing system and AIDS/HIV policy are pursued at greater length in my book, *Inventing AIDS*, op. cit.

8. At the First International AIDS Conference in Atlanta (1985), Donald Francis, of the Centers for Disease Control, presented a mathematical model which showed how the new epidemic could be stemmed if all "gay men" were tested and had sex only with people of like anti-body status. His presentation seemed absurd, ignoring that many men have sex with men who are not "gay," ignoring the efficacy of safer sex, and treating gay male sexual culture as a giant dating service where serostatus (rather than love, desire, compatibility) would be the chief selection criterion. However, this idea of using serostatus as the *condom sanitaire* permeates AIDS prevention strategies on both the individual and social level.

9. I want to be clear that heterosexualities also have local vernaculars. However in this case, users' relation to state and psychiatric policing is different since they, at least in the contemporary era, are seen as enacting variations on the sexual category viewed as normal. With the exception of extreme forms of sex-linked violence and overt child-oriented sexualities, liminal heterosexuals are largely considered "kinky" rather than pathological.

Yell When It Starts!!

Ralf Konig

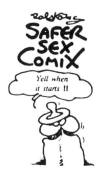

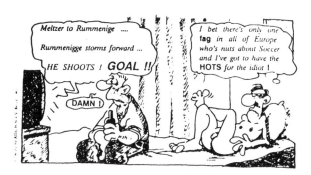

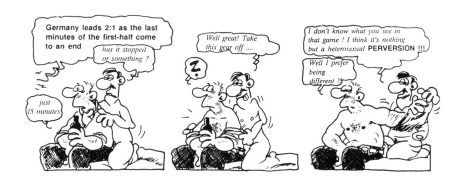

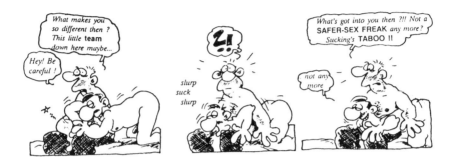

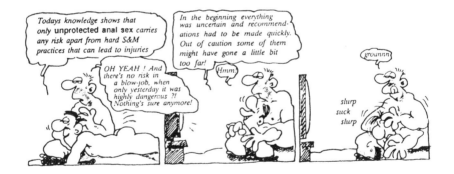

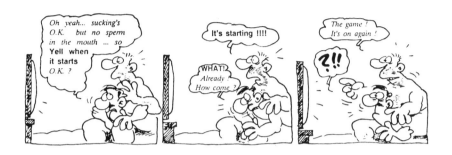

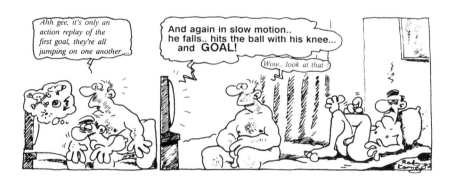

Popular Safer Sex Comix, Deutsche AIDS-Hilfe, 1987

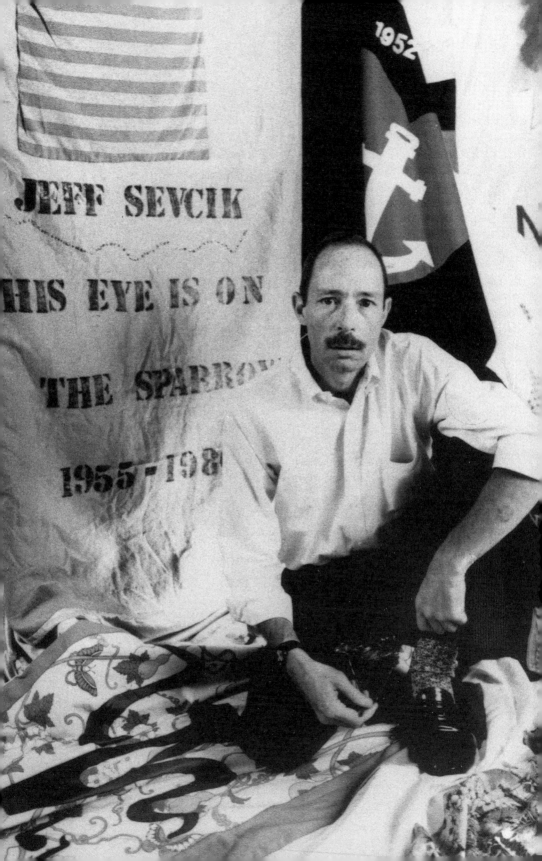

NAMING IT: LITERATURE AND AIDS

Forty Seconds of AIDS

Herbert Daniel

Deep down, I believed like everyone else: it's very hard, it's a difficult shock, it's a blow too heavy to bear, it's an earthquake, the start of a journey with no return. No one, in fact — this is what I believed — is prepared to receive news like this. At least that's what I thought until I myself received the news: you have AIDS. I got the news and it really was the start of a journey. I understood then, and not without irony, that no journey in life has a return and that life is exactly this: the possibility of an eternal second chance always lying before us. The best place in the world is here. And now.

Not that I was prepared. No one ever is. I began preparing myself, as everyone does, for living with my new conditions. Conditions for living, I repeat to make it perfectly clear, that I don't mean the circumstances of a predetermined and forcibly imposed death. I learned right away, during the health crisis that led to the severe diagnosis of my condition, that my life cannot be reduced to being defined solely through AIDS. I only have AIDS. As for what I am, I evolve, being what I am not and never was, a continuing possibility that I am from day to day, as are others.

Yet I wasn't unprepared. I was alive. I am alive. The most frightening thing, and I write these pages in protest, was the absolute unpreparedness of the doctor who gave me the news. He was unprepared. The illustrious representative of a fossilized style of medicine that has more in common with terrorism than science, was not prepared to deal with people — ill or not — he was prepared to deal with machinery, bacteria, torture, and murder.

Some stories don't seem to happen to everyone. This is one such story worth telling because it happens to many and involves a plot whose threads weave through our bodies.

I got sick. For many reasons, I didn't believe that I could have AIDS. Not the least of which was the fact that I refused to accept such a drastic hypothesis. After all, we never believe the "worst." And AIDS is always presented as the "worst thing." Besides, I didn't feel, nor do I feel now, that I could have the "worst thing in the world." There are worse things. (I have lived through worse things.

Dictatorship. The loss of freedom. Exile. Going underground. Mass murder and torture. Remember the years of authoritarianism?) I say this without wanting to take any seriousness away from AIDS, but merely to place it in due perspective. It isn't the "worst thing that could happen to a person." It is a tragic situation. It is a disease; it is not a melodrama.

Although many things about my body might have made me suspect that I had the disease, I didn't imagine it possibly happening to me — mainly because what I was seeing in myself didn't correspond to the typical "pattern" of the disease. Another thing that I have learned is that every case is a case in itself, and that the medical definition of AIDS is a theoretical generalization which must be discussed not only in terms of signs and symptoms, but also from the standpoint of the great myths of "incurability" and "fatality." I still don't mean to diminish the seriousness of AIDS. It is, for the moment, incurable. It is fatal. But it is not only that. Or more importantly, AIDS is not "essentially" that, as the prophets of fear and discrimination would have us believe.

In short, I didn't suspect that I could have AIDS because I didn't "look like" a person who was sick with AIDS. Now glancing in the mirror, I know what a person with AIDS looks like. By the way, this is an exercise that anyone can do in front of the mirror, to see the famous face facing AIDS. (I also learned that, although my "personal" case is particular to me, nothing leads me to suppose that mine is different from all the other cases. This is an epidemic. We are a multitude. We are living a story of our time. And it will be up to our time to find an answer to this story.)

In an emergency, I sought out a "doctor" (the quotes are used so as not to offend other worthy professionals, like those who treated me with such solidarity later on). I didn't know him, but I had recommendations as to his "technical competence." (A huge mistake! The technical competence of a doctor should be measured by his humanism, not by how well he has been trained to respond with conditioned reflexes. What's more, even technically he soon proved to be a charlatan. I won't say his name. There are many others just like him. He is most valuable as a symbol. Divulging his name solves nothing, since it might even lead him to believe I want to start some sort of polemic. And that might even end up adding to his vanity.)

In any event, I trusted him to tell me what evil was tormenting me. What patient doesn't make this sort of transference? During the examination, he left me seated for half an hour, naked, on the table, after taking a sample of my saliva for analysis. Dizzy with fever, with visible signs of a pneumonia that had prostrated me, I waited.

He came back, ordered me to dress and told me in three sentences that I had pneumonia of a type caused by *Pneumocystis carinii*, "a sure indication of an immunological deficiency." He was going to prescribe a medication (which he did, but in the improper dosage); afterward I was to undergo a test which would reveal the "other disease," as he euphemistically called it, that had lead me to this pneumonia. . .

Certainly, in that instant, many of the things that were happening in my body made sense to me. I didn't doubt the diagnosis. I didn't doubt (why should I?) when he told me that he had seen the protozoa. I simply felt the shock that one can easily imagine.

So, in exactly forty seconds the "doctor" gave me the news, gave me a prescription, charged me forty thousand cruzados and dispatched me from his office. Signing the check was a difficult task, mostly because I had to control my trembling hand.

(Some days later, in rather different circumstances, it was confirmed that I had AIDS, but the reason for my prostration had been glandular tuberculosis. I very probably never had the pneumonia that he had diagnosed. He very probably "saw" the P. carinii through the lens of my homosexuality, as so many "doctors" have come to do.)

Forty seconds. That was the amount of time that he gave me to absorb the news. It was sufficient time, however, to give me the horror of seeing, in that clinical indifference, perhaps a touch of cruelty; perhaps "vengeance" on me because I was a homosexual and deserved to be punished? Possibly. One can never really second-guess the sort of sexuality — or behaviour — such a "doctor" actually has.

Horror — that was exactly what I felt. Before me I had a diagnostic device, a dehumanized apparatus that could suddenly entangle me in its machinery and lead me to something even more terrible than AIDS; in the place of death as a vital experience, I faced the indignity of an empty, hospitalized death. Above all, I feared the future which that monstrosity foresaw for me. I knew that I would become subject to a series of infections and, as such, I was afraid of becoming subjected to the infernal machinery directed by this pack of dehumanizing specialists.

I have AIDS. It is a corporal experience about which I still have a great deal to say. But it has nothing to do with the illness there in the eyes of that "doctor."

I left that office deeply troubled. Forty seconds of AIDS! I had escaped. Claudio, my companion, was waiting for me out here. My friends were waiting for me. Life was waiting for me. I freed myself from the frightful disease that had killed me for forty seconds. I escaped — with the conviction that it is necessary to free other sick people from this trap. Real AIDS is something far too serious to be treated by "doctors," by that brand of medicine which AIDS came to prove has failed.

What's left is life. Forty seconds at a time. Intensely.

The Buck Stops Nowhere

Michael Lynch

What is your role as a poet writing about AIDS? How should I know? The arduous production leading to a lyric enfolds that very question. Hearing, singing, sizing, placing a line, sometimes living with it for months to see if it breathes or chokes, deciding to retain and recircle or just to chuck it out — if there are answers they are inherent and provisional, like long-term maintenance strategies during the illness.

Listing backwards, I hear in "Shit" several sonics not so audible in other of my "AIDS poems": to indict, to avenge. In a system (worldwide, national, local) which simultaneously brutalizes the ill and evades (with far more ingenuity than any lyric) responsibility for brutalization — the buck stops nowhere — one must fix one's targets where one can.

Injudicious? Perhaps. But remember this: there were well intentioned persons and benevolent rationales at Belsen too.

Shit

The ordinary props of Indian Summer:
lemongrass after the embarrassments of harvest,
off-centre pumpkins, maple leaves
like yellow watermelon, vines to prune
while leafless. Unseeing, Gram takes a walk
and David copes with diarrhea. Still sighted,
Scott checks in — our first of extrapulmonary
pnuemocystosis, Gord packs his bags

for home after weeks of no treatment
on the ward, and Ross moves into Gord's room
and Chuck moves over to Casey House.
Musical beds of a sort, but instead of them

growing fewer, we do.
A flock of birds we can't identify
shingles the emptying maples, cheeping in riot
to ease the lingering season along,

it doesn't want to go. One step at a time,
says the bird. Or was that me to Gram
for whom the smoothest sidewalk is terror.
Irregularities ahead — don't drag your feet.
He prances like a giraffe.
Try slightly longer steps, I'll warn
of any obstacle. Or was it the bird,
speaking to a summer so suddenly

terrorized it barely budges,
all the more welcome for having overstayed
its welcome. Someone in the flock
finds berries on the wall of creeping
Creeper — CHEEP! — and they all
whir out of the maples,
gorge, and empurple the walks
with diarrhea, not wine.

Now there's a novel prop, one not so frayed
as pumpkins. I pee on the crocus beds
to alienate squirrels, the only way.
But yesterday I peed too much, and today
the sun's so hot
you hold your nose to tour the mums.
We fax the forms to Bristol-Myers
and they write back by post: the forms

just changed. We resubmit by fax,
and they write back by post: they won't
accept a fax of signatures. The clinic
would courier the forms, but
the General takes two days
just to get its mail to the courier.
This program's named "Emergency Drug Release."
I take the forms myself across the street

to the courier. Death by bureaucracy.
Hospitals indifferent or hostile.
Some doctors caring, daring, kicking against
the pricks in the battle for our weal.
An interviewer asks if I use combat metaphors.
Yes, but never for the body:
too well spoken itself
to need the tongues of politics.

A yellow watermelon world, with walls
of flaming Creeper and walks of purple
streaks, and colours not available
to Gram or David, but oh the foot sees
curbs, poured concrete, lumpy asphalt,
pale-ridged interlocking brick.
I buy a durian, fearsome fruit,
rancid to smell but sweet to taste,

they say, I've never tried one.
At 4 a.m. a pain begins, wakes me
to dis-ease. When John Ward
left the General he moved in here.
Heavy diarrhea. Cryptosporidosis.
his parents would not visit,
the chairman of the board, so corporate, so clean.
When finally they came, his Mom wore shades,

a scarf around her neck, long gloves, large hat.
July. She never took them off.
They would not hire a private nurse
when he went home, and later in the General
no one to change his sheets or clean
his mess. A difficult boy, but not
deserving hours in his own cold shit.
From there it worsened.

Dr. Velland gored him with a colostomy
days before he died, alchemizing eyeballs
into pain. John knew
doctor and dad were paying him back
for fouling what they'd made:

worlds without shit, amen.
Torturing him for having loved
getting fucked in the ass by men.

Why are the sites of health and fondness
subject to greatest abuse?
Vilify the ass and cunt, vilify shit,
vilify the purple sidewalk's littering
leaves. Who sings the prostrate?
Love me, love my asshole,
even at 4 a.m. when pelvis pain
supplants November scenes.

A large truck rumbles by, breaking some ordinance.
A little wind comes up , rustling some leaves.
The furnace comes on like a respirator.
I turn through every angle. Pain persists.
I put a tennis ball between the bed and this
muscle, that, but find no point
where pressure eases pain. Philosophy's
consolations come up on the screen:

I hurt, therefore I am. From tent revivals
when I was nine and pompous
a melody sings of power,
power, wonder-working power, in the precious
blood of the lamb. Sings it again
thinking of the ancient shift from entrails
to blood, and how we shift from blood
to bowel. I am my ass. I live,

and while we live, you'll not defame this shit
without a counter-charge.
Wrap yourselves in triplicates, long scarves,
protocols or policy,
we know who you are. Our bodies want
life, our history revenge.
Your patient-management assumed
our patience. No more.

While Security sleeps we take the halls
marking with our shit
the office doors of those
few the angel will pass over.
The rest must go.
Your cleanliness, our corruption.
Your disposable plastics.
Our warm strangling hands.

African Literature:
Witness to its Time

Doumbi-Fakoly

In the environment where, since eight years now, she works, my mother has been brutally quarantined. Those whom she once called friends don't lunch with her anymore. They run from her! Her colleagues avoid her in the hallways. Her boss arranges for her not to be present at the bi-weekly staff meetings. Here, Mr. President, is where I should describe my mother's journey. My mother, you see, is a self-made women in every way possible.

— Doumbi-Fakoly, *Certificat de contrôle anti-Sida*

In order to begin to understand the role literature might play in Africa in response to social issues such as AIDS, it is first necessary to examine the African literary landscape.[1] Embarking upon such a survey, one quickly appreciates the hold the continent's historical and social evolution has on the Black writer. Symmetrical to the form of events, the thematic curve — as we shall see below — strikingly shows the continued identification of the African writer with his/her people.[2] In this respect, the minimal concern shown to such elements as a hymn to "rain and good weather" is an eloquent example.

Faced with the hundreds of expressions of misery that bleed Africa of its vitality, the Black writer's only conviction appears to be the necessity of joining the inner peace of his/her aspirations to the greater welfare of the masses. This is the reason for his/her unceasing involvement in the restoration of the people's dignity and his/her virulent denunciation of the crimes perpetrated against them, with or without their complicity. Triggering off a whole series of new developments, this multifaceted fight leads the writer constantly to readjust sights and choose different tactical weapons.

The Exaltation of the Values of the African Civilization

Redeeming ancestral values has historically been at the forefront of the active solidarity between the African writer and the African people. Misled by a colonial education system at the service of the interests of foreign domination, the Black world needed to recover its memory of the Past in order to find its true place within humanity; an exclusion that had been the result of a certain determinist miracle. It was in this environment that "negritude" made its final revival with the "New Negro" (the 1920s black renaissance in the United States) which was reiterated in *Etudiant noir*, a 1930s magazine. The Black writer of this period, whether a follower of negritude, one of its detractors, or completely neutral concerning this cultural philosophy, was unable to abstain from action in the dual claim for the right of Black People to be different and the recognition of the universality of the values of the African civilization.

The continued distance of Black people from decision-making centres has led to the relative failure of this binary demand. The disablement and lack of self-confidence of Black people, it must be understood, are the direct conse-quences of the absence of any reference to ancestral experience. In this respect, the exaltation of the positive aspects of the Black civilization is still topical. Many invitations of a *Return to the Roots* nature bear close resemblance to Birago Drop's song on the eternity of the soul and reincarnation, the Life Force and the ancestor's presence, all focal points in African thought.

> Listen to things
> More often than to people
> The way of fire is heard
> Hear the water's path
>
> . . .
> Those who are dead never left
>
> . . .
> They rest in the sleeping water
>
> . . .
> They are in the woman's breast
> They are in the newborn's cry
>
> . . .
> They are in the groaning rock[3]

A Wreath for Udomo, a novel by Peter Abrahams; Le pauvre Christ de Bomba, a novel by Mongo Béti; A Dance in the Forest, a play by Wole Soyinke; Xala, a novel by Ousmane Sembène; to name a few random examples, come within the double framework of defending and redefining tradition. The wealth of epic and historical

222

texts[4] demonstrates the same honourable desire of awakening a faithful restoration of African history.

It is nonetheless important to point out that the fight, as fierce as it may sometimes seem, to restore black people to their rightful human dimension — meaning freedom of thought and action — has never been expressed through denial of the Other. Black humanism has always been fortunate in its ability to channel revolt and protest towards the "meeting of giving and receiving," so dear to Aimé Césaire and L. Sengor.

> Men of all continents
> Holding the heavens at the end of outstretched arms
> Those who like to hear women's laughter
> Those who like to watch the playing child
> Those who like to join hands
> And form a chain
> Bullets still take off rose flowers
> On dreamy mornings [5]

The Anti-colonial Struggle

The African writer's personal conviction is that a people cannot exist without culture and that culture, by definition, is our ability to "domesticate" both nature and the cosmos allowing us, in turn, to live in harmony with them. In this way, the writer continually invites his people to pursue their rediscovery while urging them hereafter to take fate into their own hands.

In the subsequent analysis of the socio-political context, one important point stands out: no conqueror alone is able to keep entire peoples, a whole race in fact, in shackle through obscurantism and oppression. The judicial system they establish will see the same procession of defendants and accomplices march by: the colonists, broad-minded, the uprooted, and other alienated individuals.

In *Climble*, author Bernard Dadié symbolically denounces genocide in Africa at school. Fernand Oyono (*Le vieux nègre et la médaille*) and Abdoulaye Sadji (*Nini, Maimouna*) claim to produce proof of the successful alienation of Black consciousness. In *Le pauvre Christ de Bomba*, Mongo Béti presents his perception of Christian self-complacency in the same realistic manner as Oswald Mtshali in *Back to the Bush*.

> You taught me that I must not
> Kill the black bull for my ancestors.

223

You also taught me
How to feather and carve
the Christmas turkey[6]

Whereas the principle accusation of Ferdinand Oyono (*Une vie de Boy*) and Mongo Béti (*Mission terminée*) concerns the suffering inflicted on the poor, Sembène Ousmane (*O pays, mon beau peuple*) focuses attention on the obstructive tactics colonialism used against intellectuals returning home from studies abroad.

This face-off between the black writer and the alienated colonizer lasted for only a short period for the majority of African writers. Born in the 1950s (with *Coeur d'Aryenne* by J. Malonga, *Nini* by A. Sadji, *Ville cruelle* by Mongo Béti),[7] it lost its reason for existing, as independence came without warning throughout Africa. In the unliberated territories the Front would remain active for a while longer.

In the end, Agostino Neto and Ezekiel Mphahlele put away their pens and work in the warm comfort of refound liberty in Angola and Zimbabwe (formerly Rhodesia). Only a few, such as Peter Abrahams and Dennis Brutus still brandish the torch of humanism summoning South Africa and Apartheid to the judgement of history.

A Critique of the Administration of Independence

With decolonization the Black writer could have attained his/her objectives if it had brought the expected promises. But, self-rule appeared as unreal as a mirage.

The dark shadow of colonialism still hangs over Africa. The former native collaborators, now the new masters, have found it difficult to discard the old habits of the *aide-de-camp*.

The national middle class, with its blunders and baseness, now sustains the revolt of the Black African writer. Identified as the new opponent, the resulting displacement of the Front is dealt with in *Remember Ruben* by Mongo Béti with the same distinguishable cry which only recently (as in *Ville cruelle*) had been directed towards colonial rule. *Le bal des caïmans* by Yodi Karone, and *Le pacte de sang* by Puis Ngondu Nkashama must be inscribed within this framework.

This critique of the post- and neo-colonial systems is also vigorously expressed by many other writers and is far from draining all the militant energy of the African writer.[8]

In the reconstruction of the new Africa, the themes of mobilization come up again and again: social criticism — in *Tu t'appelleras Tango* by Calixte Beyala and *Une si longue lettre* by Mariama Bâ;[9] the necessary identification of youth with traditional African heros — *Amour-cent-vie* by Werewere Liking;[10] race solidarity;[11] culture shock.[12]

224

The African writer's desire to win these multiple battles necessitates a new strategy. As they increasingly gauge the scope of their role as developers of conscience, they must redefine their relationship to their people. They have acquired the certainty that it is not enough to be the "mouthpiece for the misfortunate who no longer have mouths."[13] To communicate their message, they admit that they must, above all get, under the skin of the people and attain total fusion with them, like the souls of ancestors taking possession of the bodies of new-born babies. A radical mutation of literary practice came about, character-ized by adopting a lexicology and style better capable of conveying the sensibil-ities that these writers wished to express.

Insofar as the writer presents the most representative characters often expressed in foreign languages, they now see their responsibility to best serve African thought and/or to suffer the possible contortions of circumstantial use. This is why once certain characters venture into European linguistic territories, they have all the scope to colonize phonetics (as in *Une vie de Boy*, by Ousmane Sembène). This is also why word transcription, transposition, and African turns of phrase have been so common (e.g., *Crépuscule des temps anciens* by Nazi Boni; *Le dernier de l'empire* by Ousmane Sembène; *La grève des Batus* by Animata Sow Fall; *Les soleils des indépendances* by Ahmadou Kourouma).

It must be added that the constant concern for intimate communion with the people — whose aspirations and anxieties the African writer wants above all to present — is now giving rise in some countries (for example, Nigeria, Uganda, and Senegal) to literary output in their national languages, as had already been advocated by Thomas Mofole in *Chaka*.

The advantage of this new literary trend lies in the increased accessibility to a large number of potential readers. Only increased literacy is necessary.

It is important to note, however, that despite the African writer's consistently close alignment with the concerns and desires of the people, they have curiously been absent in the general mobilization against AIDS. Two important questions emerge here: do they perceive themselves as powerless against the fate imposed by this pandemic? Or do they find it degrading to respond to the absurd Western campaign aimed at conferring African birthright on AIDS? For the time being, it seems presumptuous to seek to outline a working hypothesis when the African writer's silence is so dense that literally no impression seeps through.

My own novel (*Certificat de contrôle anti-Sida*) won't allow us to circumvent the posed questions. Alone on the African literary landscape, it seems to express an isolated feeling: the narrator's anger when confronted once again with an expression of anti-African racism, this time fed by pseudo-scientific arguments.

Whereas the African writer may have kept his/her distance, African artists (especially painters and musicians) have not been insensitive to the pandemic. Two musicians have endowed us with works of high quality, dealing directly and primarily with the battle with AIDS: Hilarion Nguéma (*Le Sida*) and Franco (*Kéba Na Sida: Fais attention au Sida*). Franco, who later succumbed to the condition, found it indispensible to warn the African youth. In his song, moreover, he calls an entire population to action: pregnant women, students, men, women, workers, bureaucrats, white-collar workers, preachers, rabbis, nuns, and others.

O AIDS, horrible condition
AIDS, darkness unforgiving
AIDS, darkness inescapable
O, this plague AIDS, which leaves medicine powerless

. . .

Infected brothers and sisters
Don't search to spitefully spread it to others

. . .

All strata of society are touched by AIDS
It can happen to anyone who doesn't protect himself

Educators, teachers, professors,
At school, in class or on the playground
Whenever you have a spare moment
Take time for an informative chat
It is part of your scholastic obligations
The latins said "a sound mind needs a sound body"

Researchers around the world. . .
Don't waste precious time fighting

Doctors, you know well how AIDS is spread
Don't show your patient that you are afraid
Don't destroy, by your words or actions, his morale
Even when he is on his last legs
For, through you, the entire medical corps will take courage
To treat this horrific disease
You, from rich countries. . .

You, arms dealers. . .

Political authorities
Use radio, television, newspapers
To inform your population about the dangers of AIDS.[14]

226

Returning now to written African literature, we notice that its evolution is not an isolated phenomenon. It has been accompanied by a disruption in the bibliographic structure, which seems to be an important element to discuss. First, it is important to identify two external factors that have been advantageous to African literary production.

The appearance of publishing houses in Africa (Cle in Yaoundé, Nea in Dakar-Abidjan,[15] Horn in Ibadan, Transition in Accra, etc.) and also outside of Africa (Présence Africaine, Harmattan and Karthala in Paris; Naaman in Québec[16]) who work to promote African authors is the most important development in the growth of Black African literary production.

At the same time that these newcomers are breaking the monopoly of European publishers, the creation of national and international literary prizes[17] constitutes a second external promotional factor, acting as a counterbalance to foreign literary prizes, that are suspected of being tainted by paternalism and "folklorism."

These conditions have allowed African writers to express their own sentiments more freely. Their bountiful cry, nourished by the sap of falsified social relationships and rigged international "friendships," gives them the inspiration that makes African literature so rich, so diverse and so masterful.

African literature has, however, developed unevenly according to genre. The original literary architecture has been noticeably modified: poetry is in the midst of a deep crisis, whereas theatre is trying to maintain its present momentum; the short story and the novel are the preferred instruments of creativity at this time.

Two particular reasons explain this change in the Black African literary landscape. The first stems from the nature of the genres and public response to them. The Black writer actually seems more comfortable in the infinitely richer world of the novel and the short story. Here s/he can create a filmic universe with as many close-ups as suits his or her senses. Concerning the specific impact on the public, theatre, without a doubt, touches only a small minority except in its popular forms such as Koté-ba (performance-party): the "illiterate" majority favour television, while poetry, unless recited as part of a play or in another show, arouses less and less enthusiasm. Potential readers appear to get something out of the escapism that the novel and the short story offer.

The second reason lies in a widespread policy of the new publishing strategy. Driven by market pressures, the publishing houses have opted for what is, at least from a management point of view, the healthiest approach: as poetry sells badly and theatre has difficulty defending its market, publishers have chosen to direct their efforts towards the distribution of the short story and, more particularly, the novel.

In this survey of African literature, two salient points remain:

1) There was a visibly united struggle before independence. When the African writers took up their pens to redeem ancestral values or denounce the impositions of colonialism and its accomplices, their cause was the liberation of all of Africa, not a single country. The general trend today is to confine the struggle within national borders as if the African renaissance were little more than fiction, and national culture lay outside the context of Black African civilization.

Using this division as a pretext, many publishers no longer hesitate to mention on book covers that it is a Senegalese, a Malagasy or a South African novel. The appearance of these national literatures, in contrast to continental solidarity, is, in all evidence, the logical consequence of the successful balkanization of Africa, something which the Black writer dreaded prior to independence. Worst of all, by narrowing their sphere of activity, national literatures have provoked a nationalist reflex in African readers whose interest appears to be limited to their own country's novels, short stories, theatre, and poetry.

2) The world of African literature is a universe where too often the hero drinks the bitter dregs of failure. Dreams — which could awaken self-confidence and help gain a better future — rarely follow reading. Is it an illusion to produce only supermen and superwomen? Certainly not. We would only like to point out that where there is an opening towards better prospects, and when the seemingly impossible is brought into the realm of the probable, imagination could help produce miracles.

In this respect, it would be instructive to reflect upon the science fiction novel and its scientific and technical implications; the spy novel and its extension into political and military strategy; the fascination of young people for Western literature where the hero always wins.

N O T E S

1. The period covered by this study is the second Africa — the colonial and neo-colonial occupation.

2. Translator's note: the masculine is used here to denote what, in the original French text, had no gender specifications.

3. Birago Diop, *Leurres et lueurs*, Présence Africaine.

Écoute plus souvent
Les choses que les êtres
La voie du feu s'entend
Entend la voie de l'eau

. . .

Ceux qui sont morts ne sont jamais partis

. . .

Ils sont dans le sein de la femme
Ils sont dans l'enfant qui vagit

. . .

Ils sont dans le rocher qui geint

4. *Soundjata*, a story by D.I. Niané; *Béatrice du Congo*, a play by B. Dadié; *Abraha Pokou*, a play by C. Nakam; *L'exil d'Alboury*, a play by C. N'Dao; *Une si belle leçon de patience*, a play by N.M. Diabaté.

5. Bernard Dadié, *Hommes de tous les continents*, Présence Africaines, 1977.

Hommes de tous les continents
Portant le ciel à bout des bras
Vous qui aimez entendre rire la femme
Vous qui aimez regarder jouer l'enfant
Vous qui aimez donner la main
Pour former la chaîne
Les balles étêtent encore les roses
Dans les matins de rêves

6. Vous m'avez appris qu'il ne faut pas
Tuer le boeuf noir pour mes ancêtres

Par contre vous m'avez appris
Comment plumer et découper
La dinde à Noël

7. With the exception of *Karim*, by Ousmane Socé, published in 1935.

8. L. Kibéra (*Voices in the Dark*, a novel); Kuma N'Dumbe III (*Kafra Biatanga*, a play); A. Kourouma (*Les soleils des indépendances*, a novel); B. Dadié, (*Mr. Thongo Gnini*, a play); A. Sow Fall (*La grève des Batus*, a novel); W. Soyinka (*Kongi Harvest*, a play); M. Sunkalow Keita (*L'archer Bassari*, a novel); M. Alpha Diarra (*Sahel, sanglante sécheresse*, a novel).

9. *Trois prétendants, un mari*, a play by G. Oyono M'Bia; *Xala*, a novel by O. Sembène.

10. *Béatrice du Congo* by B. Dadié; *L'exil d'Alboury* by C. N'Dao; *Abraha Pokou* by C. Nokan; *Soundjata* by D.T. Niané; *Amilcar Cabral*, a play by Kuma N'Dumbe III.

11. *Le sang des noirs pour un sou*, a play by Elebe Lisembe; *La décision*, a play by C. N'Doa; *L'étudiant de Soweto*, a play by Moundsé Naindouba.

12. *L'aventure ambigue*, a play by C.H. Kane; *La plaie*, a novel by M. Fall; *Sous l'orage*, a novel by S.B. Kouyaté.

13. A. Césaire, *Cahier d'un retour au pays natal*, Présence Africaine.

14. O le Sida, une terrible maladie
Le Sida un mal qui ne pardonne pas
Le Sida un mal qui n'épargne personne
O ce fléau le Sida qui laisse impuissante la médecine
. . .
Vous frères et soeurs qui êtes déjà atteints du Sida
Ne cherchez pas méchantement à contaminer les autres
. . .
Toutes les couches de la société sont touchées par le sida
Le sida peut tuer n'importe qui qui ne cherche pas à se protéger
. . .
Educateurs, instructeurs, professeurs
A l'école, en classe, pendant les vacances
Dès que vous avez un moment de libre
Consacrez-le à une causerie éducative sur le Sida
Ça rentre dans vos obligations scolaires
Les latins disaient qu'il faut un esprit sain dans un corps sain

Chercheurs à travers le monde . . .
Ne perdez pas votre temps à vous disputer

Médecins, vous savez mieux que quiconque comment le Sida s'attrappe
Ne montrez pas au malade que vous avez peur de lui
Ne détruisez pas
Par votre langage ou par votre comportement
Le moral du malade
Même si il est mourant
C'est par vous que tout le corps médical prendra courage
Pour soigner cette terrifiante maladie

Vous des pays riches. . .

Vendeurs d'armes. . .

Autorités politiques
Utilisez les radios, les télévisions, les journaux
Pour informer la population des dangers du Sida . . .

15. These two publishing houses are presently experiencing difficulties.
16. This publishing house ceased operating several years ago.
17. Grand prix de littérature d'Afrique noire, etc.

Translated from the French by Michael Bailey.

Two Songs

Michael Callen

I don't recall having much to say about my experiences . . . and song/
performance as an educational tool in the context of AIDS. People seem
to be moved by my songs.
                                        — Michael Callen, 1990

How to Have Sex in an Epidemic
Michael Callen

There across a crowded room
Stood the man of my dreams
He was a long and lean
mean sex machine
packed in tight 501 jeans
Ooooh, he looked me over
from my head down to my shoes
Then he said, "Sorry boy,
but where you been?
Ain't you heard the news?"
He said "Oh , no, I'm not crazy,
I don't take no chance
I don't kiss, I just reminisce
And I keep it in my pants"

Chorus:

Oh I'm goin' crazy
Will someone tell me what's a poor boy to do?

231

They say I can't do this
and I can't do that
Oh, I'm soooo confused
Can't it be like the fantasy?
Can't it be like it used to be?
Can't it be like the fantasy?
How to have sex in an epidemic
Without getting caught up in polemic

Home alone, late at night
Takin' matters into my own hands
Lay back, relax, betamax
playin' those
"Boys in the Sand"
Achin', Shakin'
Just a-lookin' for a little release
When in burst the P.C.
(Politically Correct)
Safe Sex and Thought Police
"Stop right there!
We've come to put you to the test
You'd better call your lawyer, boy,
you're under house arrest"

Repeat Chorus:

Oh, I miss the '70s
Things seemed so simple then
So Many men, so little time
Ah, I remember when
Where will it end my friends?
Can you tell me? Who can say?
When what is safe
and what is not
Changes day by day
Got a lemon?
Learn to make some lemonAID
Use a rubber, find a lover
in time you will discover
It's OK to get laid

Repeat Chorus:

How to have sex
How to have sex
How to have sex

The Healing Power of Love
Michael Callen & Marsha Malamet

So many things I wanna do
So many dreams still to come true
So much to give
I wanna be all I can be
I wanna keep you here with me
I wanna live

Got to hold on to life's mysteries
Can't hold out for guarantees
There are none
Together we have come this far
Don't wonder where the heros are
You are one

Be proud of all the courage you've shown
And know that as you fight, you're not alone

Life don't always go the way we planned
Sometimes, you have to take a stand
And if I stumble, can I take your hand?
And feel the Healing Power of Love
Feel the power, the power of love
The Healing Power, the power of love

And if you don't know what to say
A touch would go a long, long way
To show you care
At times I'll wanna run and hide
I may ask you to stand aside
But I'll know you're there

Cause I can feel your strength deep as the sea
I'm growing stronger as it's flowing over me

Life don't always go the way we planned
Sometimes, you have to take a stand
And if I stumble, can I take your hand?
And feel the Healing Power of Love
Feel the power, the power of love
The Healing Power, the power of love

We are all in this together
It's gonna take everything that we've got
It's up to me and you
And I know we'll do what's right
We are all in this together
Whether we know it or not
And I know we can win
If we just begin to fight

Life don't always go the way we planned
Sometimes, you have to take a stand
And if I stumble, can I take your hand?
And feel the Healing Power of Love
Feel the power, the power of love
The Healing Power, the power of love

Performance and AIDS in Zambia

Chandra Mouli & K.N. Rao

Zambia is a beautiful country set in the warm heart of the African continent. The land area is about 750,000 square kilometres and the population is about 7.5 million. The people are mainly African, of Bantu stock, and there is a rich diversity of tribes — seventy-three in all. The official language is English. There are six major local languages and over forty dialects. The influence of the "white man" and his culture have left an indelible impact on Zambian society, but traditional values, beliefs and practices are still very strong. Like many other Third World countries, Zambia is struggling hard to cope with the problems created by a severely and chronically depressed-economy.

Zambia is divided into nine administrative divisions or provinces. Our project is based in the Copperbelt province. The Copperbelt consists of a cluster of towns that have grown around huge copper mines. Large numbers of people are crammed into relatively small areas with all the attendant social problems: high levels of alcohol abuse, crime, broken marriages, teenage pregnancy, sexually-transmitted diseases, and now AIDS.

The problem is compounded by a strong population drift from rural to urban areas. As a result, within the same urban community, there exists vast differences in wealth and education; on one hand you have second-generation urban residents who are sophisticated, educated, formally employed, and fairly well-to-do and, on the other hand, recent migrants who are rustic, illiterate, unemployed or informally employed, and desperately poor.

Our health education effort has to cater to the needs of this diverse spectrum. Within the range of populations to be targeted are some audiences that are extremely difficult to reach. Peri-urban shanty township residents, for example, are a very difficult target group to reach for the following reasons: they have virtually no access to television, radio and newspapers; they are often informally employed and so cannot be contacted at the work place; their utilization of social services (such as schools and clinics) is poor; they may be unable to read information printed in pamphlets or displayed in public places.

As we have learned over time, perhaps the best way to reach these people is through traditional theatre. On holidays and weekends, when people are free from work or religious activities, huge crowds throng the townships. When a drama group presents a free, open-air performance using the street language and portraying real-life situations to highlight a problem, people can identify with it in terms of their own lives. A clever group of artists can make a strong impact on its audience.

An entire show usually lasts about one-and-a-half hours. It begins with drum beats to announce the arrival of the group. Several short, humorous skits follow, designed to hold the growing audience until the crowd builds up to several hundred strong. A play on AIDS is then presented. Depending on the size, mood and composition of the audience, a talk on AIDS may follow. Changes in attire, hairstyles, dialogue and plot depend on the venues and makeup of the audience, but the public response has more often than not been tremendously enthusiastic.

Zambians are a music-loving people. Reggae, rhumba and disco music are very popular. From the word go, we were determined to tap this powerful medium. A British music teacher who teaches at a local school helped us to produce a song containing a powerful, positive message set to a racy beat and a catchy tune. We are in the process of launching a record with a song entitled, "One woman — one man, let's start a new fashion . . .," on one side and a local language version on the flip side. This song can be played time and again in bars, restaurants and homes across the country, danced to, sung along with, hummed along with — and remembered!

Another initiative in this area is our annual AIDS song contest. The idea behind the contest is to encourage young men and women in our colleges and boys and girls in our schools to think about AIDS. One can even direct the line of thinking by giving each contest a specific theme. Previous themes dealt with prevention messages. In 1989, the emphasis shifted in response to the needs of the community, and our present campaign slogan is, "From today, do not think about dying of AIDS; instead, think about living with AIDS."

We are often called upon to give talks on AIDS at huge, open-air gatherings. Audiences would consist of men and women of different ages, from a wide range of tribal, linguistic and educational backgrounds. Here, music is a great unifier. A young church choir dressed in colourful costumes, for example, helps make a strong initial impact and bring the diverse audience together.

Early in our campaign, we realized that paper posters have only a short life span. They are ripped off, scribbled on or washed away by the rain. As a result, we have prepared and installed hoardings, sheet-metal posters and dust bins carrying health messages in strategic locations. A dust bin, fixed to a tree, in a busy urban area can carry a brief AIDS message on the front and health immunization messages on the sides.

In addition to conventional teaching materials such as books, flash cards, and

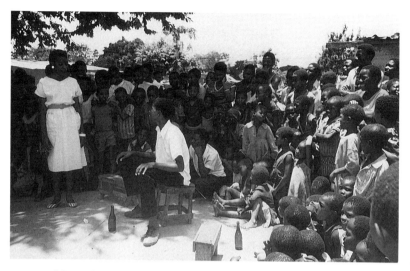

View of a performance in Zambia.

pamphlets, we have prepared special materials to meet local needs. In many parts of Zambia, facilities such as projectors, television sets, video-players etc. are just not available. More basic health education tools are needed. One such tool is our cloth flip-charts, rectangular pieces of linen with messages painted or stencilled on them by hand. A set of seven charts containing a series of messages are nailed onto a stick much like a yearly calender with different sheets for each month. The charts are mounted on a durable, portable, locally made wooden stand before use.

Finally, notebooks and textbooks used by school children in Zambia are published and distributed by a number of large companies. One such organization is the Kenneth Kaunda Foundation. In the middle of last year, we sent them a few health-education messages, requesting that they use them in any way possible. After a little groundwork, a series of drawings and slogans carrying AIDS messages was approved. They have since been printed on the back covers of 4.09 million exercise books and distributed, free of charge, to school children all over the country.

Health education in a developing country is challenging work. There is so much to be done, so many obstacles and so few resources. One could easily feel intimidated and give up without even trying. A health educator must make every effort to identify and tap the resources available within the community: the cultural heritage of the people, such as traditional theatre in Africa, ideas from other communities, the expertise of artists.

237

The AIDS Supermarket:
An Author's Ruminations

Yves Navarre

I have only what I've given.
> — *Hotel Styx*

Excerpts from Yves Navarre's contribution to a roundtable discussion on the role of writers within the context of AIDS. Montréal, June 1989.

It is hard to be a leper and carry this loathsome scourge with you,
to know that it will never heal, that there is nothing to be done
and that each day it spreads and penetrates deeper,
and being alone, enduring your own poison,
and feeling it alive, contaminating,
and dying not just once or savouring it a hundred times,
but without ever getting away from it until the very end,
the dreadful alchemy of death.
You caused this pain, by your beauty

> — Pierre de Crahon to Violaine,
> Paul Claudel, *L'Annonce faite à Marie*

I am no highwire artist, nor am I a tightrope walker; we are conceited to think that we are stronger than words. I am afraid. This evening I will not be improvising. The "unspoken": I have no idea what it means. But perhaps I know too much about it. So, I will deliver this simply, with diction and with emotion.

The moralists have been here. They stayed for a long, long time. The moralists won't be coming this way again. Perhaps this really is the true end of a decade, with its wars, organized by arms dealers; its manipulation of debts by dealers in souls. Down with the temple merchants and the advertising of suffering! Perhaps this is the decadent end of a decade after all, with its plague, its discarded marginals, its rejected, and stigmatized — victims of the cyclical return of a moral order bent on revenge.

We know everything and we don't know anything. We say everything, we say too much and we really don't know anything anymore. AIDS is over-information that has become disinformation. So much misunderstanding, so much that is mis-heard; we are now so accustomed to all kinds of horrors, to unkept promises, to manipulation of images. In the corridors of Ministries everywhere, around the world, we hope. For there is hope. Yet meanwhile, there is loafing around and dilly-dallying all the same.

This evening, you have asked for, and I quote, "a creative response to the challenge of AIDS." You appeal to better understand us, to better appreciate life and love in its various forms, to change our ways of thinking so that we become committed. We are born, once eyes are opened, committed. Either we are or we aren't.

This commitment increases, except that these events are consuming us and we are no longer able to find the words to express it. It is Yves who is speaking now, not Navarre. In the name of Alain, Jean, Alexis, Marcel, Guy, Jean-Marie and Stephan, lovers, happy lovers, friends, happy friends; every few weeks someone close departs. A day doesn't go by without the alarming death of many brothers. It leaves "patches" upon Yves' heart. On an enormous "patchwork" is written: "*Omnia amor*," "Everything is love."

A community of love was the first touched, a head-on collision: a Parisian daily newspaper ran the headline "Gay cancer." The right to be different: no. The right to indifference: yes. The feeling shared by two human beings is without difference; it is the same, the same right to emotion and, from then on, to pain. It is the same risk for everyone. With that said, "patches" are left everywhere!

Ink flows like blood. Yves remembers; Navarre intervenes. Love must be left intact; the moralists must not return. We must fall down from our high horses and fall very much in love, in order to proclaim it, but proclaim it without advertising it, bring attention to it without destroying the very essence of the lover's discourse, with all its gestures, rituals and emotions. To write these texts, this text, I have procured an ink made of blood. I want to read it with the voices of Jean-Paul, Jos, Michel and Alain-Emmanuel.

I have only my life to share.
— *Keiler*

Excerpts from *La Terrasse des audiences au moment de l'adieu* [1]

The press conference was quite an ordeal. Each group explained the results of the day's work. What did I have to say? I have since torn up my short, improvised text. I ended with "No to the AIDS supermarket." Applause. Then this woman began to shout, "this is scandalous, where is this AIDS supermarket?" "Under your feet, Madame." What are the 1,800 exhibitors of the Conference doing here? Cash? Isn't this truly the contemporary marketplace?

Afterwards, I was cornered by four journalists, eager for a quote. The fourth, a French radio journalist, pursued me: "So, you're escaping France?" I answered, in English, "Never complain, never explain." "Translate!" I translated.

The SIDART roundtable discussion, immediately afterwards, included Michel Tremblay, whom I admire, who intimidates me and who I haven't had the time to speak to; a poet from Toronto; a writer from Senegal; and a Brazilian author. Tremblay reigned, simple and sincere.

When my turn came around, I read from *L'Annonce faite à Marie*, presently playing in Montréal. Then I read the prepared text. There was a fruitful discussion afterwards. The Brazilian, a PWA (Person with AIDS), asked, "Is there life before death?" At the end, Michel Tremblay escaped behind a wall of autograph seekers before I was able to greet him. I went to dinner with Jean, G. and L., the organizer of the immense quilt exhibition in memory of the thousands of dead. I went up to my room, dead tired, with the intention of sketching down a bit of the day.

SOUL IN A SLING

Wednesday, June 7, noon. There has been a barrage of telephone calls since nine o'clock this morning. The journalist who yelled scandal when I said "No to the AIDS supermarket," has challenged me to a duel in front of the press. I can't believe it. I should have kept quiet, kept a low profile, but it was good to have spoken out yesterday. I won't be going to this rowdy encounter. I have a book signing at l'Androgyne bookstore from four to six o'clock. As Marie would say, "Take the best and fuck the rest." I give the answer to the French journalist concerning her challenge. It seems that she loves spreading terror and works for a daily that is financed by pharmaceutical labs. Henry Ford's motto will serve as my shield from now on. The terrace will now be considered dangerous territory; I wasn't able to keep my secret long enough.   Another journalist questions me

240

on the telephone. I had been warned by the SIDART organizer, so I prepared this text and read it to him:

> What trap are you trying to set for me? Sensationalism? Do you hear only what you want and create inevitable misunderstanding? I came to this Conference in response to the initiative of the SIDART group. Together with a Brazilian writer, Herbert Daniel, a poet, Michael Lynch, a playwright, Kent Stetson, a Senegalese author, Doumbi-Fakoly and Michel Tremblay. We studied the role that we are obliged to fill, not play, because AIDS is not a game, but a responsibility.
>
> We often have the concept that we are stronger than words, but words can sometimes be stronger than death. They have a therapeutic value. Thanks to SIDART, we were able to have a fruitful and fervent public discussion last night. It is true that I was invited to a press conference, which I attended in order to announce our roundtable discussion and give my opinion of the Conference. I gave my impressions about the fear I feel concerning the commerce that has been grafted onto the efforts of researchers, the passion of scientists and the willingness of artists. Yes, I spoke about "the AIDS supermarket." Do I have to explain that AIDS is not the place for competition, marketing and commerce? That's all. The SIDART group is also at the origin of the quilt exhibition, a immense work of art that speaks so much about life and death and about hope. You must see it. Thank you.

I had hardly finished reading my text when the caller asked, "Is that all?" "It's quite a lot," I answered. He hung up. Nothing. Stop.

Doubt is my one and only certainty
— Le Jardin d'acclimatisation[2]

Excerpts from an interview with Yves Navarre, Montréal, autumn 1990

I am not a homosexual writer. There is no homosexual literature. I am a writer and a homosexual. There is writing on homosexuality. To put it simply, I try "to be who I am" in my writing, "to become who I am." The person who uses "I" without being serious should beware. I don't know how many times I've repeated this over the past twenty years.

With AIDS, kissing, caressing, two bodies together are no longer the same. It is true that words have a therapeutic power. We should have discussed that power *right away* at SIDART. I didn't think of it until afterwards, out of frustration.

I don't know if there is a debate in France concerning the terms used to describe someone with AIDS. There is no fixed vocabulary. There has been no debate in France since 1789. In the "old country," unhappiness is always for the Other.

How should literature express the "unspoken"? By saying and repeating: love towards and against everything. The durability of this emotion — the indifferent emotion.

The "AIDS supermarket" certainly exists. The "vaccine" is the market of the century. Pharmaceutical laboratories, and behind them, "politics," are fighting it out. I am not attributing humanitarian intentions to them. So many doctors say this, know this, protest against it and suffer from it.

> Advertising misery is no different from its suppression
> — *Le Jardin d'acclimatisation*

NOTES

1. Yves Navarre, *La Terrasse des audiences au moment de l'adieu* (Montréal: Leméac Éditeur, 1990): 181-4.
2. Yves Navarre, *Le Jardin d'acclimatisation* (Paris: Éditions Flammarion, 1990).

Translated from the French by Michael Bailey and adapted by Ken Morrison.

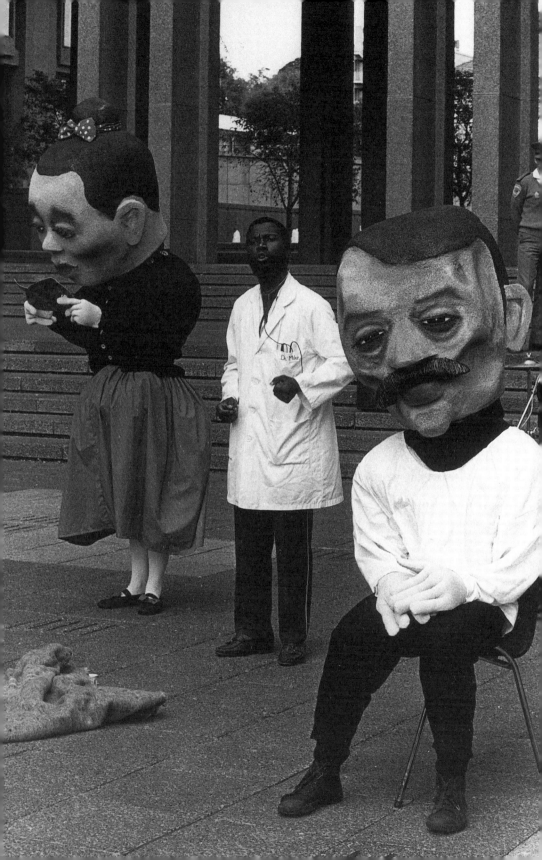

HIV AND CEREMONY: THEATRE AND TRANSMISSION

Theatre and AIDS Education in a North American Native Community

Evan Adams

The smell of burning sage slowly wafts from the stage out through the audience, as BEV slowly cleanses herself and her sleeping sister with the sweet-smelling smoke in their home on the Carston Dam Indian reserve. On the other side of the stage, in his apartment, brother SPIKE discovers a purple spot — Kaposi Sarcoma — as he dresses in stylish clothes in his city home . . . a contrast of experiences and lifestyles.

Thus begins *Snapshots*, a Canadian theatre-in-education piece about the ever more common situation of AIDS and coming home. It is based on real-life experience, inspired by a gay Native PWA's return from the city to his small community along the rugged north coast of British Columbia. He was bravely welcomed and embraced by the entire community, which cared for and loved him, and which, in the end, gave him a burial befitting a chief. This story, plus my own family's acceptance and support of me and my partner of three years, who is HIV-positive, left me with the need to share with others the tradition of caregiving and compassion demonstrated by Native people.

Tackling AIDS prevention education in the Native community has been quite difficult. Why? AIDS is seen as not only a gay disease, but a *white disease* — and an urban one at that. I personally do not believe in the efficacy of the traditional "blackboard approach," that is, education models that do not take into account cultural specificity, literacy levels and past history with formalized education. For example, the hardline assimilation policies of the residential schools have left a strong aversion to many forms of education, including formalized health promotion.

The theatre has tremendous application as an educational tool. It draws people to it, first of all, because it is a cultural event. People come who might not attend, for example, an AIDS prevention education workshop. Also, in the Native community, there is a precedent for its use. In a traditional setting, Native children learn ideas, customs and morals through stories and allegories told in legends and dance. Even today, complex issues like AIDS, that involve questions of sex, death, morality, etc., simply cannot be reduced to the blacks and whites of "do/do not," "right/wrong." Misunderstanding, fear, childishness — are all hinted at in looking at AIDS through story. An image of pain is followed by one of compassion, then of hope or misery. Coming to terms with AIDS (or homosexuality or abandonment, etc.) is a journey. Theatre is the easiest and most effective way to see the path clearly.

Snapshots also allows us to see Native people on stage. Native audiences are pleased to finally see images of themselves created by one of their own. Likewise, the play is about young people as seen by young people — the playwright and actors are all twenty-three years old or younger. This makes it of interest to them.

This success at having a high level of audience identification, however, does not come only from feeding them images of themselves. (The play has been tremendously successful with non-Native audiences too.) The power of this play is that it dares one to identify with the characters whether or not one is young, Native, gay or living with AIDS.

People rarely see or speak about AIDS, sex or dying. *Snapshots* allows them to do just this. It also models behaviour that is safe, sensitive, sympathetic and actively concerned. This is important. The everyday person is not learning to deal with AIDS effectively on a personal level. They can identify with the sisters' varying reactions: surprise, denial, fear, anger and eventual acceptance. Perhaps it is summed up by an observation from one member of an audience: "They are humans; life and death is the same, whether you are gay or not."

SNAPSHOTS

The Characters

SPIKE is a young, gay Native man with AIDS. He lives in the city and is trying to come to terms with his lover's death a short time earlier.

Younger sister, COCO, is a streetwise young woman living on the reserve. She's an IV-drug user and is accustomed to going out on the town and picking up men, without acknowledging that this behaviour puts her at risk for AIDS. Her brother, Spike, is her "best friend" and because of this, she finds his diagnosis and prospective death difficult to bear.

BEV is the elder sister. She leads a more traditional life on the reserve. She is pregnant and single; caring, yet short-tempered; no-nonsense and capable, despite her bad leg. She has had much to overcome, but still lives her life as fully as possible, especially for the sake of those who need her strength.

Scene 1

[MUSIC]

[LIGHTS up on both sides of the stage. Enter BEV as COCO sleeps on the livingroom couch in their home on the Carston Dam Indian Reserve. Enter SPIKE, stage opposite (in his urban apartment), wearing underwear, wiping his face with a towel.

In their respective homes, both do their morning rituals. BEV "smudges," SPIKE peers into the mirror, combs his hair, etc., then begins to dress. The smell of burning sage slowly wafts from the stage out through the audience, as BEV slowly cleanses herself, then her sleeping sister, in the sweet-smelling smoke. On the other side of the stage, brother SPIKE discovers a purple spot — Kaposi Sarcoma — as he dresses in stylish clothes.

BEV exits and returns with a cup of tea and gently awakens COCO, who, hungover, slowly sits up. BEV gives COCO the tea and sits down quietly with her. SPIKE is also sitting, head down. All freeze, then BEV gets up and exits.]

[BLACKOUT]

Scene 2

[Up SPOTLIGHT on SPIKE]

SPIKE: Dearest Sister Coco,

You ever had one of those days? You ever had your life flash in front of your eyes — yeah, really! You ever heard of Kaposi Sarcoma? It's like a little explosion under the skin . . . It ain't very pretty, and in this game, it ain't whether you win or lose, it's how you look. So I guess my life isn't that great.

Yes, I have been angry with you — you know, those of us with "the big disease with the little name" get ignored often enough, let alone for you not to stay for Michael's funeral. Yeah, you saw some pretty bad stuff with us, Coco, but I thought you'd stick around . . . we could have had a toast to the end of his life. We could have had some fun for a change, like when we first came to Vancouver and before all this began . . . But we'll talk about it, Coco, cuz, you see, I'm coming home.

I guess that's where you are anyway — at home, I mean. Since you haven't been around here for a few days and by the two hundred bucks I found on the counter, I figured you must've gone back. Thank you for the money. I know better than to ask you how you got it . . .

Hey, you remember when we were kids, that old lady who used to stand on the wharf? She had hair out to here (gesturing with his hands) and her only job was to make rude comments at all the Indians who went by? Remember that day you got her so mad that she dropped her purse and all these little, white pearls fell out across the boards and between the cracks? Chichiye gave you a lickin' that day. She said, "That lady, she may be old and she may be crazy, but you don't treat sick people that way." I remembered her today, scrambling in the rain to pick up her pills even as they dissolved in her hands. I remember just how ugly she could be. You understand what I'm tryin' to tell ya, Coco? We'll talk about it. You say hello to "Sarge" for me, huh — I mean our sister Bev. You know I love you.

Your Brother, Spike.

[LIGHTS out]

Scene 3

[COCO strikes a match in the darkness, LIGHTS come up slightly. She sits with SPIKE's letter open on her lap. She lights a candle and goes over to the ghetto blaster. She pushes in a tape; LOUD MUSIC begins to play. Enter BEV with cleaning stuff.]

BEV: What are you doing sitting in the dark? [BEV turns on the lights.] You should be helping your dear old sister. [BEV throws a rubber glove that she's been wearing at COCO, hitting her.]

COCO: Hi Bev.

BEV: [Turns music off, blows out candle] So Coco, d'you have fun last night? I heard you come in pretty late. Indian poke. [BEV pokes COCO's head with her duster to get her attention.]

COCO: God! Big ears! I went down to the pool hall with Pinki and Bernadine, met a coupl'a guys. You know. You gonna go out tonight?

BEV: No —

COCO: What am I talkin' about? 'Course you're not gonna go out tonight.

BEV: [BEV sits down with COCO] I have to head up to Redonda.

COCO: How come?

BEV: Don't you know? Aunt Doll's youngest girl got herself pregnant, and she wants to go and quit school.

250

COCO: So, what's wrong with that? The best things in life ain't learned in school, you know. Sounds like she knows that already, ungh?

BEV: Aunt Doll wants me to go up there and talk some sense into her. She don't have to go off to work. She's got a big family, they'll look after her and the baby. Us Indians, we gotta stick together. Might stay there a coupl'a days, make sure everything's okay.

COCO: Fourteen-year-old, knocked-up Indian chick. Sounds like a traditional kind of girl to me, ungh, Bev?!! You know us Indians, we gotta stick together!

BEV: Ah, you're sick.

COCO: So where's the Dad?

BEV: Shit. How many Indian guys you know stick around? They're all the same, sweet-talking rabbits, all of them. The Indian man who's of any use to a woman is a thing of the past. Don't hunt, don't fish, don't know how to look after a woman, let alone kids of their own . . . all they know how to do is drink and sleep and eat . . .

COCO: And suck and lick and smooch . . .

BEV: Yeah, right. What a man's best at only lasts ten minutes . . .

COCO: Ten minutes? I wish!

BEV: . . . and we've gotta spend the rest of our lives payin' for it. Did we get any mail?

COCO: Uh-huh. You know what's funny? How all the bills come at the same time.

BEV: Can I have my mail?

[COCO hands over a couple of envelopes, but pockets SPIKE's letter with the yellow envelope. BEV, as always, notes everything.]

BEV: Bills. Damn bills. [She turns and stares at COCO.]

COCO: Stare! Bug eyes! What have I done wrong now, ungh?

BEV: What have you done right?

COCO: Yeah, right.

BEV: D'you get any mail?

COCO: Yeah. [pause] Got a letter from a friend from Vancouver. He's, ah . . . you know, doin'. . . all right . . .

BEV: A friend from Vancouver, huh? That's funny. I remember givin' Spike yellow stationery before he moved to Vancouver. Haven't heard from him though. And what's even funnier Coco, is you've been home three weeks now and you haven't mentioned one word about him. How come?

COCO: I'm sure he's okay . . . spreadin' his love and happiness everywhere. Listen, I'm gonna fuck off now, okay?

BEV: [sarcastically] Yeah? Well have a good time!

[They get up at the same time, COCO to put on her jacket, BEV to put away her cleaning things. COCO begins to exit, stops and turns back.]

COCO: Eh, Prego?
BEV: If it's money you want, forget it! I gave you my last twenty bucks last night! You better start makin' your own way 'round here. If you think . . .
COCO: I don't want your money! I'm tryin'a tell you somethin'. Sit down! [pause] Sit down . . . [BEV sits] It's . . . ah . . .
BEV: You're pregnant! Ee mutl! You don't have to be afraid to tell me that! I been tryin' to figure out why you come home from Vancouver so sudden. Now I know why. But let's get one thing straight. I don't want no asshole comin' 'round here makin' trouble for me . . .
COCO: Bev, I'm not pregnant!
BEV: [pause] You're not?
COCO: Nope.
BEV: Oh.
COCO: Why don't . . . why don't you come out with me tonight? [COCO gets up and turns the music on again.] C'mon, we'll act like a bunch a' white chicks, we'll put lipstick on!
BEV: I told you! [She turns the music off angrily.] I have to go to Aunt Doll's tonight!
COCO: What's the matter? You scared?
BEV: Scared? Scared a' what?
COCO: Scared someone's gonna touch you?
BEV: No!!
COCO: Scared someone's gonna kiss you? [She makes a loud kissing sound.]
BEV: No!
COCO: Scared someone's gonna squeeze your boobs, ungh?

[COCO playfully honks one of BEV's breasts and runs away. BEV, lame and pregnant, cannot catch her, but swings a hand at her anyway.]

BEV: Stop that kind of talk, I told you!
COCO: How you gonna catch any fish if you don't go fishin'?
BEV: You're a woman!
COCO: What's that got to do with anything?
BEV: Everything! You have to respect yourself! I try so hard to walk a straight road and here you are acting like some dirty dog in the ditch. Geez, if your mother could see you now!
COCO: Well, she can't, can she? [pause] I'm tryin' to tell you somethin'.
BEV: [suspiciously] What?

COCO: It's about Spikey.

BEV: What about Spike?

COCO: Well . . . he's a fag, ungh, and . . .

BEV: A what?!!

COCO: . . . you know, a cocksucker . . .

BEV: You're just tryin' to get me mad, aren't you? Well, just stop it!

COCO: It's no big deal! I thought you knew — you practically raised us . . .

BEV: Just stop it! Just go back to your sleazy bars, to your sleazy life! You think you can talk to me like that, talk about your own brother just to get to me?!!

COCO: It's no big deal! It could get worse.

BEV: You really want to hurt me! Well, go ahead, just punch me, I know you want to! [pause] I don't want to hear any more of your bullshit! You talk to me properly or you get out of this house!

COCO: You gonna come with me?

BEV: Just get! Go!

COCO: Fine!

[Exit COCO, then BEV. LIGHTS OUT]

Scene 4

[LIGHTS up on SPIKE)

SPIKE: Dearest Sister Coco,

Today, I found some hope . . . today, I found some hope in a room full of skeletons and death. I went to an AIDS support meeting, on palliative care. Some of those guys, they must weigh about a hundred pounds. Michael used to go to them. They ask you to check in. "Hi, my name is Spike and I have AIDS." Fuck. I remember when Michael was given his death sentence, when the doctor said, "I'm afraid you have AIDS." Michael gave away all his things, wrote out his will — hell, he even arranged his funeral! — and he waited. Eight months he waited. Eight months he stopped living and wasn't dead yet. And I swore that if it ever happened to me, I wasn't going to do it that way.

So I'm sitting on the bus tonight, thinking about "living with AIDS," and this abscess in my tooth finally breaks. There's blood and pus everywhere, running down the front of my jacket. And I'm laughing! What a dramatic way to die, huh, in a pool of blood and pus, on a bus going across town?

And did I tell you? I'm not coming home. I'm going to live my life the way I've always lived it — right here, in the city. I got no more fight, no more going out and looking. It's all gonna come to me in the end anyway. So be happy for me — today I found some hope. And I'll be seein' ya . . . maybe.

You know I love you.
   Your brother, Spike.

[LIGHTS out, SPIKE]

Scene 5

[LIGHTS up as BEV enters holding a photograph of SPIKE]

BEV: So, Spike, I know now that you're gay. But why? Is it because I made you do the dishes? Or is it because I made you do the laundry? But I told you, you have to be responsible. I told you. Oh, what's the use? This picture isn't working. [She sits the photograph upright on the couch, towards the audience.] Spike, is it my fault? What did I do wrong? Why me? Why you? I wanted you to be an engineer. I wanted Coco to be a nurse. Why can't you be someone I recognize? Now I feel like I don't know who you are. [She turns and notices a book placed in front of the photograph by COCO, who has already entered and exited. She goes over and picks it up.] "Loving Someone Gay." Oh, that Coco, she can be so sneaky. Why couldn't she give it to me herself? [Exit BEV. LIGHTS out]

Scene 6

[LIGHTS up on SPIKE in mid-conversation]

SPIKE: I used to dream about being a hero once, when I died. But then, I used to want to be a sex bomb, to walk into a room and set everyone dreaming. When I was really little, the nuns used to make me want to be a saint. But that was a month of Sundays ago.

   I was thirteen years old in 1981. I grew up in the age of AIDS. And, ooh baby, look at me now! I'm a chorus girl in this cheap melodrama of second-rate, dying Camilles. Everybody's dying, or hurting or fighting . . . and there ain't no heroes anymore! Ain't much difference 'tween the corpse that's made its peace or one that died screamin' bloody murder.

   I think about the millions of Indians who died before me . . . smallpox, whooping cough, tuberculosis, [pause] alcohol. We survived. Have you seen us, still trying to exorcise our demons, care for our crippled and maimed, secure our sanctuaries so we can be left alone to heal the damage perpetrated against us?

   You ever wonder what the gay man of the future's gonna be like? He's gonna grow up amongst a bitter, ragtag group of survivors, burying men at

254

the same time as he's learning to kiss 'em. He'll be just like me. And that scares me. You don't think I was born like this, do you?. Do ya?!!

[LIGHTS out, SPIKE]

Scene 7

[LIGHTS up on COCO sitting, eating milk and cookies. Enter BEV with gun and hunting gear on]

COCO: You're getting too big to go hunting, Bev.
BEV: Well, if I wait for you to get food, we'd starve.
COCO: Someone's gonna mistake you for a bear!
BEV: A nice, good-lookin' brown one.
COCO: Eeee! D'you get anything?
BEV: A coupl'a rabbits. They're hanging out in the shed. I'll skin 'em later.

[BEV sits down to her knitting]

BEV: Coco, you were the last one to see Spike. Tell me, how is he? COCO: He's doing okay.
BEV: Where does he live? What's his house like?
COCO: He's lives in this great big apartment in a tall, concrete building.
BEV: Hmph. Does he eat well? Does he do his dishes? Of course he does his dishes, I taught him how.
COCO: God, you want to know if he does his dishes?
BEV: Where does he work?
COCO: He works downtown. Just go to the city and see for yourself, he's got plenty a' room.
BEV: I thought you said he had a . . . you know.
COCO: A lover?
BEV: Yeah, a . . . lover. Michael? [pause] Tell me about Michael.
COCO: What about Michael?
BEV: What's he like?
COCO: Michael's . . . Michael's white.
BEV: (pause) And?
COCO: I don't know why he stays with him.
BEV: Why? Cuz he's sick? [NO ANSWER] You said he has AIDS, didn't you?
COCO: Who?
BEV: You.
COCO: Me? I don't have AIDS.

255

BEV: No, you said Michael has AIDS.

COCO: Ah, yeah. It was gettin' pretty bad when I left.

BEV: So why aren't you there helping him? You were in the city.

COCO: Cuz I'm here on the reserve.

BEV: You ran away, didn't you?.

COCO: I didn't run away, I took a bus.

BEV: You can give your body away easy enough. But givin' away love is different, isn't it? You couldn't give in the end.

COCO: That's what you think. Spikey's different now. He wears this bright-coloured clothin'. He's got all these expensive pictures done by Indians hangin' on his walls. He talks real big. He don't need me there to remind him where he's from.

BEV: Do you believe everything you see? 'Course he needs you.

COCO: Yeah, what about what I need?

BEV: Selfish.

COCO: Shut up, Bev. God, I remember when we used to smile around this house. I'm sick of tryin', Bev. What's the use?

[Exit COCO. LIGHTS out. Exit BEV]

Scene 8

[MUSIC]

[LIGHTS up, both sides of stage]

[SPIKE contemplates a suicidal pill-overdose but decides otherwise. COCO quietly drinks from a beer bottle, drunk and unhappy, on the other side of the stage. No words are spoken. SPIKE throws the bottle of pills on the floor. Exit COCO. SPIKE begins to leave, turns around, picks up the bottle of pills and pockets it as he exits.]

Scene 9

[Enter COCO wearing high-heels, to position downstage. She addresses the audience.]

COCO: I remember the first time I fucked a guy.

[Enter SPIKE to position downstage, opposite COCO]

SPIKE: The first time I made love with a man, I think I was about eighteen.

COCO: I fucked a lot a'guys.

SPIKE: His name was Michael. Michael used to say to me, "If all Indians are like you, it's no wonder the Europeans stayed."

COCO: You know, all they want is sex, just when it's hard, they want to come inside you . . . Not one of them got to know me.

SPIKE: These days, I feel really beautiful. I live my life up here [gesturing], all my noblest intentions. Sure, I made some mistakes, broke some rules . . . who hasn't? I remember breaking my first rule, I went into Coco's room one day when she wasn't home. She had these black high-heeled shoes. I put them on and I walked around the room . . . and I took them off. Ugh! How can you live a life in those things? But I learned something! Not that I liked wearing women's clothes, but that I could put high-heels on and it wasn't the end of the world. And I found out I could love a man and it wasn't the end of the world. I have AIDS. It's still not the end of the world, not even for me. I have to believe that.

COCO: You know, the very first time was when I was twelve. It was in my own room, with my stepfather. You know, the nice one. I liked him, but he fucked me, he fucked me around. The only person who really knows me is Spikey and I wish that the last time I saw him in the city I wasn't so goddamned screwed up and shot up that I could have told him I loved him, you know. But now he's gotta go and get AIDS. He's gonna leave me. Why the fuck you gonna die on me, you bastard?!!

SPIKE: Before Michael died, he was sufferin'. I held his hand and I said, "It's okay. You go through that door, Michael . . . I'm just seein' you to the door." He said "Don't cry, don't cry." "I love you, Michael." "I love you, Spike."

COCO: I don't feel too beautiful these days, you know. The only time I do feel like me is when I have my high-heels on. That's when I feel set free.

[Exit COCO and SPIKE. LIGHTS out]

Scene 10

[LIGHTS up on BEV as she sits looking at a photo album. Enter COCO with can and can-opener]

COCO: Hi, Bev.

BEV: Oh, hi.

COCO: What you doin'?

BEV: I'm looking at some old pictures.

COCO: Damn can. [nudges BEV and hands over the opener and the can]

BEV: Coco, how many times have I told you, spam you use the opener, corned beef has its own key. It's probably at the bottom of the cupboard.
COCO: That's too bad. I was gonna make "Coco's Potlatch Special," loved by Natives everywhere. Hungry?
BEV: Not anymore.
COCO: [COCO sits down beside BEV and laughs] That's you! Look at your hair!
BEV: Looks like it was cut with a bowl, doesn't it? Aah, look at the dress you've got on. That's mine! Well, it *was* mine.
COCO: Hey, that's Hallowe'en, ungh?
BEV: Yeah, you look great as a witch.
COCO: Look, there's us the next year when me, you and Spikey dressed up as Charlie's Angel's! Remember?

[They point imaginary guns, shake their hair and yell, "Freeze!" simultaneously and laugh.]

BEV: Oh yeah, remember that time —
COCO: Remember, remember we were running across that meadow and Spikey fell down Mabel's big hill and twisted his ankle and we had to carry him home! He was such a big baby! [They laugh.]
BEV: He's always been a bit sensitive.
COCO: Such a wuss!
BEV: And those bad Timothy boys went and took all his candy —
COCO: Well, there were twelve a' them.
BEV: . . . and I had to give him my candy.
COCO: You were getting too fat anyway.
BEV: And you kept teasing me with yours.
COCO: Yeah, that was funny.
BEV: I just love this because you get to watch them grow up. Yeah. And this is my favourite page. Well, there's a favourite — I, I've got a favourite page that you're on, just you . . .
COCO: Ah-huh.
BEV: And look, there's the wharf at Redonda where Aunt Doll lives. Look at her big fancy car! Remember she took us for a ride just after Momma died!
COCO: And we laughed the whole way!
BEV: Funny, it made me feel better. She had a little grey dog . . .
COCO: What was its name?
BEV: C-C-Chlorox? No, not Chlorox . . .
COCO: Kotex?
BEV: Kotex! I remember: Chloxtuk!

COCO: Chloxtuk? Are you sure?

BEV: Yeah, it means Furry-With-A-Big-Mouth. She still talks about that dog. It was psychic, you know. Remember we used to go pick huckleberries up there. Chloxtuk was in the kitchen once, just staring at the cupboards over the sink. I was there. Slowly, one of the cupboard doors opened all by itself and Chloxtuk started barkin'. I told Aunt Doll she must have rats or something but she said, "Oh, no. That's Chloxtuk's way of lettin' you know she's hungry. [turns the page]

Look, there's that old lady who used stand on the wharf! Remember?

COCO: Yeah, I remember her down there, actin' like she was Queen Elizabeth. Maybe she was one of those white ladies who wanted to sleep with a real Indian chief.

BEV: She was a hooker.

COCO: A hooker? On a wharf?

BEV: Yeah, she used to work the fisherman from all over Desolation Sound.

COCO: Oh that dirty dog . . . I wonder whatever happened to her.

BEV: Oh, she's probably someone's sweet granny somewhere. [Getting up] Well, I should start getting things ready. I gotta do those dishes and clean the bathroom, there's so much work to do. You never know when Spikey might decide to come home. What should I do first?

COCO: He's not coming home.

BEV: What are you talking about? C'mon, quit joking around. I don't like your jokes anymore. You always cry "Wolf," then I don't know if you're joking or if you're just being Coco.

COCO: He's not coming home.

BEV: You never stop . . . just stop it . . .

COCO: He wrote me a letter. [pause] He has AIDS.

BEV: In that book you gave me, there's a part on AIDS. Is it all true? [COCO nods]

BEV: Damn book. Tell me no . . . not my baby brother . . .

[BEV cries. After much waiting, COCO goes over to hug her and leads her from the stage. LIGHTS out]

Scene 11

[Enter SPIKE. LIGHTS up]

SPIKE: Sometimes, in my dreams, my grandmother comes to visit. She's just an outline against the wall. I remember the first time she came to see me . . . "A blond stranger comes into your life," she said. "Keep him. I tell you this because you're so stupid you'll ignore him otherwise. He'll be weak, but he's the one you've been looking for." I said, "No, Grandma. I don't want someone weak. I want someone strong, to protect me." "Strength," she says, "belongs only to women." I said, "No Grandma. Men are strong, women are weak." She just smiled. I believe her now.

That blond stranger was Michael. Our destiny was not to live happily ever after — it never is, you know. Have you figured that one out yet? But death is a destiny. It isn't a failure.

I've tried so hard to be brave, Grandma, but this battle has been so dirty and bloody . . . I've done my best . . . [sings a few bars from RANGIPUKOHU KOHU]

Sounds like an Indian song, ungh? It's Maori, from New Zealand. Michael and I always wanted to go to New Zealand. Some people say the Maoris are our long lost brothers and sisters. That's reason enough for me to go there.

[Exit SPIKE. LIGHTS out]

Scene 12

[LIGHTS up on COCO and BEV in mid-argument]

BEV: I've tried so hard-

COCO: That's what's wrong with you. You try too hard.

BEV: I work from dusk to dawn. That's the way I was taught.

COCO: Yeah, you work from dusk to dawn for other people!

BEV: You drink from dusk to dawn.

COCO: Yeah, I'm havin' a good time.

BEV: You call that a good time, you don't even remember half of it? You call that living?

COCO: Oh, excuse me! I think I'll mop the floor. I'm living! I think I'll polish the furniture — I'm so fuckin' alive.

BEV: You live in a bottle.

COCO: At least it's *my* bottle.

BEV: What do you mean?

COCO: *My* bottle. *My* life. Get it?

BEV: You're screwing around with my things in my own house. Puttin' cigarette burns in my couch . . .

COCO: Screwing around?!! [pause] Screwing around? At least I have fun when I screw around. For you, it's right down to business. Pop that baby out of your no-nonsense biscuit and skip the best part.

BEV: I have a fine life.

COCO: You're lonely.

BEV: I haven't been alone for seven and a half months now. I have enough love for ten kids if I wanted. But it's only gonna be the one and I'm quite happy about it. I'm going to be a good mother, no doubt about it.

COCO: Good mother! Yeah, right. We left home cause we weren't happy!

BEV: And you're happy now? You sure came runnin' back, didn't you, Sweets? How long were you gone in the city? How long did you last out there on your own, Coco?!!

COCO: It was paradise compared to this place!

BEV: I did the best I could. If you guys wanted to leave it was your choice. There was nothing I could do to bring you back.

COCO: You just don't get it do you, how much you take over our lives? Where else can we go but the city? At least we get to decide our own lives. All your traditional values . . . "tradition" is just another word for rules. There's a whole world out there that doesn't care if I change my panties or have kids or dress up and play Pocahontas when the moon is full. I get to decide what I want. And so does Spikey. And he's not coming home.

BEV: I didn't do nothing wrong. I did the best I could. Everybody leaves. Momma left. Spikey left. All the elders are leaving. Then maybe you and me.

COCO: Fuck you.

BEV: Chichiye used to say that nothing is forever. White people, they're always lookin' for eternity, but nothing ever lasts. Time's always gonna win, every second that goes by never comes back. You tell me that's a winning game.

COCO: So you gonna spend the rest of your life lookin' after other people?

BEV: That's what I'm here for. What's you're excuse?

COCO: I'm here for a good time, not a long time!

BEV: You're just usin' up good air if you're not makin' this world a better place.

COCO: You really think you make a difference? Not to Spikey.

BEV: You could have made a difference and you didn't!

COCO: So who's better, you or me? I left Spikey behind, Spikey left you. We're all gonna end up with nobody in the end anyway.

BEV: Yeah? You sure got that right, Sister!

[Exit BEV]

COCO: Bev?

[LIGHTS out]

Scene 13

[Enter SPIKE. LIGHTS up]

SPIKE: Faith is what separates us from the animals. Men will always only believe what they want to believe. I see my own people take their secrets, put them in seashells and bury them deep in the sand. I see them take their troubles and blow them to the wind. I see them put their fear into pouches around their necks. But keeping is a white thing.

Me, all that's been left to me is a little bit of hope and my dreams. And these I give to you. I put them in a seashell and I bury them deep in your heart. I hope you keep and honour them for a while before you give them away again. Ee mutl! Ee mutl!

[LIGHTS out]

Scene 14

[MUSIC]

[Enter BEV as COCO sleeps on the livingroom couch. Enter SPIKE with his suitcase to his side of the stage. BEV "smudges," SPIKE packs a few things, looks in the mirror and says good-bye. Exit SPIKE. BEV slowly cleanses herself, then the sleeping COCO, in the smoke. Enter SPIKE. They look at each other for a moment, then BEV blesses him with the smoke. He is warmly welcomed, first by BEV, then by COCO when she awakens. BLACKOUT]

END

From the more than one hundred and fifty evaluation forms of the play filled out during its tour in the Yukon Territory in Canada, Lisa Tremblay, the AIDS Information Co-ordinator, concluded in her report to the Federal Centre for AIDS that, "Everyone appreciated the play for its realism, its sensitivity, and its sincerity . . . Many remarked that it was a moving portrayal of a person living with AIDS.

"Most people felt that they would be more compassionate and empathetic towards PWAs (Persons with AIDS) now than they would have been before. Many, as well, acknowledged that they would have fewer fears in regard to casual contact with, or caretaking of a Person with AIDS."

Ms. Tremblay further concluded in her report that the play was helpful in four ways: it provided information about AIDS; it developed a consciousness about risk; it challenged prevailing negative attitudes towards gays and it promoted compassion and understanding for Persons living with AIDS.

Empathy is the overriding sentiment experienced by people after seeing the play, whether they are AIDS educators (as at the Second International Symposium on Innovations in AIDS Education in Cameroon), support workers and PWAs from across Canada, or Native people of all ages and nations.

All in all, the response from audiences was overwhelmingly positive. The play's emotionality and message of caring and respect created an atmosphere of trust that opened and supported active learning. Not only this, it challenged negative stereotypes of gays, PWAs and Native people and endeavoured to change attitudes and responses that prevail in relation to AIDS.

In all honesty, the Howie Gaw'nit Players have been quite amazed at the overwhelming reaction to the play since we began touring in April 1989. Perhaps it is simply a story that needed to be told.

On Warm Wind in China

Kent Stetson

Warm Wind in China was first produced in 1988 in Halifax, Nova Scotia, Canada after having been workshopped at Playwrights Workshop in Montréal. Since then it has been produced in both French and English in various locations in Canada.

In the Bedrooms of the Nation

"The state has no place in the bedrooms of the nation." With these words in 1966, Canadian Minister of Justice Pierre Elliott Trudeau and Prime Minister Lester B. Pearson unwittingly invited Canadian gay men to come out. Gay liberation in Canada preceded America's Stonewall (considered by many to mark the beginnings of the modern gay movement). We began not by violent confrontation but by negotiation and legislation. Perhaps it came too easily. We took our rights for granted, worked quietly (by comparison) within the system and it seemed we'd gained ground.

But like our American cousins, we had barely drawn our first breath of fresh air when we noticed we'd moved out of the closet into a ghetto. With political determination and help from increasing numbers of enlightened individuals, we began to dismantle the ghetto walls. We hit our stride and it felt good. It seemed basic rights accorded citizens of civilized societies might soon be ours.

Then AIDS struck, and stronger, higher walls arose around us with alarming speed. Stone by stone, rumour by rumour, death by bone-chilling death, we found ourselves encircled. Terrible social cruelties emerged. Teachers and health care workers lost jobs, men too weak to care for themselves lost friends, relatives, apartments — basic human rights and needs were snatched away without a second thought.

We were blamed, maligned and persecuted as though the terrible calamity we suffered was of our own creation. The virus became more important then the humanity it destroyed. We were on our own. We rallied and, informed more by compassion than fear, we began again. Stories of gay male heroes emerged as the

264

walls of the AIDS ghetto began to crumble. And in the struggle we began to redefine ourselves.

Excerpt from WARM WIND IN CHINA

DAVIS: Tell you what. I'll give you everything I've got. We'll fight this thing together.

SLATER: We can't win.

DAVIS: We can't give up. The longer we fight the better our chances. We'll go to Paris . . .

SLATER: [rising] . . . we'll sell the house, the cars, the furniture. Then burn my clothes. We'll put all our possessions in three back packs and move to France, you and Matt and I. The great Canadian hippie trip revisited. Between visits to the clinic, we'll bum around Europe. We'll go to Lourdes for smart drinks. That'll be fun eh? We'll walk the Seine, hear the accordion players, stand in the light of the rose window in Notre Dame. A family portrait. In red.

DAVIS: It's mostly blue.

SLATER: What's mostly blue.

DAVIS: The Rose Window.

SLATER: Why do they call it rose?

DAVIS: The shape.

SLATER: Oh. One day we'll go to the Louvre. You can park me on crutches, in front of Klimt. Or Goya. That's where you'll leave me. You'll come home and sell the tavern, meet someone else. Then you'll send Matt to live with his grandparents on the Island where my name hangs in the air like dust in the attic. And that will be that. [He retrieves two small photographs, returns to DAVIS and squats.] Here we are on the side lawn beneath the lindens. Dad, me, and Uncle Edwin. Father, son and son of a bitch. That's Dad with his arm around me. See the rope? One end of the hammock. Summer evenings he'd roll in after a hard day's work in the fields and I'd sleep, swinging under the lindens, warm in the evening breeze. 'There's always a breeze on the Island'. The smell of his sweat made me feel safe. I remember the day it became the scent of yearning. We were perfect. [ocean sounds become present for a moment — gulls, wind, surf] It is that boy, Davis. Not some medieval poet, not your pal the tavern keeper. It is me. Andrew David Slater. Thirty-two years old. Educated beyond use. Lost in my prime. I finally started to feel good about myself. Stopped blaming. Stopped regretting. One regret. You weren't the first man, the only man to look back. Don't let me die by myself.

DAVIS: [He embraces his lover.] I fell in love with you the minute you said my name. It was your voice. And those eyes. Your eyes. [SLATER settles in

DAVIS's lap, closes his eyes.] Remember the farm? I never forgot the things you told me that day. I swore I'd never leave you. You didn't believe me. But I'm still here, Slater. I'm still here. I don't want you to die. Slater? How are we going to tell Matthew?

SLATER: [He stirs.] Huh? What time is it?

DAVIS: I don't know. Three thirty-four.

SLATER: Oh. [He moves, resettles, then rises.] He's got that party.

DAVIS: There's lots of time.

SLATER: [surveys beach] What a mess. Who did his?

DAVIS: I don't know. Some asshole.

SLATER: Fun guys will do anything for kicks.

DAVIS: Fun times don't come cheap.

SLATER: Too many cooks spoil the broth.

DAVIS: Virtue is its own reward.

SLATER: I dreamed you gave me everything I need. It's beautiful here.

DAVIS: Yes. Come on sweetheart. Let's go home.

[gulls, wind, surf. END ACT 1]

Warm Wind In China is dedicated to friends and lovers and those who seek to understand. The play is many things to many people. It was written as a bridge piece between the gay and straight communities of my generation. The first act takes place on a Nova Scotia beach. Slater has taken Davis there to tell him he has AIDS, and to extract three promises. He wants Davis to raise his ten year old son Matthew. He needs assurance that Davis will not let Matt become a ward of Slater's father, Jack. And he needs to hear Davis promise that he will not leave him. This promise is particularly hard for Davis. Slater has hidden his physical condition from him. Slater is afraid Davis will forsake him.

DAVIS: I am in this too. You made decisions that are going to affect me for the rest of my life and never even consulted me. You just stewed and fumed and took it out on Matt. Look what you've done to me. Why shouldn't I just turn tail and run?

SLATER: Because I love you.

DAVIS: Cut the crap. You were willing to sit there and watch me drown. No one can go through what you've got to go through but yourself. If you think that gives you the right to stomp all over people, go right ahead. But by Christ, Slater, you won't stomp all over me. You owe me you son of a bitch.

SLATER: I owe you?

DAVIS: You owe me everything you've got.

SLATER: I owe you sweet fuck all.

DAVIS: You owe me respect. If you want me to protect Matt, you give me what I need.

SLATER: I'm giving you the finest thing I have. I'm giving you my son.

DAVIS: I need you, Slater, to forgive me, Davis. [silence] We are screwed. [begins exit]

SLATER: [coiled, on the sand] It stinks. The whole thing stinks. Davis. Please. Help me.

DAVIS: [returning] Slater. [tries to uncoil him. SLATER is rigid] Slater. Slater, look at me. [SLATER can't] Slater! [firm] Look at me. [He can't] I promise I won't leave you.

In the Bedrooms of Town

Act Two takes place in the intensive care unit of a Nova Scotia hospital. Slater is unconscious when his parents come from Prince Edward Island to tend their son and claim his boy. For the first time in his life, Davis is forced to fight a battle that requires a personal vision informed by issues beyond basic self-interest. Davis needed a force of equal or greater strength against which to test himself. I chose to match him with Slater's parents. I wanted to say to my straight friends, "This is what we are going through. We need you more than ever, and we need you on our terms. Here they are." I wanted gay men to understand the scope of the rift that was forming, to appreciate the danger inherent in the plague mentality. Society was fashioning masks and we were being fitted. A masked human being is featureless, easy to diminish, easy to destroy. The first step had been taken. Our contributions were ignored, the brilliance of our struggle demeaned. Our heroes were becoming "non-persons." Straight society attempted to confiscate AIDS, and with it the dignity of a community facing terrible trouble with strength and dignity. We had to come to terms with homophobia before we came to terms with AIDS.

I wanted to fix the dilemma we faced in time, to solidify my position and do what I could to prevent my/our backslide into doubt and self-blame. I needed to reassure myself and others that we were right before, right to claim a place of power and respect in society, that we must hold fast, build on what we had achieved, continue our own journeys of self-discovery for our own good and for the safe passage of those we love.

It soon became clear, to my surprise and delight, that *Warm Wind in China* also spoke, and continues to speak, to my parent's generation. It appears to provide an accessible metaphor, symbols and vocabulary to people in a moral dilemma; their children are dying and there is nothing familiar for them to cling to; no clear route into this foreign, threatening world. In Act Two, scene two, Davis confronts his lover's mother, Elna Slater, after her husband Jack has fled their son's seizure. Davis knows that he must win her support and affection if he is to succeed in carrying out his first promise to Slater — that he will keep Matthew from the dysfunctional family Slater himself barely survived.

In his hospital room, Davis has been comforting Slater behind the curtain, which he opens as Act Two, scene two begins. Elna Slater sits nearby.

ELNA: I have been sitting here listening to you comfort my son, Mr. Davis, and I don't mind telling you that I am mad as hell. I am furious. What you did to us was brutal and cruel.

DAVIS: It was our decision, not mine.

ELNA: I don't care whose decision it was. It was wrong. How long has he been like this?

DAVIS: He told me three months ago.

ELNA: You should have taken him home to us.

DAVIS: We discussed it. He wouldn't go.

ELNA: What if he doesn't come out of this coma?

DAVIS: I think he will.

ELNA: What if he doesn't? I will never be able to speak to my son again.

DAVIS: He didn't want to see his father.

ELNA: I could have driven over myself and taken care of him. He told that woman at the desk I was dead.

DAVIS: He's afraid . . .

ELNA: I know what he's afraid of. They're both afraid of the same damn thing. They'd fight and wrangle each other into the grave rather that talk about it.

DAVIS: Mrs. Slater I am well prepared.

ELNA: You sound as though you've armed yourself for war. We are his parents, Mr. Davis, his family.

DAVIS: Matt and I are his family.

ELNA: He is my son. I bore him.

DAVIS: I love him. I am losing him.

ELNA: I have no taste for games.

DAVIS: Either do I.

ELNA: Then why do you insist on playing this one?

DAVIS: This is no game. I have a commitment to your son. And grandson.

ELNA: You think I have no place here, Mr. Davis?

DAVIS: That's not for me to say.

ELNA: I'm no stranger to loss.

DAVIS: You've never lost a mate.

ELNA: Have you lost a son? [near SLATER's bed] How old are you, Mr. Davis?

DAVIS: Thirty two.

ELNA: You were never married?

DAVIS: No.

ELNA: Have you got something against women?

DAVIS: Of course not.

ELNA: Or are they just . . . out of reach.

DAVIS: I fell in love with your son. And he fell in love with me.

ELNA: Well. I must say I find all this very odd. Two men and a boy.

DAVIS: I don't know how things are in Morell, P.E.I., Mrs. Slater? I thought people were different here.

ELNA: People are pretty much the same no matter where you find them.

DAVIS: So it seems. Matt was accepted as the kid with two fathers. We dealt with the nasty stuff, which wasn't often. We made sure of that. You taught school for years. You know the politics.

ELNA: Eighteen years of grade ten English. I know the politics all right.

DAVIS: They called a special PTA meeting. A week early. I never gave it a second thought. We went.

ELNA: You went together?

DAVIS: We are a couple. We go everywhere together. Especially where Matt's concerned. Slater does committee work. I coach little league. People admired us — all very broad-minded and upwardly mobile. People began to arrive — people who'd partied at our house, people whose houses we'd visited. Friends. I thought he looked great. I guess it was only by comparison. They'd come over to say hello and you could see it happen in their faces. Soon we were sitting alone in a room full of strangers. Empty chairs all around us. They started talking about kids biting each other and getting infected. I lost it. The last thing I remember is Slater herding me out of there, me yelling "Matthew is not a dangerous child!" Now Matt's in a new school, I'm fighting for my job. And Slater's breathing oxygen so pure it destroys the tissues that absorb it. [silence]

ELNA: Where are you in your family?

DAVIS: What?

ELNA: Oldest? Youngest?

DAVIS: I'm the youngest of three.

ELNA: The youngest is the sweetest. Where are your folks?

DAVIS: Bridgetown. In the valley.

ELNA: Do you see them?

DAVIS: Yes. We go down whenever we can. Weekends, mostly. holidays.

ELNA: How do they feel about you?

DAVIS: They love me. They love us all. Especially Matt. They treat him like . . .

ELNA: Like a grandson?

DAVIS: Like one of the family.

ELNA: Do you have a first name?

DAVIS: Carlyle. I prefer Davis.

ELNA: [She moves to SLATER later.] I thought I heard him call. Now I don't want to touch him.

DAVIS: You're perfectly safe.

ELNA: I am his mother.

DAVIS: Go on. Take his hand. [She does]

DAVIS: You think this is happening because of me.

ELNA: It certainly isn't my fault.

DAVIS: There was infidelity. We aren't certain.

ELNA: Well. That's something we don't have to worry about. Normal people don't die of infidelity.

DAVIS: There's always murder.

ELNA: I mean in natural circumstances.

DAVIS: So do I. You think Slater and I aren't natural?

ELNA: Davis, don't jump on me. I am not small-minded. I am simply trying to understand. Men. You're hard on us, but by God you're brutal with each other. He began treating me like an ornament fragile, too delicate to handle. And his father started treating him, I don't know . . . cool. Kept us both at a distance.

DAVIS: Mrs. Slater. He doesn't blame you for anything.

ELNA: Bearing children is nothing. Raising them is having living strips of flesh torn from your back. Nobody knows how to be a parent. You pour your dreams into them until you're damn near empty. They become strangers and skulk through the house as though there were landmines beneath the broadloom.

DAVIS: [light laughter] Sorry. That's exactly the kind of thing Slater'd say.

ELNA: What?

DAVIS: Landmines beneath the broadloom.

ELNA: Really. I wish I could share your pleasure. Just know I'm afraid I can't. What about Matthew?

DAVIS: He's okay. He's a fine boy.

ELNA: Yes. His letters are wonderful.

DAVIS: Like his grandmother's.

ELNA: You've read my letters?

DAVIS: I help Matt answer them. I guess we've had a secret correspondence going for years.

ELNA: Did you read what I wrote Andrew?

DAVIS: He read bits to me. I feel I have an unfair advantage.

ELNA: How's that?

DAVIS: I know you better than you know me.
ELNA: Did you read Andrew's replies?
DAVIS: No.
ELNA: Then we are even.
DAVIS: Slater wrote about me?
ELNA: You were more of a presence. Someone other than Matthew he . . . of
    whom he was fond.

Elna's journey has begun. She recognizes an essential humanity in Davis, and his
importance in the life of her son, a life that had become a distasteful mystery.
Davis has what he needs — her curiosity. It is the first step and he responds.

In the Bedrooms of the Family

Jack is a much tougher case. There is something in the standard father/son
relationship that a gay child threatens in a profound way. Bum-fucking, no doubt,
is an essential part of it. The notion of the anus as sex organ is not a popular one
with straight men, though anal intercourse is evidently more common in
heterosexual relationships than straight society cares to admit. The greater
problem appears to be one of power, or more correctly, the abuse of power.
Guardians of patriarchal values, most often ignorant men, they have inherited
extraordinary power over other men, women and children. They do not earn
this power, nor, clearly, are they divinely equipped to administer it. They perform
it rather with a minimum of insight. They are generally authoritarian and thereby
limited. They use traditional tools of subjugation, ridicule and finally the threat of
violence. When the question of Matthew's future must be confronted, Slater's
father shows his true colours.

JACK: What about your new buddies.
DAVIS: What new buddies?
JACK: Someone like that Arnold. I mean you guys and kids. If Matt was a girl it
    would be different.
DAVIS: Arnold is into men, not boys. We leave that to married men and straight
    relatives.
JACK: You're treading on dangerous ground.
DAVIS: Uncle Edwin still live next door? [silence] You're terrified of me.
JACK: Scared of a faggot? Not too god-damned likely.
DAVIS: You don't mind a bit of lisp and swish, but if a guy looks you in the eye

and says, 'I love your son the way he needs to be loved,' it all goes to ratshit.

JACK: What Andrew did with his life is his own business.

DAVIS: When I met Slater he was throwing himself at every man who came along.

JACK: That's none of my concern.

DAVIS: He was looking for you.

JACK: He knew where to find me.

DAVIS: So he thought. That party at the farm. The whole family gathered under the lindens on a Sunday afternoon in July.

JACK: You watch your step, Davis.

DAVIS: You went looking for your brother. It took a while, but you found him all right. In your brand new warehouse on a pile of burlap bags with your twelve-year-old son.

JACK: I went to your tavern. Men dancing, handling each other, kissing. Drunk as lords.

DAVIS: t's a gay bar Jack.

JACK: I might be just an ordinary guy, but I got some rights left too, you know.

DAVIS: Yeah, well so do I. And in spite of what you think of him, so does your son.

JACK: I love my boy.

DAVIS: You told him he could be anything he wanted.

JACK: He turned queer.

DAVIS: He was born gay.

JACK: Don't try and pawn this off on us.

DAVIS: Slater was a perfectly normal gay kid until you turned your back on him.

JACK: Gay gay gay. I'll be damned if you'll ruin my grandson.

DAVIS: I'm not taking any more shit, Jack.

JACK: Then we'll see you in court.

DAVIS: You let Edwin go and took it out on Slater.

JACK: That's a lie.

DAVIS: I heard this story in his nightmares for years. I believe every word.

JACK: What kind of man are you?

ELNA: I never could fathom your affection for that man.

JACK: Ed is my brother.

ELNA: Andrew is our son.

JACK: You stay out of this.

ELNA: What did you say?

JACK: I said stay out of this.

ELNA: Andrew said you beat him.

JACK: I never hit that boy. I may have given him a shake, but I swear to God I never beat my kids.

ELNA: Why would he lie?

JACK: He wouldn't talk to me. What was I supposed to do? Staring at the ground. Wouldn't look his own father in the eye. You got it all buggered up, boyo. He was hiding something from me that I couldn't handle and it turns out I was right.

DAVIS: Something you were afraid you couldn't handle?

JACK: That's not what I said.

DAVIS: That's what I heard.

JACK: I said something he couldn't handle.

DAVIS: You couldn't handle.

ELNA: That's what you said, Jack.

JACK: Where were you when he was staring at the ground?

ELNA: In the house wondering why we couldn't talk to each other.

JACK: I put Ed on the road and that was the end of that. Then Andrew decides he's going to make a career of it. I'm not blind. I knew what was going on that day you and him took off for the woods.

DAVIS: We made love.

JACK: I don't care what you fellas do. Just don't cram it down my throat.

DAVIS: He asked me to take him. There on the farm. It had to be there. And I did. I took off his clothes, he lay on his back on the moss . . .

ELNA: Davis, don't.

DAVIS: You asked.

ELNA: Not in front of Jack.

DAVIS: He put his feet on my shoulders and I leaned over, my hands on either side of his head and I kissed him.

ELNA: Davis . . .

DAVIS: You've had people you love inside you — your children, your husband. Soon we were moving, lost in each other. I watched a cloud lift from behind his eyes. He told me he loved me and I knew I loved him. We were perfect.

ELNA: Davis. How could you?

DAVIS: I love your son the way he needs to be loved.

ELNA: That's not what I meant and you know it.

JACK: I tried to respect that boy after what happened. He was ashamed and I was ashamed for him. Besides, he was getting too close.

DAVIS: He got too close to the back of your hand.

JACK: He was smothering me.

ELNA: He worshipped the ground you walked on.

JACK: I asked him what happened. He told me alright. He told me he liked it. Yes I hit him. I hit him once in my life with the back of my hand and that was that. And don't you come onto me with that holier-than-thou bullshit.

DAVIS: You deserted him when he needed you most.

Society requires images of gay men that are twisted and bitter. Fathers require sons to reflect themselves. They support these sons with all the rites of passage acceptable to late twentieth century mores: straight sons get the family car, or a car of their own; straight sons are taught basic social standards regarding male/female relationships; straight sons are prepared to accept the mantle of patriarchal power. When straight sons mate it is a time for celebration. When gay sons mate it a time of shame, fear and retribution. And if a gay child is preyed upon by a patriarch, it is the boy who is punished.

DAVIS: Now. Let's put this thing together. Begin at the beginning.
SLATER: My father.
DAVIS: What will he do?
SLATER: What they all do.
DAVIS: What?
SLATER: He pulls you under and holds you until you suffocate.
DAVIS: Hold it. No more double talk. Take your time. Tell me exactly what to expect.
SLATER: I'm telling you. He grabs you by the throat and pulls you in.
DAVIS: Slater. Come on . . .
SLATER: He takes a mirror. He holds it up to you. Then just as you are getting a sense of who you are, his fist smashes through from behind, he grabs you by the throat and squeezes until you're out of breath. He'll pull you in.
DAVIS: Stop it!
SLATER: He tells me to put it back, put the mirror back together. See? Then he grinds it with his heel. Thousands of grains of glass. I don't know why he'd do that. He tells me to put it back the way I found it. The way I found it. I do my best. I can't. I'm just a kid. Dad won't look at me. I stare at the ground. Can't talk to him. Can't talk to Mom. Can't talk to anyone. Then Ed comes back from Boston or Toronto and it starts all over. It happens again and again and again and it hurts. And it makes me sick. I loved him. Now Ed calls me the little faggot in front of Dad. And Dad doesn't do a God-damned thing about it. [SLATER lies contorted in pain. A *cri de coeur* escapes him. It is primal.]

In a city with a population of 1,000,000, there are 100,000 gays. In a city of 3,000,000 persons, 30,000 are gay, etc. Canada's gay and lesbian population exceeds 2,000,000 people. Gay men have straight friends who want to help. Many have reasonable relatives who open themselves when love is required. Like us, they need reassurance. And we need their help.

The need for positive gay art grows. The theatre remains a potent venue where groups of people struggle together toward truth and enlightenment. The best

274

theatre challenges and illuminates. The very heart and soul of human experience lives on stage. Theatre can reassure, it can open small minds and elevate the human spirit.

One truth that effects 20 million gay North Americans is clear. Our lives are considered less important than those of our straight brothers and sisters. Because of who we are, society feels no requirement to honer our suffering.

Theatre shines a light on this ignorance, this terrible unkindness. And it is here we begin to celebrate our heroes. Davis prevails against Jack. He will retain guardianship of Matthew. He leaves an opening for Jack, who begins to perceive a way to the truth of his dying son's essential humanity. But Davis's greatest victory is within. He discovers a clear path forward for himself, a path that will honour his lover and his lovers future as embodied in the boy Matthew. And most significantly, Davis sets his foot upon a path that will deepen his love of himself.

Act Two, Scene Five

[ELNA and JACK are seated on the couch in a pool of light. JACK's back is to the audience. DAVIS is seated on the bed, SLATER in his arms. The respirator hose and mask have been removed. The heart rate gradually speeds up.]

DAVIS: I took Matthew to the beach this morning. It was warm, the water still. A perfect mirror. He felt a breeze. He said it was you. Was it you Slater? Or just a warm wind in China? We had fun, Slater. For the first time since you got sick Matt and I had fun. He's a fine boy. I'm proud of him. [He listens to the changing heart monitor rhythm, holds SLATER close.] Your father took him shopping. He wanted a new suit. And a white shirt. And a tie. [He buries his head in SLATER's shoulder.] Dear God. My heart is breaking and mending itself at the same time. You're going to fly right out of this room, Slater. Bound elsewhere. Toward the light. I'm sticking with you. I'm sticking with you 'til the end. 'Til the beginning. 'Til . . . [The heart-rate monitor speeds to a blur, stops.] Oh, Jesus. I love you, Slater. I always will. [He rocks SLATER like a child. In the silence he looks in his lover's face and sees that it is finished. He lowers SLATER gently to the bed. A light kiss.] Go to the light.

[A wind chime sounds in the far distance. Fade to black.]

CURTAIN

Puppets Against Aids

Mike Milvase with Gary Friedman

Excerpts from an interview with Gary Friedman, 1990

After studying with the late Jim Henson in 1987, often discussing the possibility of putting together a project looking at indigenous traditions of puppet and mask theatre in Southern Africa, Gary Friedman and friends formed a group to research the idea for a trial period of six months. This eventually lead to the formation of the African Research and Educational Puppetry Program (AREPP).

"We decided to select projects of local relevance around which to work," recalls Friedman. "Some of these initial topics proposed were women's rights, child abuse, agriculture, nutrition, the environment and so on . . . AIDS was chosen because at that time nothing was being done in AIDS education in Southern Africa at all. After consulting various people, we embarked on our first long-term project."

Much of the work of AREPP revolves around follow-up workshops to performances in collaboration with community and development agencies. "We are working closely with organizations like PPHCN's (Progressive Primary Health Care Network) AIDS Forum and through SACC (South African Council of Churches) which are both progressive grassroots organizations. We teach simple skills of building puppets from junk materials and waste, putting together a simple puppet show and then teaching people how to use the medium of puppetry to put a message across," states Friedman.

In 1990, AREPP worked with communities such as The Soweto Concerned Youth and the University of Zululand. They toured Zululand, Namibia, the Transkei and the Eastern Cape, the Western Cape and the Transvaal. Shows vary from one venue to another. Although the larger show can draw crowds as many as 3,000 at a time, the smaller show is more cost effective and portable.

To the obvious question of "why puppets?" Friedman becomes both philosophical and pragmatic. "I've been a puppeteer from a very young age. I have always felt it to be a strong visual metaphor. The puppet is one step removed from the human being, so puppeteering is not as threatening as using a human actor could be."

"People can identify with the puppets because they are larger than life, sort of fantasy characters. And the large puppets can be seen by many more people at a time. It is also a lot more attractive. For me the first function of the puppet is entertainment. The public is grounded and then you can put a strong educational message across. We use large grey puppets because they do not represent any one race or cultural stereotype. Often people ask which race gets AIDS and we tell them 'the human race.' The white homosexual sector were the first to have AIDS and are relatively well-informed already that we do not have to do much education there. In Africa AIDS is essentially a heterosexual problem but we stress that everybody is at risk."

What we have to do all the time is target the show in terms of our audiences. When we do it for adolescents, we stress different things to when we do it for adults. The same goes for urban and rural differences. If it is a street performance then it is more of a general show. Before we do a show we speak to people in the community. We find out what the key words are; for instance in Zimbabwe we couldn't use the word penis or vagina and in Shona there is no word for it. Shona people use the word "kutsi" which means "down there." So you would say "down there man" and "down there woman" to indicate the respective sexual organs. You have to be quite sensitive to all this because every community has specific words and different ways of putting things across.

The whole notion of safer sex seems to be a difficult concept to get across in Africa, particularly because the condom is often seen as foreign. As Friedman puts it, "The condom has always been linked in South Africa as a political thing, a tactic used by the government to limit the black population. The same situation happened in Zimbabwe: the condom has various stigmas. It has been used as a family planning device and now it is being used to save lives. It is difficult to convince people that you are not part of this government scheme to stop blacks from populating. It's a very sensitive thing. The one way to overcome this is to work through credible community leaders, so that you are seen in a serious light and people take the message seriously.

The only real way to combat the AIDS problem is to work through credible people and a grassroots approach. This is the World Health Organization's strong recommendation. The government didn't do its research. Now the whole thing has got out of hand. It should be worked through television, radio and on all levels. The message needs to come across and be reinforced as much as possible."

The African National Congress (ANC) has more recently taken up the AIDS issue. "This is very important," says Friedman, "if leaders of the ANC stand up at rallies and start saying put down your AKs and pick up a condom, it will help a lot. It needs to be pushed on all sides by all politicians, not just the ANC. Things can't be left to a post-apartheid society. There won't be people left if it's put on hold!"

Some evaluation and epidemiological research has registered an improvement in the knowledge and in the intended behaviour change which indicates the message is getting through. "We still encounter myths about AIDS, however, such as: you can get AIDS from kissing, from a lavatory seat; AIDS came from the back of a comet tail, a plot by the Russians to destroy the Americans and vice versa; AIDS was acquired by having sex with green monkeys; AIDS is a disease that the South African government has imported to destroy the blacks. It is part of the "victim—blaming" syndrome, which we're so desperately trying to overcome!"

On the Road with PUPPETS AGAINST AIDS

The following extracts are taken directly from the AREPP Report on their 1990 Namibian Tour. Two weeks of performances and workshops are given as examples of their work.

The schedule comprised thirty-six presentations of *Puppets Against AIDS* and the distribution of 30,000 AIDS comic brochures and condoms. Most programs, except those presented at schools, were supplemented with condom demonstrations and the showing of AIDS information videos, which proved very effective back-up material to presentations. A two-day Puppetry and AIDS Education workshop in Katatura Township, Windhoek, was also conducted.

Presentations were made in schools, military installations, town squares, clinics and mine hostels throughout Namibia. The languages used were English and Afrikaans, with simultaneous translation into Herero, Ovambo and Nama-Damara. The puppets text was also translated into the local languages, to the great amusement of the crowds.

On August 27, we drove to Rehoboth, starting at the Vooruitsig Secondary School in the morning for about 1,500 high school pupils. After lunch, we had a record attendance of 2,500 high school pupils in the town hall from five local schools. Later that afternoon we again performed in the town hall, to local residents (mainly parents). Although not many questions followed, a good response was felt from the small crowd.

On August 28 and 29, we held a two day Puppetry in AIDS Education Workshop for seven members of Platform 2,000, a local theatre group at the People's Place in Katatura township, outside Windhoek. The first day was used to polish up on AIDS education skills, which the group already possessed, since they had

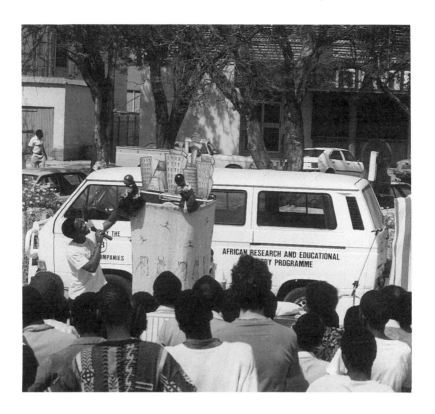

A street performance with the small puppet stage, *Puppets Against AIDS*.

previously worked on an AIDS play. We also wrote short scenarios, which we would later adapt to use with the puppets. Later in the day we gave a performance at the Zoo Park in Windhoek to show students how we conducted our puppetry program. The second day was spent doing puppet and object manipulation/animation exercises and showing examples of different puppetry techniques. Thereafter we performed the AIDS scenarios with simple glove puppets.

On August 30, we drove to Okahandja, were we performed at the Okahandja Secondary School in the morning to about 800 pupils. At the school we were approached by the local school inspector who asked us about our response from other schools in Namibia. Apparently at this particular school, which had never had any previous sex education, fifty-eight girls had left in the past seventeen months, due to teenage pregnancy. The children inquired about where they could get condoms, and many appeared to be sexually active. (According to the local sister at the clinic, by 4:00 p.m., the clinic's condom supply had run out, due to the school children lining up for condoms after school.)

At lunch time we performed outside the Okahandja Town Hall and in the evening at the local Military Base to the new Namibian forces and their British Army training instructors. Questions lasted for about ninety minutes and were simultaneously translated into three languages. (During interviews with members of the Okahandja community after the performances, many felt that the UNTAG forces, who had previously spent the last year in Namibia, during preparations for independence, were spreading sexually transmitted diseases and AIDS. They had apparently been paying local women and even school girls for sex. These men were apparently not tested for HIV before they came to Namibia and their largest contingency had occupied the Okahandja/Windhoek areas.

On August 31, performances were held, once again at the Zoo Park in central Windhoek. These was covered by an NBC (Namibian Broadcasting Corporation) television news team.

On September 10, we performed out morning show at Otjikoto Secondary School to about 800 pupils. After the teachers left the venue, there were questions for more than one hour. This proved to be very positive. Many questions involving discrimination and blame came up, especially from adolescent audiences.

In the afternoon, we performed at the single-sex hostels of the Tsumeb Corporation Limited (TLC) mine in Tsumeb. The program took place in their dance arena to a very enthusiastic crowd of men of all ages, which lasted until dark. (More complaints were received that condoms should be made directly available at the mines, instead of the men having to approach the female nurses at the local clinic).

On September 11, we drove to Grootfontein, which, before independence was used as a military base for the South African Armed Forces fighting SWAPO in northern Namibia. Now the military base has been occupied by the new Namibian forces. In the morning, we performed at Fridrich Awaseb Junior Secondary School to 288 pupils. (Again there were complaints about the availability of condoms from the local clinic. Too many questions were being asked as to why the pupils wanted condoms!)

In the afternoon we drove to the military base, where about 600 soldiers of both sexes attended our program. The performance went ahead on the field under a sweltering Namibian sun. With sweat pouring down our faces, we fought to get the message across! We then drove down through Otavi to distribute AIDS brochures at the local clinic and then on to Otjiwarongo.

On September 12, we travelled to Okakarara in Hereroland West, where we spontaneously performed at the Okakarara Technical College and Secondary School to an audience of about 400. Another extremely hot place, where the heat made the puppeteers' fingers swell and blister.

On September 13, the final day of scheduled performances, we presented our program to audiences in Otjiwarongo: first, outside a rural market, and again at lunch time in the town square on the lawns. The first performance attracted two schools of about 1,500 people and the second about 500.

On the way back to Windhoek, before the long haul home, we passed through Omaruru, giving out brochures at the local clinic, municipal offices and doctor's rooms. We then drove to one of the most isolated areas in the Damaraland desert, Spitzkoppe, where we distributed brochures and condoms to the local Red Cross, clinic and school. After an accidental meeting with representatives from the Swedish and Namibian Red Cross Societies at Spitzkoppe, we drove back to Windhoek, before leaving for Johannesburg on September 16.

Plays For Living: Reflections on Live Wire

Robert Metcalf & Helen Smith

MOM: [sits right] It's all arranged, with the loan and what we save, it'll be enough. If you get your grades back up, and keep them up — and I don't mean straight A's necessarily.

ETHAN: Good, Because that's not me.

MOM: But above average, regular — that's you. Right? If you'll just let yourself be a regular guy, instead of a superman. [Gently pushes ETHAN off "sofa" with feet] Deal?

ETHAN: Deal. [They toast with their "mugs" and sip "cocoa."]

MOM: Good night. [exit right]

ETHAN: 'Night. [To audience] I stuck to the deal, except that somehow, no matter what, I always had to keep up with Larry. I hid the pressure from everybody, by doing everything. I kept my grades up, so Mom didn't press me about my late hours. I did my job, never missed a day. And by the last two weeks of school, just before finals [Sets "mug" down right of "sofa"] when I stood to make it or blow everything — I was running out of fuel.

— from *Live Wire*

Problems and Successes in New York
Robert Metcalf

Plays for Living (PFL) gives dramatic voice to compelling social problems by developing and producing original stage and video plays about critical issues related to family, community, health, and work. Each half-hour drama is written by a professional playwright, developed with a panel of authorities on the subject, and tested before target audiences. Each story is open-ended, serving as a springboard for post-performance discussion.

282

PFL presents an issue in a dramatic format without necessarily advocating a singular point of view on that issue. The topics that we discuss in these plays tend to be controversial, difficult to view objectively and fraught with emotion. PFL's objective is not to foster debate, but rather to encourage discussion. We are in a partnership with our audiences that depends on mutual trust. The audience trusts us to be fair and comprehensive in our writing and staging of the play, and we trust the audience to be open-minded and to approach their post-performance discussion in the spirit of cooperation and compassion.

About LIVE WIRE

Nowhere is this more true than in the case of *Live Wire*, our play by Bruce Peyton, dealing with AIDS awareness and prevention for teenagers. *Live Wire* is intended to demystify the disease, to make facts available, and to present characters with whom the audience can identify. It tells the story of one young man who contracts the HIV virus through needle sharing and his attempts to persuade his loved ones to take responsibility for their own health.

Since June 1989 when the New York production of *Live Wire* premiered, we have performed it over thirty-five times for audiences ranging in age from teen to late middle-age. The responses have been as varied as the make-up of the audiences, but nearly all have been extremely favourable.

An observation by one young woman in her teens convinced us that we had in large measure achieved the goal we had set for the play. She said, "I don't think you can understand a disease unless you know somebody who has it. I don't know anyone with AIDS, but now I *feel* like I do."

The ability of our younger audiences to identify with the characters in *Live Wire* is of paramount importance. For the play to be effective, the audience members must realize that they are very much like those characters, that they face some of the same pressures and dangers.

A play can be useful for a wide variety of audiences with differing needs. While the play is targeted primarily at teens, the reactions of a number of adult audiences have been positive in another way. Various social workers and health care professionals have stated that *Live Wire* has helped them reach out to their younger clients; particularly those at risk. They seem to see in the characters a reflection of the teens they work with every day.

Finally, the reactions of parents to *Live Wire* have been along the lines of how to protect and educate their children with regard to AIDS; what they should tell them, how to broach the subject, etc. The play serves to focus their attention on the subject, in some cases to clarify their understanding of the disease, and mostly to reinforce their concern for their own kids.

ETHAN: [To the audience] And speaking of the sex lady, you may notice a striking resemblance between her and Mom. That's because what you've seen is what we've got, in terms of actors. [MARTIN, LARRY, and SANDY ENTER and sit on floor, LARRY down stage right, SANDY and MARTIN down left, facing upstage] So use your imagination, okay? This is not Mom. This is Mrs. Richards, the lady from the health department. [Sits on floor, right.]

[The two pairs represent the two different classrooms. The "sex lady," played by MOM, takes her place up centre between the two "classrooms" and immediately begins her talk directed at middle-schoolers MARTIN and SANDY. She mouths the words; we hear only ETHAN and LARRY. ETHAN has fallen asleep on LARRY's right shoulder.]

LARRY: Ethan. [Nudges him. No response.] Ethan. [Nudges him again. No response again.] What's wrong with you, man? [Knocks him over.]
ETHAN: Somebody just woke me up is what's wrong with me. You know all my tricks — including sleeping with my eyes open.
LARRY: [sarcastically] I recognized your snore.
ETHAN: You're kidding.
LARRY: [snickering] Just keep awake.
ETHAN: Take notes, okay, Larry? Tell me if there's anything I should know. You're the ladies' man. Nothing she said before has ever been of any use to me. [beat] I can't believe I just told you that. I was kidding. I didn't mean it. I'm a sexy guy, I need to hear this. [He goes back to sleep.]

[Immediately the Sex Lady turns from the middle-schoolers to the high-schoolers, and now we can hear her talk. At the same time, SANDY and MARTIN freeze.]

SEX LADY: Ethan.
ETHAN: [surprised] Present. [Larry snickers.]
SEX LADY: Yes, I know, dear. Sleep on your own time. This could save your life.
ETHAN: Yes, ma'am.
SEX LADY: Can you name one of the three ways?
ETHAN: Three . . . ways?
SEX LADY: . . . that AIDS is transmitted. Name one way, one kind of behaviour.
[LARRY whispers from behind him.]
ETHAN: Sex.
SEX LADY: More specifically . . .

[another whisper from LARRY]

ETHAN: Sexual intercourse.

SEX LADY: Correct. Especially, unprotected sexual intercourse. Meaning? Lawrence?

Larry: Without using a rubber ... uh ... condom?

Problems

There are problems connected with *Live Wire*. Few, however, have to do with the play itself, but more often than not, they have to do with Marketing. PFL's performance list currently consists of thirteen plays that range in subject matter from prejudice and discrimination among teens to death with dignity and living wills. Of the thirteen, two of the hardest to "sell" are *Live Wire* and *The Survivors* which deals with teen suicide prevention, despite the fact that this at a time when both problems are epidemic in our part of the United States. The difficulty in booking these plays could be chalked up to production problems (bad plays) except that audiences who have actually seen the plays are almost universally enthusiastic.

The problem with the *The Survivors* is relatively simple to grasp. There is a significant body of opinion, some of it impressively informed, that suicide is a subject best not discussed with children and teenagers. Those who believe this are, we suspect, in the minority, but the notion that seeing a drama about someone who is at risk of suicide could lead a young person to commit suicide himself or herself is a frightening one. Add to that the highly litigious nature of our society, and one can understand (if not agree with) a decision by the school principal based on nightmares about losing one of his students to suicide after seeing a performance of *The Survivors*, not to mention being sued by the grieving parents.

Live Wire is a more complicated case. When we were first staging the production in June of 1989, we were concerned by reports of a widely held view in the African-American community that AIDS was strictly a gay/white disease, and therefore, black teens need not concern themselves with awareness and prevention. Since a large percentage of the target audience would be urban African-American teens, we decided to cast the production entirely with black actors. This was not a decision based on uninformed expectation. A number of our clients in previous seasons had told us they would not book *Just One Step*, our play about children who live with parental alcoholism, unless at least part of the cast was black. It was too easy, they felt, for minority youngsters to dismiss the ideas in the play if only white actors were performing. The same would be true, we reasoned, of an AIDS awareness play.

However, at a showcase of *Live Wire*, a black educator was concerned that the all African-American cast perpetuated the attitude that AIDS is a black/ghetto disease.

In support of this assertion, at an all-white school in New Jersey where we had performed many of our plays in the past, the teachers found that *Live Wire* was our least successful effort. They felt their students, although at risk, did indeed perceive AIDS as a black/ghetto disease and therefore they did not need to be concerned with prevention.

In other words, our solution to one problem resulted in a backlash from other quarters. But rather than filing these responses under Sometimes-You-Just-Can't-Win and forgetting them, we are now experimenting with multi-racial, non-traditional casting in *Live Wire*, as we have with our other plays.

What is very clear from these reactions is that the issue of AIDS has a very high denial quotient. If audiences are given an excuse to believe that the ideas expressed in the play do not apply to them, they *will* believe it.

This still does not answer the question, "why is it so difficult to book this play?" We have come up with some possible explanations:

- Homophobia. It seems the opinion of many educators that any discussion of homosexuality with students will be taken as condoning homosexual activity, and that is something they are unwilling to do.
- By the same token, some of the same educators are uncomfortable with any aspect of sex education, particularly the use of contraceptives. They feel that by discussing the use of condoms with students, they are giving their tacit approval to widespread sexual activity. This is a particularly incongruous attitude in light of the fact that Dr. Joseph Fernandez, the New York City Schools Chancellor, has not only mandated AIDS education in all city schools, but has submitted a plan to distribute condoms free of charge to any student on demand.
- For some, there is still a religious taboo where contraceptives are concerned.
- Sexuality and death are subjects that many adults find difficult to discuss with each other, let alone with children. It is, after all, adults who book the plays, not kids.

Because of Plays For Living's mission, it would be irresponsible of us to produce an AIDS awareness and prevention play without including a discussion of all the above sensitive subjects. Consequently, having *Live Wire* in our repertoire gives us both great satisfaction and great frustration.

It is enormously satisfying when a school principal calls to book a performance as the centrepiece for his/her school's Wellness Day program; when a parent who has just seen a Corporate Employee Assistance Program performance asks for information kits to take to the next PTA meeting because he is concerned with the lack of AIDS education at his children's school and plans to demand that *Live Wire* be presented there; when a Health Care Professional or Social Worker reports that her young people were enthusiastic about the performances and several have approached her for private counselling.

It is equally frustrating when a principal asks us to remove any mention of condoms or homosexuality before his students see the play. (*Live Wire* is performed as written or not at all.) It is especially frustrating when we look at our performance records and realize that we are only reaching a small fraction of the young people who are at risk in our community.

ETHAN: [struggles to recover a modicum of self-control] Look, I'm sorry, Sandy. But you gotta understand, Larry is . . .

SANDY: [crosses centre to ETHAN] Larry is your best friend. Was.

ETHAN: I don't want that guy messin' with my sister! I know that guy. I've spent my life bein' jealous of that guy.

SANDY: You believe all his bragging. That's what guys do with each other — they brag. But I know him. And I know he's telling me the truth when he says he hasn't been with anyone else for a year.

ETHAN: [crosses left, below sofa. MARTIN crosses right] That's not the point. A year doesn't matter. It's his whole life that matters. And there's a lot of messin' around back there. The point is . . .

SANDY: The point is you're jealous, ETHAN. Like you said, you always have been. [crosses down left to "window." Opens it] Larry, wait! I'll be down in a minute.

[SANDY crosses right to get "coat" from "wall hook" and puts it on.]

ETHAN: Where are you going?

SANDY: Larry and I are spending the night at his parents' house. [crosses centre to ETHAN] Mom thinks I'm staying with a girlfriend. We were going to ask you to vouch for us.

ETHAN: Sandy, how can I?

SANDY: Tell Mom whatever you want. It doesn't matter. It's my life I'm living. [tries for the door]

ETHAN: [stopping SANDY] Right! So don't take any chances with it. Larry's been around, Sandy. Wait till he gets tested.

SANDY: Why should he get tested?

ETHAN: Because if you sleep together, it would be a first for you, but not for him. Don't you understand — you could get AIDS!

SANDY: [Wrenching herself from ETHAN's grip, running for the door.] Nobody I know has AIDS!

ETHAN: *I* have it! [SANDY stops dead. MARTIN moves toward
ETHAN. Beat.]
SANDY: What?
ETHAN: I have the virus, at least.
MARTIN: Ethe, how?
ETHAN: From a needle, a long time ago. Just like Larry could have it from sex
    . . . even from a long time ago.
MARTIN: [softly, stunned, pained] But you look fine.
ETHAN: I am fine, for now.

Why LIVE WIRE Works

We must keep in mind that the sensitive nature of AIDS and its related issues is the very reason that live drama is the ideal format for their presentation. Theatre is a communal experience and necessitates cooperation. A group of people, perhaps with little in common, who may be apprehensive about the subject matter and very reticent about voicing an opinion, spend half an hour sharing a performance — a story that has been brought to life before them. Vague ideas have been brought into focus; characters have been fleshed out; a plot has unfolded. The individuals in the group have been entertained together, and at the end of that half-hour they stand on a tiny patch of common ground. The discussion that follows often brings out thoughts and feelings that would not have emerged without the benefit of the "springboard;" the group has relaxed with both the material and with one another.

In a very real sense, the very fact that AIDS is not easily discussed makes it a perfect subject matter for Plays For Living, in that facilitating the exchange of ideas is what we are all about.

A Performance Tour of *Live Wire* in Chattanooga
Helen Smith

Background

In September 1989, alarmed at the rapid rate at which Tennessee teenagers were contracting AIDS and eager to combat it through effective preventive education, a staff member of the Chattanooga-Hamilton County Health Department's Minority AIDS Prevention Program contacted Family and Children's Services (FCS), Plays For Living's Chattanooga Affiliate, inquiring whether a script existed on AIDS prevention for teens. For several years, FCS productions of PFL's half-hour dramas on timely and significant social issues had proven very effective in stimulating audience thought and discussion in Chattanooga. The Health Department felt that the use of these plays to address the topic of AIDS seemed a most effective way to get vital information to Tennessee's teenagers. A review of the *Live Wire* script and its accompanying discussion guide convinced the Health Department staff of the appropriateness of this vehicle for meeting their objective.

Chattanooga's High School of the Performing Arts and Chattanooga CARES, a community-based group providing AIDS resources, education and support were invited to join the collaboration. It was understood that the Family and Children's Services' Plays For Living staff would coordinate the venture and its Youth Services Division would work with the Health Department and Chattanooga CARES in developing and implementing an effective follow-up format to the play.

Tour Description

The target group for *Live Wire*'s audience were eighth-graders in Chattanooga Middle Schools. It was hoped that an educational impact about AIDS might be made on these young people *before* most initiated sexual activity.

The actors participating in the tour were recruited from the student body of the High School of the Performing Arts. The play was performed daily for a period of two weeks, reaching all ten Chattanooga middle schools. Participating schools were urged to avoid, whenever possible, scheduling the play in a facility whose large size prevented the intimacy between performer and audience. Intimacy is a critical element to an effective Plays For Living performance. Instead of gyms or auditoriums, the use of school libraries, choir rooms, etc., was suggested. Two performances for the public at large were also given at a local community theatre on a Saturday afternoon.

The format for follow-up discussions included one representative from each of the sponsoring agencies. All persons from the collaborating agencies who participated in leading the follow-up discussions were required to attend a workshop on effective techniques for facilitating discussions.

All performers were required to participate in two workshops held during the rehearsal period. One workshop focused on "facts and fiction" regarding AIDS transmission. The second explored the psychological impact on carriers, their friends and families. Both workshops addressed the aspect of peer pressure and teens. All discussion leaders were encouraged to attend at least one rehearsal of *Live Wire*.

Learning on the Road

All performances proceeded as planned except for the fact that with each successive presentation, the teen performers became increasingly active participants in the follow-up discussion, enthusiastically offering their own insights and attitudes. This unanticipated "bonus" greatly enhanced audience participation, as the eighth-graders were able to relate comfortably to older teens and to shed much of the self-consciousness and reticence with which they initially approached the forum.

The student actors became increasingly comfortable with the subject of AIDS and their sense of responsibility "to participate as peers in the post-performance discussion" demonstrated that "a large amount of clear, unambiguous information had been received and retained," according to the director of the High School for the Performing Arts.

The Chattanooga-Hamilton County Health Department reported that after the second presentation of *Live Wire*, four teenagers presented themselves to the HIV Counselling/Testing Clinic at the Health Department, stating that they had seen the play and wished to have more information on HIV and the antibody test.

The staff of Chattanooga CARES had expressed the conviction that up to thirty percent of the current population of persons with AIDS (PWAs) in Tennessee were infected with HIV as teenagers. It had been noted that, although the majority of teens are aware that "high risk" behaviour can lead to infection, mere knowledge about behaviour is not enough. They believed education programs such as the *Live Wire* project were imperative to help teens learn to assert themselves in situations which could lead to transmission of the HIV virus.

A few months after the Middle School tour, an additional performance was presented in Nashville, Tennessee at the conference of the Tennessee Network of Youth and Family Services. Audience response was excellent, and encouraged the belief that the performance might lead to replications of this project throughout the state.

It has been decided to make one significant change in the presentation format in the future. As a result of our observations about the effectiveness of teen actors in stimulating audience involvement, it was decided to invite the teen performers themselves to initiate follow-up discussion. Each performer will come prepared with at least one provocative question with which to open discussion and promote audience participation. The adult discussion facilitators will continue in their capacities as "experts."

This amended follow-up should promote even more effective discussion with our young audiences, demonstrating clearly and dramatically the extraordinary impact effected when AIDS prevention information is theatrically presented *to* teens *by* teens.

Play On

Godfrey Sealy

As a playwright, I feel it is my obligation to write plays that would lead towards possible positive change. I have toyed with a lot of social issues. I say toyed because I really enjoy myself doing this, sometimes much to the consternation and criticism of others. And why not, why must the waters be always calm. The most passionate issue for me was, and still is, AIDS. In 1987 I wrote a play, a drama, about the topic and for a number of reasons it took me over a year before it was produced. I think it must have been some sort of landmark in the history of Trinidad and Tobago theatre; no one wanted to touch the play. In all honesty, however, there was much public ignorance on the subject; people were not quite sure how exactly AIDS was contracted. After the play proved successful and became internationally acknowledged, the public realized that theatre in itself was definitely not a way to catch AIDS.

Education is most difficult where AIDS is concerned and it was quite obvious that no matter how many posters, pamphlets, booklets or flyers you print, no matter how many lectures, workshops, focus groups or symposiums you hold, there will be a certain sector that will not grab the true essence of the AIDS scenario. Educators themselves haven't tuned into the true essence, they too often remain clinical in their approach and refuse to be emotionally affected by the impact of this disease.

People like myself therein continue to strive forward in an attempt to give the public the opportunity to be part of this whole scenario — to live out the cause and the effect, to laugh, to cry, to sympathize, to console, to feel.

Sometimes you don't want to upset the public by giving them too heavy a piece. AIDS is already a heavy topic. It touches obvious issues like death and illness, but also many other important but subtle issues like love and relationships.

In Trinidad and Tobago, very few people see beyond the illness and death. The mere mention of love and relationships creates a kind of mind-blowing experience for the layman; you might call it culture shock. Yes, we tell people, persons with HIV and AIDS have healthy relationships with other people. A healthy relationship should not be determined only by the serostatus of a person and their partner.

I wrote *AIDA, The Wicked Wench of the World!* with the intention of appealing to the gay community. Gay people in this country don't know where they are at. Most of them lead a precarious life, torn between uncertain love affairs, hopelessly in search of an image suitable to the stringent homophobic society in which we live.

"Whores," as we call ourselves (at least the ones who have escaped from the moral society with some sense of humour), had not had a drag show in years and I know that they would love nothing more than a little excitement. I created a burlesque that was both fun and informational, at the same time about AIDS (with regards to discrimination and safer sex) and about gay relationships (especially in the face of AIDS).

Everyone loved it, even the straight people in the audience. Trinidad has a tradition of carnival where everyone dresses up and where men don women's clothing in satirical splendour much to the pleasure of everyone who loves nothing better but to get into the act.

This gave me the idea to adapt the script, make it amenable to a heterosexual public and use it as carnival street theatre. It became what we would call an *ole mas* band and paraded in the streets. Placards were used to express various messages, as is done in traditional *ole mas*. Once the band had attracted a large enough audience we would stop and perform. *AIDA* became a very successful venture. In allegory, it showed many people that out of the most trying times one can still find love and compassion.

Extract from AIDA, THE WICKED WENCH OF THE WORLD!

Caught in the swirl AARON saw a bright light and thinking it was the passage back he entered. He was now absorbed into the land of hope where he came upon the GOOD FAIRY.

FAIRY: What is your problem my child?
AARON: I am lost and cannot find the way.
FAIRY: Fear not. You have found the Way.

[And she began to explain to him why he had felt a certain way and that instead of running away from his situation he should learn to cope with it. In time he would find what he was looking for, nothing came before its time. She also told him that he should not worry but use his experiences as symbols for growth. She advised him that in his search to find himself that he must first search within himself and that only then will the truth be revealed.]

AARON: What about the red noses? And why were people without them treating them in that way?

FAIRY: Those people with the red noses are symbols of change. A change that will give meaning to life itself.

AARON: I don't understand.

FAIRY: All you must understand is that not all change is bad and that all negative reactions to this change must be made to be positive.

AARON: How do you do that? Is it not natural for people to react in this way to something like this? I am confused.

FAIRY: Don't be.

AARON: Then what can I do to help?

FAIRY: Well, you can help me prepare this here which I call the Antidote for ignorance.

[And she began to make her potion. Into her Teflon pot, she put a measure of self acceptance, two tablespoons of compassion, a dash of understanding, a lot of support, with education for flavour. She stirred it to the right consistency and just before she was finished she sprinkled a bit of love and commitment which she got from AARON. With the Antidote finished, she put some into a pretty bottle and was about to hand it to AARON.]

AARON: Why me?

FAIRY: Because I think that you are responsible and caring enough. And to besides, have you looked into a mirror lately?

AARON: No.

[And the GOOD FAIRY handed him a mirror. To his great surprise, he too had a red nose].

AARON: But, how?

FAIRY: Does it really matter now that you know what you know now?

[And with a shrug on his shoulder and a smile on his face, AARON was about to leave when the GOOD FAIRY stopped him.]

FAIRY: Oh, I forgot to give you one important thing. [And giving him a pair of rubber gloves she said:] Put these on. They will protect you wherever you go.

Scene Four

And so in the flash of an eye, the GOOD FAIRY was gone and AARON was whisked back into the land of Now, with its commotion and turmoil. He wasted no time in administering the Antidote to everyone. Of course, some didn't want to take it but with much persuasion, AARON finally managed to give it to everyone.

At first, it seemed as though nothing was happening and AARON was starting to give up hope when things started to change.

All of a sudden, the hustle and bustle stopped and people seemed now to have more time for each other. And relationships started to develop. And the people without the red noses stopped shunning those with red noses and made friends with them. And Aaron made a new friend without a red nose to whom he gave rubber gloves and whom he told about the GOOD FAIRY and what she had taught him. And they became close and learned to love each other and so did everyone else. And everything seemed better in the land of Now.

(Image of AIDA laughing in the background)

END

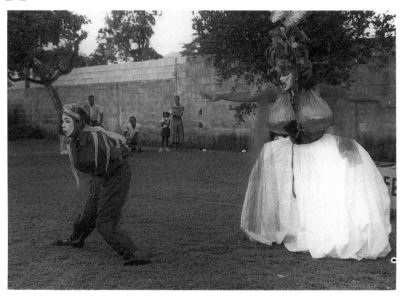

Aida, in *AIDA, The Wicked Wench of the World.* Performance in Trinidad.

Notes on the Challenges of AIDS Education

Alan Richardson

> All pain is shattering, but when it is shared, at least it is no longer a banishment.
>
> — *Simone de Beauvoir*

I.
Compassion

is our only hope

to reverse the pain
the social stigmatizing,
and sense of banishment

that presently surround
all aspects of AIDS
in our societies . . .

the compassion inherent in teaching is rarely found in its content

but rather

in the ways and means
used to communicate

the material
and how those ways
and means relate

to the actuality of
the subject material
in day to day

experience.

2.
In our AIDS education work we have found both traditional theatre and generally accepted teaching practices were useful only to that point of creating an environment of shared facts. But neither traditional theatre, with its dependency on illusion and behaviourism (that ultimately intensifies individualism), nor teaching practices linked so tightly to the authoritarian imparting of information (that ultimately intensify our awareness of sickness rather than health), were entirely adequate:

neither theatre
nor teaching

in their present form

could instill that profounder

awareness of the interconnectedness

of life in its

human

natural

or aesthetic forms

that is the root of

compassion.

3.
Consequently, in our AIDS education endeavours, we at Trinity are more in the process of exploration and discovery at this time, rather than a company touring an aesthetic product to various audiences.

Ostensibly, we have three so-called presentations for the public: *Face to Face* (for youth), *AIDS in the Workplace* (for adults), and *Teaching to Learn* (for educators). In reality, the first two are a series of provisional scenes on various aspects of sexual education, relationships, and social issues.

The scenes are provisional because they are continuously being changed and adapted depending both on us and on our immediate audience; new scenes are being created in response to growing awareness . . . (*AIDS and Women, Multiculturalism and AIDS*).

our aim is to renew
theatre practice in the immediacy
of the "street" encounter

and not in tinkering
with theatre aesthetic
or subject matter.

As such the audience member has much more to do with content and style than traditional theatre techniques allow.

Therefore, the practice of a growing "catalogue" of scenes responding to when, where, and whom you are playing was inevitable in our explorations, and this practice seemed particularly appropriate to the issues of AIDS and sexual education, since they are issues that are at once both intensely personal and public.

4.

Teaching to Learn is a series of live presentations, workshops, and videos for educators. They are based on the premise that we are all learners, and that we should pay more attention to teaching *how* to learn rather than *what* to learn. This approach can help the professional educator avoid that appearance of alienation or indifference endemic to much of modern institutional life.

This stance is to be avoided, particularly in AIDS education since there has been, already in Canada as elsewhere, an enormous amount of alienation in our society, bigotry — both overt and subtle — and neglect given to both persons with and the issues related to AIDS.

That bigotry was, and is, present in sexism, gender discrimination, authoritarian education systems, and workplace inequities, to name a few; the neglect was and is omnipresent — so much so, that, from time to time in our work, we have wondered whether any serious education program past that of perfunctory information-sharing could be mounted.

This bigotry and neglect has all to do with our refusal to deal with AIDS in terms of personhood and intimacy — in plain talk, these are men and women like ourselves who are dying, and not vocal minority members or social misfits, approachable only through pity or our charity.

5.

Once you have the confines of the traditional theatre stance, whether in one of our cultural "palaces" or a school auditorium, you must pay attention, first, to your strategy for how and where to encounter your audience — in essence all the world becomes your stage — and secondly, to the pursuit of that possible intimacy and atmosphere capable of promoting personhood. Both become key matters in the organization for performances, as well as constructing the scenes, and lead ultimately to a confrontational stance with audiences, but one free of threat, of guilt mongering, of condescension or the subtle advocacy of bankrupt "lifestyles."

Members of the ensemble, consequently, spend time making connections in the community where the series of presentations will take place. These connections can be performances of trial scenes and discussion, but also interviews with involved business people, board level educators, unions, teachers, and students.

6.

A typical trinity "presentation" is made up of a variety of elements: monologues, audience/performer "exercise" sections, traditional theatre scenes portraying behaviour, choral narrative patterns, participation duets that the performers take into the audience, and learning scenes meant to initiate audience reaction.

The following excerpt is from a "Learning Scene" section in *Face to Face*. It contains a brief choral narrative preface and a learning scene portraying a mother and daughter attempting to discuss sexuality — and would be followed by an audience discussion concerning how all of us might learn to *share* information without "characterizing" it with our sexual stereotypes or "colouring" it with our fears and hesitations.

The scene is presented without set or costumes, and was performed at SIDART in Montreal, in June 1989, by Sarah Richardson (age ten) and Louise Deniset.

Learning Scene

it's becoming

increasingly obvious

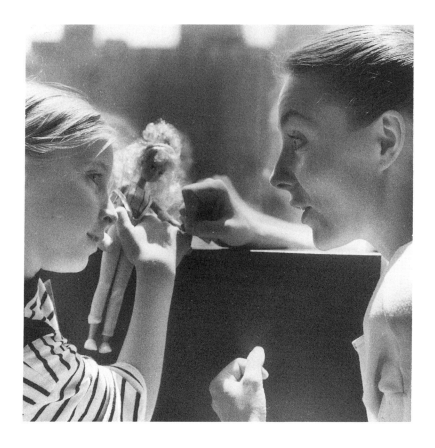

Louise and Sarah in *Face to Face*, Trinity Theatre of Toronto.
Photo: The *Montreal Gazette*.

to all of us

that learning

is sharing

regardless of age differences
or cultural biases
or role and status

becoming a person means
learning to share

your experiences and life stories

your insights and points of view

and through that sharing
knowledge of how the world
may look to someone else

I think back for instance

to when I was ten

when I was first beginning
to discuss matters of sex
with my Mother
I'll be the child?

I'll be the Mother . . .

Scene One

LOUISE: Sarah?
SARAH: Bonjour maman!
LOUISE: Ah te voilà
SARAH: Me voilà
LOUISE: Veux-tu t'asseoir?
SARAH: J'aimerais mieux rester debout

LOUISE: Moi, j'aimerais mieux que tu t'asseois — Assis!

SARAH: [to audience] When Mother talks like that she either has something
serious to say -

LOUISE: [to audience] Oh, why did I do that, why?
Pourquoi j'ai fais ça?

SARAH: and I get very afraid inside

LOUISE: this shouldn't be so hard. C'est difficile.

SARAH: or something simple she's going to make hard

LOUISE: Sarah this is a very easy, really . . . I wanted to talk to you today about
what is sometimes called "the birds and the bees"

SARAH: the birds and the bees?

LOUISE: or in other words sex . . . now this is an area —

SARAH: the drone honeybee is designed to explode after it mates

LOUISE: Comment?

SARAH: Monsieur Lemieux nous a raconté ça en classe.

LOUISE: I see . . . [to audience] why is this so hard?

SARAH: [to audience] and I know lots of stories
about spiders who eat their mates —
I just said that
about the bees
because I'm scared! J'ai peur!

LOUISE: I learned awkwardly, why must I pretend now to know all?

SARAH: Mom I didn't mean to throw you off track

LOUISE: Oh, you didn't throw me off track, it's just that —

SARAH: Oui?

LOUISE: Où est-ce que je commence? There are certain things about us that
are natural, and therefore very good, and which can give us great joy, mais
. . . cependant . . .

SARAH: Cependant?

LOUISE: Perhaps we should start with the parts of the human body . . . [LOUISE
goes on.]

SARAH: [to audience] I'm scared because . . .
when you've taught me the parts of the body
what do I know?

LOUISE: Je ne le sais même pas moi, c'est pour ça que j'en parle en termes
biologiques.
Do I know what
kind of person I should be.
Est-ce que je sais, moi?
Adults seem to imply some
serious meaning but

you never say what
that is!

to say the truth, I was
brought up to take care
of myself physically, but

my sexuality was
something I was to

understand in relation to
a man, and not myself . . .
pas pour moi.

C'est à des moments
comme ceux-là où j'aimerais
plutôt jouer

et certainement on
pouvait jouer avec

et découvrir son
sexe, mais le jeu dans

ces cas n'est pas
très amusant
mais absolument
jamais l'associer
avec le plaisir

is that growing up? when
things that gave you
pleasure don't anymore?

oh my goodness, what
have I done? she looks
so glum! Sarah!
SARAH: Oui maman!
LOUISE: Excuse-moi, we all have to go through learning the biological facts, and
it requires a balancing act inside because the truth is le sexe est une chose
merveilleuse . . . it's a beautiful and wonderful *thing!*

SARAH: *thing?*
LOUISE: which has certain do's . . .
SARAH: Oh no!
LOUISE: and certain don'ts
SARAH: I thought so
LOUISE: attached to it [LOUISE goes on . . .]
SARAH: those do's and don'ts
   scare me even more —

   Après que je les ai appris,
   qu'est-ce que je vais savoir?

   that a relationship
   with another person
   is a set of rules
   you must follow?
LOUISE: Now we're closer,
   now we're
   communicating.

   and that getting closer
   to another person someday
   depends on how you
   follow these do's and don'ts

   she'll learn for herself, but I'll be there if she needs me.

   and you hear about
   them in so many
   different ways —

   and I'll answer her

   perhaps I'll just ask, *maman?*
LOUISE: Oui, Sarah.
SARAH: Parle-moi du Sida.

[a long pause]

AIDS Prevention on Stage

Pierre Berthelot

The dramatic arts, when looked at in relation to other mass communications media, manage to serve an educational purpose without losing specificity or emotional integrity. Two stage-performance experiments, both taking AIDS prevention as their subject, emerged from a desire to touch the emotional universe of perspective target audiences. The premise of our work was that an open heart is the foundation of all learning.

An analysis of these two educational shows on AIDS — a play, *Unknown in our Comic*, and a stand-up comedy routine, *Sister Nunsex* — illustrate this point. Both were born out of the solitude I felt working in an environment governed by rationalism, the health and social service system, and from my theatre experience, wherein I learned that messages addressed directly to the heart have a great impact.

I had already noticed one glaring fault in AIDS prevention campaigns: they appeared to do little more than constantly bombard people with slogans and cognitive messages. In order to demonstrate to the people around me that there were other methods of informing people about AIDS, I turned to a group of professional actors who were interested in doing "something" in the area of AIDS.

UNKNOWN IN OUR COMIC / INCONNU DANS NOTRE BANDE[1]

The background material we used to develop our play moved the actors: anonymous letters written by professionals about their fears concerning AIDS. I had used them as case studies in training sessions on the issue. Reading these letters helped the actors, some of whom were relatively unfamiliar with AIDS, to realize that it is a problem for all, including the non-infected. Together we decided to focus our attention on characters not infected by HIV, but affected directly by AIDS because of being close to someone who was infected.

The Creative Process

We made a decision — to base our work on an emotional approach, to touch the audience using theatre, our chosen form of expression. The theatre's human dimension and the absence of any intermediary seemed well adapted to a public that had become blasé about electronic communications. We chose to present a family of "ordinary" people, whose language, concerns, relationships were as close as possible to those of young people. We felt it best to avoid, as much as possible, an extreme dramatization of the experiences of people with AIDS. This extremism, so dear to other media, has the effect of distancing viewers so they cannot discern any common points between the presentation of a dire situation and their own experience.

Because we were aiming our play at a young audience, we focused on the discomfort of those close to a person with AIDS (named Christian), rather than on Christian himself. He only appears at the end of the play, at a point when he has developed a serenity the others do not yet possess. There is no reflection on negative clichés (queer, drug addict, sex maniac), or on the more gruelling aspects that often confront people with AIDS (extreme thinness, facial Kaposi lesions, isolation and rejection).

To keep emotional pathways open, we refrained from making obvious value judgements, preferring to show each character's reactions as legitimate. We also tried to avoid the trap of many "educational shows" that communicate unmotivated information messages. The didactic angle could not follow directly upon the heals of the theatrical component: messages about AIDS symptoms and safer sex were simplified and conveyed through the dramatic situation.

UNKNOWN IN OUR COMIC

Pierre-Louis, a fifteen-year-old, and his Uncle Christian have shared a common passion for several years: comic strips. One writes the text, the other draws the pictures. This great complicity leads them to dream about publishing their last work, which recounts the adventures of Frankie and Donayod, two men travelling aboard a spaceship, on a mission of undetermined duration over which they have no control (an allegory for the relationship between the two creators).

Our protagonist, Pierre-Louis, communicates by cassette with Christian, busy with his job away from home; they meet, however, at each important step in the project. The teenager's parents, Claude and Jacqueline, are somewhat jealous of this relationship, but they don't withhold support for their son's creative endeavour. Pierre-Louis' sister, Geneviève, has put all her adolescent hope into a future career in show business.

306

At the beginning of the drama, Pierre-Louis informs Christian by tape-recorded message that he is beginning to get tired of his increasingly long absences. Through the intermediary of the parents, in the meantime, we learn the true reason behind Christian's long absences: he has AIDS.

For the time being, Christian would rather not see Pierre-Louis. Consumed with fear and at the mercy of their own prejudices, Pierre-Louis' parents hide the truth from him. In the end, by listening in on one of their conversations, he discovers the reason his uncle is absent from his life.

A family crisis ensues. Jacqueline tries to convince her husband not to reject his brother. At the beginning Claude is outraged, but over the course of the play he changes. Finally at the end of a clumsy conversation, he even offers his son some condoms.

CLAUDE: So many things have been going through my head these last few days . . . I've been thinking a lot about you and your friend Marie-Michèle, about Geneviève too. Love can be so beautiful. . . . [He hands Pierre-Louis a box of condoms.] . . . Here . . . I didn't know how . . . umh . . . I, here. God, I feel so stupid! A father giving this to his son.

Pierre-Louis and his sister later have an intimate conversation about sexuality and contraceptives:

GENEVIEVE: Shit. It's got to the point where we have to use condoms because of old boyfriends . . . They really get people into a panic with all of this AIDS stuff. Besides, I hate condoms. It takes away my inspiration. And I'm not alone either. My boyfriend hates them too. Everyone hates them.
PIERRE-LOUIS: Well, if you wanted to, you could make it part of "foreplay." You could make a game out of it.
GEVEVIEVE: A game. Have you ever tried that?
PIERRE-LOUIS: Umh . . . well, no. But, I'm going to.

Pierre-Louis is terrified of losing his best friend. The comic strip serves as an outlet: an outsider appears on the space ship and threatens Frankie's life. In one of the last scenes of the play, Pierre-Louis and Christian have an emotional reunion:

PIERRE-LOUIS: I thought you'd have gotten thinner; that your skin would be all blotchy and that you would hardly be able to walk.
CHRISTIAN: You must have been afraid of seeing me again.
PIERRE-LOUIS: I'm happy. You don't look sick. But what do you think you can do?
CHRISTIAN: Simple things with the people I love, like we could continue our project . . .

INCONNU DANS NOTRE BANDE

This play was written in 1989 by five professional actors from Québec City and performed by them at the Fifth International AIDS Conference in Montréal as part of SIDART. It was presented there on three occasions. We wanted to develop a play that would perhaps then tour schools.

Statistics show that Canadian adolescents are quite badly-informed, and feel little personal concern, about HIV and AIDS. Moreover, they convey many of the older generation's prejudices towards those infected.

Our goal was to reduce the distance between adolescents and AIDS: to make them realize, first, that HIV is a risk to be confronted and, second, that those already infected are no different from other individuals. We wanted them to know about means of HIV transmission, to take a serious look at prevention methods and to help them develop a more understanding attitude towards those infected.

In pursuit of these objectives, the show was developed to help set things in motion, preparing a favourable atmosphere for communication between students and their parents or teachers. Dialogue is imperative, but our hope was only that we would touch them deeply enough to help open up the lines of communication.

Impact Evaluation

After each performance at SIDART, the audience was invited to exchange views with the creators and fill out an evaluation questionnaire. Their answers tested whether we were successful in attaining our objectives concerning knowledge, attitudes and the theatre's ability to reach an audience on an emotional level. Basically, an impact study undertaken by three researchers from the Laval University School of Social Services leads us to believe that the final result was true to our original intentions.

The Short History of the Play

The play was performed on two other occasions in Québec City in 1989. The first performance was before an audience of social workers, the second before adult educators (parents, teachers, school principals) and young people. Both experiences provoked a similar reaction.

The play was not performed again — essentially because professional fees were an expense which schools, with their budgetary and educational priorities, were not prepared to pay, and governments felt that school boards should pay all of the costs. There was a proposal to make a video recording of a performance: distribution costs would have been much less and, like other electronic media, it would have been more convenient for teachers to use. But this would have altered the effect completely. To us, the idea of simply transposing the medium without altering treatment demonstrated a glaring lack of understanding of the production's essential strength.

Despite a few mishaps and difficulties along the way (complexity and cost of the production, actors' lack of availability), the choice to do stage performance was perfectly relevant to our intention to promote prevention. We could both visit people in their own environments, and relate to them in language they could understand, enabling us to win them over.

Public health administrators should allocate as much money to artists as to scientists: we could put much more emphasis on research into original ways of conveying our message. It is extravagant to subsidize epidemiological research at hundreds of thousands of dollars a shot, if it always leads to the kind of intervention — cold and intellectual — that leaves most people untouched and indifferent.

Stand-up Comedy

Presented three times in 1989/90 in gay bars in Québec City and at a colloquium of francophone AIDS prevention community organizations in Paris, this stand-up comedy routine was commissioned by MIEL-Québec (a community-based AIDS organization in Québec City) as part of a fundraising activity.

The Target Audience

It cannot be said that, in general, male homosexuals are not concerned about AIDS. This is, in fact, quite the opposite of the situation with adolescents. The homosexual population was the first and hardest-hit group in North America to contract the disease. So many gay people have seen their friends and lovers suffer and die from AIDS. More than eighty percent of those who are seropositive or living with AIDS in Québec are homosexual men. It is an ever-present spectre on the homosexual scene.

If self-identified gay men don't protect themselves against HIV, it certainly isn't because they haven't heard enough about it. It is common for a homosexual to know more than ten people who have died of AIDS or are living with it. Gays, moreover, were pioneers in creating organizations for self-help and the fight against AIDS. The problem has become part of daily life: posters, pamphlets, magazine articles and fundraising drives all keep people in contact with the reality of this problem.

Yet, despite all this preventive work, still more is needed: the available safer sex information is not uniform; younger homosexuals feel less concerned; drugs and

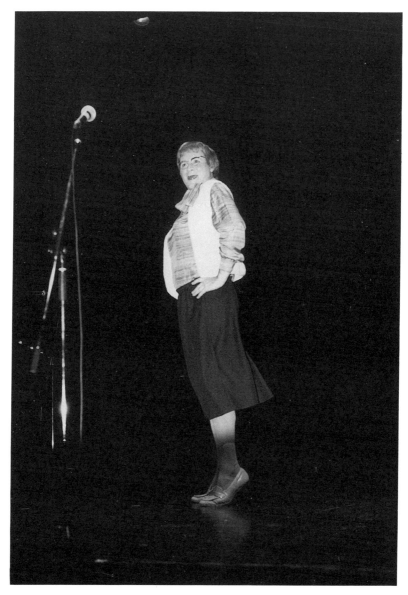

Pierre Berthelot as *Sister Nunsex*, performed at Re-Voir le Sida,
Montréal, 1991.

alcohol hinder consistency in safer sex practice. There is also a saturation effect caused by the omnipresence of the problem.

Gay Objectives

The main objective was to extend the preventive work already underway, but from a different perspective than that taken with young people. In this case, convincing people does not consist of sensitizing them to a new problem, but rather in keeping them open to a frequently repeated message so painful that people often prefer not to hear anything about it, especially in an entertainment environment.

Persistence is important in promoting safer sex behaviour; the challenge was to make it as palatable as possible and to find a way of getting a message across again. Humour seemed most appropriate, since it allows relative distance from the lived realities that are so painful close up.

Who is Sister Nunsex?
(and what is she doing on the table?)

Sister Nunsex is a strange character: a good nun who decides to found a religious order dedicated to AIDS prevention after her job retraining in physical education and sexology. Homosexual men are her mission. She has opened a health club where she leads a weekly "Aerobics Mass" for their benefit. She also gives safer sex seminars in bars, passing on information using direct, somewhat crude language. She asks questions and talks about specific sexual acts and risks, all within the frame of reference of laughter-as-empowerment. Punchlines punctuate the text:

> Oral sex is low risk. But, if you do swallow sperm, it doesn't make it any safer if you swallow a condom afterwards.

> Penetration without a condom is as dangerous for your health as jogging on the "Capitale autoroute" . . . using poppers . . . at rush hour.[2]

The Creative Priestess

In order to understand this routine, it must be seen in context. The organizers of the fundraising event, an auction in a gay bar, wanted to include an educational segment on safer sex. The choice of location seemed incompatible with this type of activity: a noisy bar, drug-and alcohol consumption, people who had come to do their part to fight AIDS, but in a fun atmosphere not meant for discussion. We wanted to share their solidarity, but definitely not with gloomy faces. We wanted to laugh and charm these people and help them to better live with sorrow. The "bio-medical conference" was immediately ruled out. In stepped Sister Nunsex. Anyone familiar with the commercial homosexual subculture knows importance of the drag show.[3] Without doing a psychoanalysis of this phenomenon, let's just say that many people enjoy watching men strut around on stage trying to act like glamorous, popular female singers and stars. A transvestite basically conveys a female Hollywood stereotype. It is part of the "folklore" of the gay bar.

Sister Nunsex was inspired by the "man-disguised-as-woman" principle, a caricature of transvestism. The transvestite's intention may be to look as much like a woman as possible, but Sister Nunsex wants to look as much like a man "disguised as a woman" as possible. This character is the opposite of glamorous: she wears a doubleknit skirt, thick nylon stockings and a track suit — calculated bad taste. Some people burst into knee-slapping laughter; others turn red with empathetic embarrassment.

Most gays are aware of the church's double standard around the issues of AIDS and homosexuality: both oppressing their sexual preference and giving support to people with AIDS. They see a paradox we felt was important to raise, even exaggerate, exemplified by an athletic, crude-talking, sexologist-Nun who works in gay bars. The content is simplified and crude with a campiness familiar to and cultivated by gay subculture.[4] The rhythm of the interaction between the actor, the audience and the music, creates a party atmosphere.

The Impact and the Compact

This routine was presented on three occasions in Québec City gay bars. People found it indisputably funny and amazingly educational. The safer sex information was taken from the document published by the Canadian AIDS Society "Safer Sex Guidelines," a consensus of community and medical expertise. Comments we received demonstrate that the monologue met its objectives of arousing and maintaining people's attention, communicating information, and making people laugh.

To date, no university has shown interest in doing research on Sister Nunsex. Although she would be flattered by such an offer, it wouldn't be worth it as she has a mission. She would also like to say to anyone who will listen, that there are two things she really loves: to give conferences in bars and to be invited to international conferences. A note to those who aren't interested: there is a lot of Nunsex in the world.

Playing for life

These two educational vehicles for AIDS prevention, *Unknown in our Comic* and *Sister Nunsex* have several points in common. First of all, each has the objective of educating a specific target audience; one relatively unconcerned, the other saturated. In the first situation, we created characters that young people could feel close to. In the second, we presented a character that allows people, through comedy, to keep a distance. In both situations, the sensational and dramatic messages usually associated with AIDS were avoided. The play presented simple people and showed a warm, productive relationship between a young person and an adult whose life is threatened; the stand-up routine succeeded in turning the serious into the seemingly frivolous, while conveying its message through humour.

In both cases, there is an emotional appeal: those who were previously unmoved by the problem shed tears; those who were to close to it, roared with laughter. There was also room for audience participation. People were asked to get involved — during post-performance discussions of the play, and in *Sister Nunsex*, during the show itself.

Although there were selected cognitive messages, we didn't try to say everything. We found it best to get to the point, without detailed study, through common language and terms people are familiar with. We were not giving a lecture; the didactic aspect was almost imperceptible. As vehicles, the characters shared a common language with, and belonged to the same culture as the audiences they were speaking to. In the play, there are young people who like comic strips and music, who are preoccupied with their sexuality but, like their parents, are embarrassed to talk about it. *Nunsex* reflects different aspects of the gay-bar subculture by presenting a man disguised as a woman, a nun no less, who is comfortable enough with sex to joke about it. AIDS prevention can and should emanate from the heart, and use an appropriate medium for its target.

NOTES

1. The name of the play in its original version, conceived collectively and signed, Richard Audé. Translated here as *Unknown in our Comic*, it is a play on the word *bande*, at once a reference to comic strip and to gang (clan).

2. The Québec City central multiple-lane freeway.

3. An evening of cabaret-style performances, many of them consisting of female impersonators.

4. In her famous essay, "Notes on Camp," Susan Sontag described the essence of camp as "love of the unnatural: of artifice and exaggeration . . . [a] sensibility . . . a private code . . . among small urban cliques [which] converts the serious into the frivolous."

Translated from the French by Ken Morrison.

"AIDS and the Reconceptualization of Homosexuality" by Dennis Altman is reprinted from *Which Homosexuality: Essays from the International Scientific Conference of Gay and Lesbian Studies* (GMP Publishers, London and Utigerveij, An Dekker/Shorer, Amsterdam, 1989).

An earlier version of "Seduced and Terrorized: AIDS and Network Television" by Paula A. Treichler appeared in *Artforum*, October 1989, pp. 147-51.

"Flesh Histories" by Tom Kalin is reprinted from *Views*, vol. 11, no.3. Summer 1990.

"Media Health Campaigning: Not Just What You Say, But the Way that You Say It!" by Jon Baggaley is reprinted from *AIDS Prevention through Health Promotion: Facing Sensitive Issues*, WHO AIDS Series 10 (Geneva, World Health Organization, 1990).

"Do It! Safer Sex for Girls and Boys Comes of Age" by Jean Carlomusto and Gregg Bordowitz was first printed in *Outweek* magazine, August 28, 1989. "Reflections on Safer Sex Porn" is a transcript of the author's presentation at the New York International Film Festival of Gay and Lesbian Film, 1990.

Yell When It Starts! by Ralf Konig. Copyright Deutsche AIDS-Hilfe, Berlin, Germany.

"Forty Seconds of AIDS" by Herbert Daniel is reprinted from *Vida Antes Da Morte / Life Before Death* (Rio de Janeiro: Jaboti, 1989).

"How to Have Sex in an Epidemic" by Michael Callen from the Album *Purple Heart*, copyright 1987 Tops 'n Bottoms Music. "The Healing Power of Love" by Michael Callen and Marsha Malamet, copyright 1987 Tops 'n Bottoms Music and Malamution Music (BMI).

Excerpts from *La Terasse des audiences au moment de l'adieu* (Leméac, Montréal, 1990), by Yves Navarre courtesy of Editions Leméac, Montreal, 1990. Excerpts from *Le Jardin d'acclimatisation* by Yves Navarre courtesy of Flammarion, Paris 1990.

Excerpts from *Warm Wind in China: A Play in Two Acts* (Montréal: Nu-Age Editions, 1989) by Kent Stetson were reprinted by permission of the author and the publisher.

ILLUSTRATIONS: xiv – Courtesy of Blair Robbins; 11, 15 – reprinted from *The Columbian Exchange: Biological and Cultural Consequences of 1492* and *Ecological Imperialism: The Biological Expansion of Europe, 900-1900* by Alfred W. Crosby; 35 – courtesy of the Canadian AIDS Society; 44 – courtesy of Douglas Crimp; 48 – photo by Robin Holland, courtesy The New Museum of Contemporary Art, New York; 51, 52, 55 – courtesy of Douglas Crimp; 61, 65, 68 – photos by Jan Zita Grover; 72-75 – photos of Miasme/Hyène et la Valve, 1988/89, by Martha Fleming and Lyne Lapointe; 76 – from *Christianity, Social Tolerance and Homosexuality*, by

John Boswell (University of Chicago Press, 1980), photo courtesy of the British Museum; 78 – from a Barnum and Bailey Circus poster; 80, 81 – (lower image) "Methodus plantarum sexualis" by Linnaeus, courtesy of the British Museum; 86 – photo by Leena Randvee, courtesy of John Greyson; 90, 91 – still photo courtesy V Tape; 100 – photo, *Toronto Sun*, courtesy Monika Gagnon; 106 – courtesy of Paula Treichler; 110, 115 – still photos courtesy Jon Baggaley; 122 – photo by Rand Gaynor, courtesy Tom Kalin; 124, 127, 133 – courtesy Tom Kalin; 138, 142 – still photos courtesy of Paula Treichler; 158, 162 – photos by Gabor Szitanyi courtesy of American Playhouse Theatre; 170 – courtesy Wieland Speck; 178, 183 – still photos courtesy of Jacques Perron; 187, 189 – still photos courtesy of Wieland Speck; 194, 195 – photo by Philip Hannan; 207-209 – photos by Jacques Perron, comix courtesy of Deutsche AIDS-Hilfe, Berlin; 210 – photo by Joe Dimaggio courtesy of Direct Cinema Ltd.; 237 – photo by Chandra Mouli; 244 – photo by Gisele Wulfsohn, courtesy of AREPP; 279 – courtesy of AREPP; 295 – courtesy of Godfrey Sealy; 300 – photo, *Montreal Gazette*, courtesy Trinity Theatre of Toronto; 310 – photo by Ken Morrison, courtesy DGLQ.

MIKHAËL ELBAZ is professor of Anthroplogy at the University of Laval in Québec City.

RUTH MURBACH is professor of Law at the University of Québec at Montréal. Her published articles include "Le grand désordre: le Sida et les normes," *Anthropolige et Sociétés*.

ALFRED W. CROSBY currently teaches in the American Studies Program at the University of Texas, Austin, Texas. He is author of *The Columbian Exchange: Biological and Cultural Consequences of 1492* (Greenwood Press, 1972) and *Ecological Imperialsim: The Biological Expansion of Europe, 900-1900* (Cambridge University Press, 1986).

NORBERT GILMORE is professor in the Department of Medicine at McGill University and a member of the McGill Centre for Medicine Ethics and Law, and Associate Director of the McGill AIDS Centre. He is also Senior Physician and member of the Division of Clinical Immunology of the Royal Victoria Hospital and of the Immunodeficiency Unit of the Montréal Chest Hospital. He was Chairman of the Canadian National Advisory Committee on Acquired Immunodeficiency Syndrome (NAC-AIDS) from 1983 to 1989.

DENNIS ALTMAN is the author of several books including *AIDS in the Mind of America* (Anchor Press, 1986). He teaches politics at La Trobe University, Melbourne, and is vice-president of the Victoria AIDS Council.

DOUGLAS CRIMP is an art critic and AIDS activist. He has taught at various institutions including Princeton University, California Institute of the Arts, Cooper Union and is currently visiting professor at Sarah Lawrence College lecturing in Gay and Lesbian Studies. For thirteen years he was an editor of the journal, *October* where, in 1987, he edited the special issue entitled "AIDS: Cultural Analysis/Cultural Activism." He is also the author (with Adam Rolston) of *AIDS Demo Graphics* (Bay Press, 1990).

JAN ZITA GROVER edits *Artpaper* in Minneapolis. She has written about the cultural politics of AIDS for *Afterimage, Exposure, High Performance, October, The Women's Review of Books*, and anthologies in the U.K. and the U.S. She curated *AIDS: the Artists' Response* (Ohio State University, 1989. Available for $2.50 plus postage from Wexner Center for the Arts, 1440 N. Main Streeet, OH 43201-1226, U.S.A.).

MARTHA FLEMING & LYNE LAPOINTE are visual artists. The work of art around which they structured their performace for SIDART, *Miasme/Hyène et La Valve,* was conceived as part of EAT ME/DRINK ME/LOVE ME, an installation put together at the invitation of the New Museum of Contemporary Art (New York, 1989/90) which proposed a quest for sites of pleasure, for the expression of pleasure, and for the acknowledgement of pleasure for women, inside the rigid cultural institutions that are available to us. With Creative Time, they produced a second site project in New York in 1990. The project, *The Wilds and the Deep*, concerns the rapport between the brutality of colonial methodology and the origins of museum collection and display.

JOHN GREYSON is a Toronto-based film/video artist. His current film, *The Making of Monsters*, won the Gay Teddy Bear Prize at the 1991 Berlin International Film Festival. He is currently developing a murder mystery musical about Patient Zero, the Air Canada flight attendant accused of bringing AIDS to North America.

MONIKA GAGNON's writings on feminism and Canadian art have appeared in numerous magazines, anthologies and catalogues. She is currently co-editor of *Parallelogramme* magazine in Toronto

TOM FOLLAND is a writer and curator. He recently organized the exhibition *Commitment* for The Power Plant in Toronto, which explored the relationship between activism and art. His article, "Representing Acquired Immune Deficiency" appeared in *Vanguard* magazine.

JON BAGGALEY is professor of Education at Concordia University in Montréal and Director of the University's M.A. Program in Educational Technology. He has co-authored books including *Dynamics of Television* (Saxon House, 1976) and *Psychology of the TV Image* (Saxon House, 1980). He has consulted on media health campaigns in Canada, Britain, Norway and Africa.

TOM KALIN is a film/videomaker living in New York. He has worked at AIDSFILMS, a non-profit education company for the last two and a half years. He is also a member of the AIDS activist collective Gran Fury. His current film, *Swoon* is about the infamous boy-killers, Nathan Leopold Jr. and Richard Lode.

PAULA A. TREICHLER teaches at the University of Illinois at Urbana-Champaign in the College of Medicine, Institute of Communications Research, and Women's Studies Program. She is the co-author of *A Feminist Dictionary* (1985) and *Language, Gender and Professional Writing* (1989) and has published widely on the AIDS epidemic.

SIMON WATNEY is a writer and critic based in London, England. He is a member of the Health Education Group of The Terrance Higgins Trust, and is the author of numerous books and articles. His most recent book is *The Art of Duncan Grant* (John Murray Ltd., 1990).

PRATHIBA PARMAR is a writer and filmmaker living in London, England. Her film credits include *Emergence* (1986), *Reframing AIDS* (1987), *Sari Red* (1988), *Memory Pictures* (1989) and *Khush* (1991).

BERNARD ARCAND currently teaches Anthropology at the University of Laval in Québec City. He has authored publications examining the representation of Amerindians in curriculum textbooks in Québec. He has recently published a book on pornography, *Le Jaguar et le tamanoir* (Boréal, 1991).

JEAN CARLOMUSTO is coordinator of video production at Gay Men's Health Crisis, New York. She began the "Living with AIDS Show" which airs each week on cable television. She frequently collaborates with Gregg Bordowitz to produce a wide variety of AIDS activist video tapes. She is a founding member of DIVA TV (damned interfering video activists), as well as a member of Fierce Pussy, a group of lesbians producing materials designed to fight lesbian invisibility. She has recently completed *L is for the way you look*, and is currently collaborating on *Not Just Passing Through* a videotape about lesbian herstory

GREGG BORDOWITZ has been assistant coordinator of Audio Visual Production for Gay Men's Health Crisis, N.Y. since 1988. He is also a founding member of DIVA TV and Testing The Limits Collective. His has collaborated on many AIDS activist videos including *Target City Hall* (1989), *Safer Sex Shorts* (1990), *An Informed Approach to HIV Testing* (1990), and *Thinking About Death* (1991).

WEILAND SPECK is a filmmaker and assistant organizer of the Panorama section of the Berlin International Film Festival. His films include *Westler: East of the Wall* (1985). His series of six videos for SAFER SEX PROMOTION are available from: SPECKFILM & VIDEO, Grainauer Str. 11, D-1000 Berlin 30.

CINDY PATTON is Manager of Community Education, AIDS Action Committe, Boston. Her writings on AIDS include *Sex and Germs* (Black Rose Press, 1988), and *Inventing AIDS* (Routledge, 1990). She is co-author with Janis Kelly of *Making It: A Woman's Guide to Sex in the Age of AIDS* (New York, 1987).

RALF KONIG is a well-known cartoonist. He has produced comics for the general public, for youth, and for gay men and lesbians. His comic strips have been published by leading German publishers.

HERBERT DANIEL is co-founder and editorial coordinator for the Brazilian Interdisciplinary AIDS Association (ABIA). He has written three books about AIDS since 1983; *Jacrés e Lobisomens* (1983); *Alegres e Irresponsaves Abacaxis Americanos* (1986); and *Life Before Death* (Tipographia Jaboti, 1989).

MICHAEL LYNCH was a Toronto writer and AIDS activist. Since 1981 he was editor of the *Gay Studies Newsletter*, and was a writer for *The Body Politic* between 1973-1984. He founded both THE AIDS MEMORIAL and AIDS ACTION NOW! in Toronto in 1988. He is the author of a collection of poems, *These Waves of Dying Friends* (Contact II Press, 1989). Michael worked tirelessly to establish The Toronto Centre for Lesbian and Gay Studies.

DOUMBI-FAKOLY is an author whose books include *Morts pour la France*, (Editions Karthala, 1983); *Le Retaite Anticipé du Guide Suprême* (Editions L'Harmattan, 1984); *Certificat de contrôle anti-Sida* (Editions Publisud, 1988).

MICHAEL CALLEN is a founding member of several groups and coalitions for and with people living with AIDS. A prolific writer and a singer-songwriter, he is editor of *Surviving and Thriving with AIDS* (People Living With AIDS Coalition, 1988).

CHANDRA MOULI and **K.N. RAO** work with the Copperbelt Health Education Project in Zambia.

YVES NAVARRE has written an autobiography and many works of award-wining fiction. His works include *Le Jardin d'acclimatisation* (Editions Flammarion, 1980) and *La Terrasse des audiences au moment de l'adieu* (Leméac, 1990).

EVAN ADAMS is an actor and playwright. He is artistic director of the Howie Gaw'nit Players, Vancouver, and is a member of the National Native Role Model Program in Kahnawake, Québec. He acted in *Lost in the Barrens* which won an Emmy in 1991.

KENT STETSON is a playwright and screenwriter. He has recently completed a triology, *The Survivors Cycle*, on parental abuse which includes *Warm Wind In China*, *Queen of the Cadillac* and *Sweet Magdelana*. He is curently working on a film adaptation of *Queen of the Cadillac* and a new play, *Just Plain Murder*. He currently teaches at McGill University, Montréal.

GARY FRIEDMAN is a puppeteer. After studying at l'Institute National de Marionette, he studied with the late Jim Henson who helped begin the Puppets Against AIDS project with **MIKE MILVASE**.

ROBERT JOHN METCALF is the production manager of Plays for Living. He has acted on film, television and stage and has taught acting, stage combat, movement and voice at the Center Stage Conservatory in Baltimore and the Utah Shakesperean Festival.

HELEN SMITH is currently the coordinator of Volunteers and Plays for Living at the Family and Children's Services of Chattanooga, Tennese.

GODFREY SEALY is a playwright and AIDS educator living and working in Port of Spain, Trinidad. In addition to several successful plays and performance pieces, he has signed an award-winning AIDS video and contributed to several books including *The Third Epidemic*.

ALAN RICHARDSON is the artistic director of Trinity Theatre in Toronto which he founded in 1982. He teaches at York University and has developed projects on AIDS Education, Drug and Alcohol Abuse, and Workplace Issues.

PIERRE BERTHELOT is an actor and social worker living in Québec City. He works at the Québec City District 3 AIDS Prevention Centre.